Birth, Distress and Disease

T0281658

This volume examines the role of steroids and peptides in the regulation of pregnancy and pregnancy outcome, and their long-term effects including possible influences on adult-onset diseases. During pregnancy the placenta acts as a central regulator and coordinator of maternal and fetal physiology, and of the onset of labor, through its production and regulation of steroids and peptides. Perturbations to this regulatory system can result in poor pregnancy outcome, such as preterm birth and low birth weight. These in turn are linked to diseases in later life. Intriguingly, many of these regulatory actions of steroids and peptides also occur in the brain. The induction and suppression of peptides by steroids appear to be the key to regulatory function in both brain and placenta. These various interweaving strands, linking basic sciences with obstetrics, are all reviewed in depth here producing a fascinating account of an important area of materno-fetal medicine.

Birth, Distress and Disease

Placental–Brain Interactions

Edited by

Michael L. Power

Smithsonian National Zoological Park
Washington DC, USA

American College of Obstetricians and Gynecologists
Washington DC, USA

and

Jay Schulkin

American College of Obstetricians and Gynecologists
Washington DC, USA

Georgetown University School of Medicine
Washington DC, USA

National Institute of Mental Health
Bethesda MD, USA

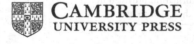

CAMBRIDGE
UNIVERSITY PRESS

CAMBRIDGE UNIVERSITY PRESS
Cambridge, New York, Melbourne, Madrid, Cape Town, Singapore,
São Paulo, Delhi, Dubai, Tokyo, Mexico City

Cambridge University Press
The Edinburgh Building, Cambridge CB2 8RU, UK

Published in the United States of America by Cambridge University Press, New York

www.cambridge.org
Information on this title: www.cambridge.org/9780521182676

First published 2005
First paperback edition 2010

A catalogue record for this publication is available from the British Library

ISBN 978-0-521-83148-2 Hardback
ISBN 978-0-521-18267-6 Paperback

Medical disclaimer
Power and Schulkin
Birth, Distress and Disease
HB ISBN 978-0-521-83184-2

Every effort has been made in preparing this book to provide accurate and
up-to-date information which is in accord with accepted standards and
practice at the time of publication. Although case histories are drawn
from actual cases, every effort has been made to disguise the identities of
the individuals involved. Nevertheless, the authors, editors and publishers
can make no warranties that the information contained herein is totally
free from error, not least because clinical standards are constantly
changing through research and regulation. The authors, editors and
publishers therefore disclaim all liability for direct or consequential
damages resulting from the use of material contained in this book. Readers
are strongly advised to pay careful attention to information provided by
the manufacturer of any drugs or equipment that they plan to use.

This volume is dedicated to the students and young (and not so young) scientists we confidently predict will extend and improve on the research presented here.

We would also like to acknowledge and thank certain individuals for the personal contributions they have made to one of us (JS): E. E. Krieckhaus; Ellen Oliver; and Stanley Schulkin.

Michael L. Power, Ph.D.
Jay Schulkin, Ph.D.
November 17, 2004

Contents

List of contributors

Andrew Bisits
Mothers and Babies Research Centre, John Hunter Hospital, Newcastle, NSW, Australia

John R. G. Challis
Departments of Physiology, and Obstetrics and Gynaecology, University of Toronto, CIHR Group in Fetal and Neonatal Health and Development, CIHR Institute of Human Development, Child and Youth Health, Canada

Eng-Cheng Chan
Mothers and Babies Research Centre, John Hunter Hospital, Newcastle, NSW, Australia

Vicki Clifton
Mothers and Babies Research Centre, John Hunter Hospital, Newcastle, NSW, Australia

Elysia Poggi Davis
Department of Psychiatry and Human Behavior, University of California, Irvine, California, CA, USA

Amanda J. Drake
Endocrinology Unit, University of Edinburgh, Western General Hospital, Edinburgh EH4 2XU, UK

Kristine Erickson
Molecular Neuroimaging Branch, National Institute of Mental Health, Bethesda, MD, USA

Pasquale Florio
Department of Pediatrics, Obstetrics and Reproductive Medicine, University of Siena, Siena School of Medicine, Siena, Italy

Warwick Giles
Mothers and Babies Research Centre, John Hunter Hospital, Newcastle, NSW, Australia

Laura Glynn
Department of Psychiatry and Human Behavior, University of California, Irvine, California, CA, USA

Calvin J. Hobel
Department of Obstetrics and Gynecology, Cedars Sinai Medical Center, Los Angeles, California, CA, USA

Megan C. Holmes
Endocrinology Unit, University of Edinburgh, Western General Hospital, Edinburgh EH4 2XU, UK

Sam Mesiano
Mothers and Babies Research Centre, John Hunter Hospital, Newcastle, NSW, Australia

Timothy J. M. Moss
School of Women's and Infants' Health and the Women and Infants Research Foundation, University of Western Australia, Western Australia

John P. Newnham
School of Women's and Infants' Health and
the Women and Infants Research
Foundation, University of Western Australia,
Western Australia

Richard Nicholson
Mothers and Babies Research Centre, John
Hunter Hospital, Newcastle, NSW, Australia

Felice Petraglia
Department of Pediatrics, Obstetrics and
Reproductive Medicine, University of Siena,
Siena School of Medicine, Siena, Italy

Michael L. Power
Department of Conservation Biology,
Nutrition Laboratory, Smithsonian's National
Zoological Park, Washington DC, USA
Department of Research, American College
of Obstetricians and Gynecologists,
Washington DC, USA

Curt A. Sandman
Department of Psychiatry and Human
Behavior, University of California, Irvine,
California, CA, USA

Louis Schmidt
Department of Psychology, McMaster
University, Canada

Jay Schulkin
Department of Physiology and Biophysics,
Georgetown University School of Medicine;
Clinical Neuroendocrinology Branch,
National Institute of Mental Health; and
Department of Research, American College
of Obstetricians and Gynecologists,
Washington DC, USA

Jonathan R. Seckl
Endocrinology Unit, University of
Edinburgh, Western General Hospital,
Edinburgh EH4 2XU, UK

Deborah M. Sloboda
School of Women's and Infants' Health and
the Women and Infants Research
Foundation, University of Western Australia,
Western Australia

Roger Smith
Mothers and Babies Research Centre, John
Hunter Hospital, Newcastle, NSW, Australia

Suzette D. Tardif
Southwest National Primate Research
Center, San Antonio, TX, USA

Wylie W. Vale
Peptide Biology Laboratory, Salk Institute,
La Jolla, California, CA, USA

Pathik D. Wadhwa
Departments of Psychiatry and Human
Behavior, and Obstetrics and Gynecology,
University of California, Irvine, California,
CA, USA

Alan G. Watts
The NIBS-Neuroscience Program and
Department of Biological Sciences,
University of Southern California, Los
Angeles, California, CA, USA

Tamas Zakar
Mothers and Babies Research Centre, John
Hunter Hospital, Newcastle, NSW, Australia

Preface

In the summer of 2002, a small one-day conference was held at the offices of the American College of Obstetricians and Gynecologists in Washington DC. The purpose of the conference was to consider the implications of the intriguingly converging research areas of peptide regulation by steroids in both brain and placenta, and how these research findings might enhance our understanding of the physiological processes of human gestation and parturition. An important subtext of the discussion was how events and processes at the beginning of life can affect health and well-being decades later. Among the participants were both clinicians and basic scientists; the research presented concerned both human studies and comparative research on animal models; the perspectives examined ranged from clinical medicine to evolutionary biology.

Our understanding of the physiological and regulatory processes that underlie the timing and progression of labor and delivery remains incomplete. Perhaps the most graphic indication of our inadequate understanding of this fundamental biological process is the current lack of accurate and effective clinical tools to either predict or prevent preterm birth. In the USA, the rate of preterm birth continues to rise, and half of preterm births are classified as idiopathic.

Progress is being made, however. A key paradigm shift is replacing the idea of the placenta as a largely passive organ mainly responsible for delivering nutrients to the fetus with the concept of the placenta as a metabolically active, transitory endocrine organ that serves as an important central regulator of maternal and fetal physiology. The placenta is now known to produce a wider array of steroids, peptides, cytokines and other regulatory molecules than does any other organ in the body, except possibly the brain.

In the mid-1980s, independent groups, some working on the brain and others on the placenta, made important discoveries regarding the differential regulation of one such neuropeptide, corticotropin-releasing hormone (CRH), by cortisol. Previously, the received view was that CRH release and production was negatively restrained by cortisol; the paradigmatic example of this was the negative feedback system of the hypothalamic–pituitary–adrenal axis. It turns out that in several areas of the brain (e.g. central nucleus of the amygdala, bed nucleus of the stria terminalis) and in the placenta, CRH release and production is induced by cortisol. Neural CRH is important in the induction of adaptive behaviors in response to conditions where high alertness and metabolic effort are appropriate (e.g. dangerous, fear-inducing situations). Placental CRH appears to play an important role in human gestation, fetal development and parturition, possibly either reflecting or serving as a gestational 'clock'. Although initial enthusiasm for placental CRH as a predictor of preterm labor has been tempered, recent research has suggested that it, indeed, may have clinical value (Wadhwa *et al.*, 2004).

This volume was inspired by the talks and discussions that occurred during the meeting in Washington DC in the summer of 2002. We strove to put together a book that reflects the diversity of research relevant to understanding neural and placental physiology, their intriguing similarities, and how these diverse lines of research can contribute to understanding human biology and improving health. We could not include all relevant areas in a single volume, and we apologize to our colleagues and other scientists whose work is not represented here.

REFERENCE

Wadhwa, P. D., Garite, T. J., Porto, M. *et al.* (2004). Placental corticotropin-releasing (CRH), spontaneous preterm birth, and fetal growth restriction: a prospective investigation. *Am. J. Obstet. Gynecol.*, **191**, 1063–9.

Introduction: brain and placenta, birth and behavior, health and disease

Michael L. Power[1] and Jay Schulkin[2]

[1] Department of Conservation Biology, Nutrition Laboratory, Smithsonian's National Zoological Park, Washington, DC, USA; Department of Research, American College of Obstetricians and Gynecologists
[2] Department of Physiology and Biophysics, Georgetown University, School of Medicine; Clinical Neuroendocrinology Branch, National Institute of Mental Health; and Department of Research, American College of Obstetricians and Gynecologists, Washington DC, USA

This book focuses on the production and regulation of steroids, peptides, and other regulatory factors by the placenta and by maternal and fetal organs, especially brain. These regulatory factors play vital roles in the maintenance of pregnancy, the timing and onset of labor, fetal growth and development, especially the programming of fetal physiology, and maternal and fetal neural function and regulation. The maternal–placental–fetal axis is an important target for research into the regulation and control of human pregnancy. A subtext of the book is the role of maternal–placental–fetal interactions in the onset of disease and disability, especially from preterm birth and fetal programming of physiologic systems that lead to adult onset diseases, such as diabetes and hypertension. The book addresses the relationships among glucocorticoids, neuropeptides (primarily corticotropin-releasing hormone, CRH), maternal nutrition, psychosocial 'stress', fetal growth and development, the onset of labor, and subsequent effects on health and behavior of infants, children and adults (Figure I.1).

The placenta is not just a conduit of oxygen and nutrients from the mother to the fetus. It is not a passive organ, but rather it is very metabolically active. It metabolizes 40–60% of glucose and oxygen extracted from uterine circulation (Gluckman and Pinal, 2002, 2003). The placenta produces a large number of 'information' molecules, such as biologically active steroids and peptides that serve to regulate and balance maternal and fetal physiology (Petraglia *et al.*, 1990). Once stimulated, placental hormones act on the placenta itself, and enter the maternal and fetal circulation. They act as endocrine, paracrine, and autocrine factors, to control the secretion of other regulatory factors that play functional roles in the growth, development, and maturation of the fetus, and likely have significant regulatory functions in maternal physiology and in the timing and onset of labor. Alterations in placental peptide and

1

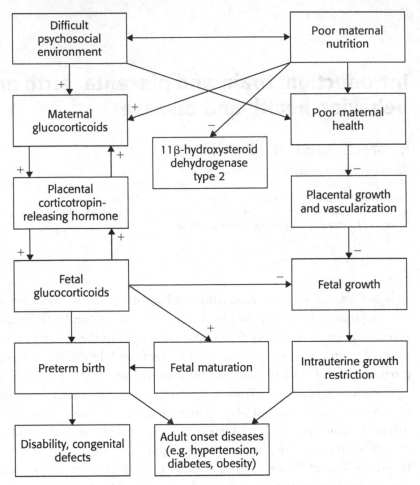

Figure I.1   A simplified schematic of the effects of maternal environmental on birth outcome

steroid production and regulation will have significant effects on fetal growth and development, and can lead to intrauterine growth restriction (IUGR), and/or deviations from the normal progression toward parturition leading to preterm birth.

Many of the hormones produced by the placenta are also produced by and are active in the brain. For example, CRH, cortisol, oxytocin, vitamin D, and catecholamines are found in cells within the placenta (Petraglia *et al.*, 1990), and in the brain. This has led some experts to suggest that the placenta performs regulatory functions that are similar, or at least analogous, to ones normally ascribed to the central nervous system. In other words, that the placenta becomes a central regulator of maternal and fetal physiology.

The first chapter of this book by Felice Petraglia and colleagues, introduces the reader to the broad array of brain, pituitary, gonadal, and adrenocortical hormones

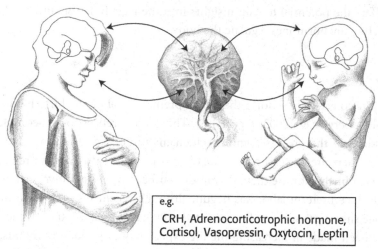

e.g.
CRH, Adrenocorticotrophic hormone,
Cortisol, Vasopressin, Oxytocin, Leptin

Figure I.2   The placenta acts as a central regulator of maternal and fetal physiology. It produces numerous peptide and steroid hormones that are also produced by and function in brain. These molecules can have endocrine, paracrine, or autocrine effects

produced by the placenta and other gestational intrauterine tissues (fetal membranes and deciduae). These peptides, steroids and monoamines are, for the most part, chemically identical and as biologically active as their hypothalamic/gonadal counterparts. Petraglia and colleagues suggest that the human placenta may be considered as a (transient) neuroendocrine organ, and a central regulator of maternal–placental–fetal physiology (Figure I.2).

Consider growth hormone (GH) production during human pregnancy. In humans, from 24 weeks gestation to parturition, maternal pituitary GH declines (and becomes effectively nonexistent). Biologically active GH-V, produced by the placenta, is secreted into maternal circulation, and appears to serve as a replacement for pituitary GH. GH-V is not regulated by GH-releasing factors, but is suppressed by elevated maternal glucose. The function of GH-V is not completely understood, but it likely serves to induce relative maternal insulin resistance, and encourages reliance on lipolysis for maternal energy metabolism (Lacroix *et al.*, 2002).

Thus, in this instance the placenta performed a role in the regulation of maternal physiology that before pregnancy was coordinated by the central nervous system. For the developing fetus, many hormones that will eventually be produced by fetal organs are, by necessity, first provided by the placenta. The placenta is also the most likely source of factors that stimulate the cascading steps in the labor and birth process. The placenta is a central regulator of maternal and fetal physiology, ensuring appropriate physiologic milieus for normal growth and development of fetal, placental and maternal tissues necessary for successful reproduction. As such, it offers the potential to gain insights into the role, function and mechanisms by which many hormones regulate the body.

Preterm birth

Despite considerable efforts, the rate of premature labor and birth has not declined (Goldenberg *et al.*, 2003; Figure I.3). This largely reflects our incomplete understanding of the processes and mechanisms underlying the timing of labor and birth. There are, as yet, no accurate diagnostic criteria to predict preterm labor or preterm birth. Nor are there therapies that have been definitively shown to delay birth once preterm labor has begun, although recent research regarding progesterone shows promise (da Fonseca *et al.*, 2003; Meis *et al.*, 2003). Clinical advances have been made in increasing the life expectancy of premature infants; but these infants still face a life of increased risk of early death, disability and disease (Regev *et al.*, 2003).

In their chapter (Chapter 2), Roger Smith and colleagues briefly review the astonishing variety of processes observed in mammalian pregnancy. There does not appear to be a single path to parturition among mammals, nor does there appear to be a single pathway leading to labour in humans, suggesting a fail-safe system. Smith and colleagues stress that a good understanding of the normal physiology which determines the timing of human birth is necessary to understand the

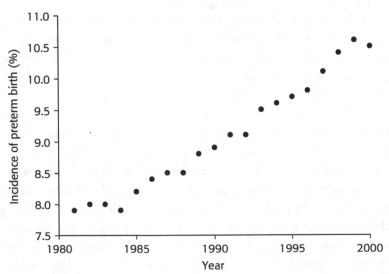

Figure I.3   The incidence of preterm birth in the USA from 1981 to 2000. Data from Goldenberg *et al.* (2003)

disturbances that occur in pathology leading to preterm birth. They review recent evidence for a number of factors involved in human parturition, including CRH, but especially the role of progesterone receptors in the final pathways of human myometrial activation.

Michael Power and Suzette Tardif review the effects of maternal nutrition on pregnancy outcome, and consider some of the possible metabolic signals involved. Epidemiologic studies and animal experiments support a role for poor maternal nutrition in preterm birth and IUGR. In developing nations, protein-energy malnutrition is, unfortunately, still a significant factor in adverse pregnancy outcome. In developed nations, excess food intake (and insufficient energy expenditure) leading to obesity and type 2 diabetes is a more significant factor, although micronutrient undernutrition (e.g. folate, calcium, vitamin C) can adversely affect pregnancy outcome. The roles of CRH, leptin and the insulin-like growth factor system in pregnancy outcome are considered.

An important subtext in this chapter and also in the chapter by Smith and colleagues is the possible role of CRH produced by the placenta in normal and pathologic pregnancy. Soon after the isolation and characterization of hypothalamic CRH by Vale and colleagues (1981), CRH was detected in maternal serum during pregnancy (Sasaki et al., 1984). The CRH gene was subsequently shown to be expressed in the human placenta (Grino et al., 1987), and to be the source of the maternal (and fetal) serum CRH. Several groups documented the pattern of increasing serum CRH concentration in normal human pregnancy (Goland et al., 1986; Campbell et al., 1987; Laatikainen et al., 1987; Sasaki et al., 1987), and the marked elevation of CRH in pregnancies complicated by multiple gestation (Warren et al., 1990) and pre-eclampsia (Laatikainen et al., 1991). Women destined to give birth prematurely exhibited both elevated CRH (Warren et al., 1992) and a precocious rise in CRH (McLean et al., 1995; Hobel et al., 1999; Leung et al., 2001; Figure I.4).

The evidence strongly supported an important role of CRH in the progression of human pregnancy to parturition. Subsequent research has supported that hypothesis, but the possibility that CRH could serve as a simple, reliable clinical marker for pregnancies at risk for delivering preterm has not panned out (McLean et al., 1999; Inder et al., 2001; Ellis et al., 2002). This may be partly explained by evidence showing that CRH has autocrine, paracrine, and endocrine actions, and may contribute to pregnancy via multiple pathways. For example, CRH may perform an autocrine, or paracrine function in the human chorion that assists in regulating prostaglandin concentrations via production of 15-hydroxy prostoglandin dehydrogenase, and thus may contribute to myometrial quiescence (not stimulation) during most of the pregnancies (McKeown and Challis, 2003).

From the comparative and evolutionary perspective, CRH remains a prime candidate for research into the regulation of human pregnancy and fetal development.

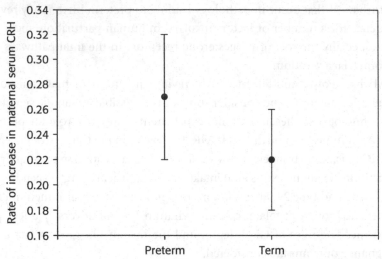

Figure I.4   The rate of increase in maternal serum CRH concentration is greater in pregnancies destined to deliver preterm (adapted from Leung *et al.*, 2001, with permission). Data are the means and 95% confidence intervals

Anthropoid primates are the only species known to produce placental CRH during pregnancy (Robinson *et al.*, 1989; Bowman *et al.*, 2001). Understanding this apparently unique anthropoid primate adaptation may be key to understanding the normal course of human pregnancy, and metabolic disruptions of pregnancy. This will likely require the further development of nonhuman primate models of human pregnancy, fetal development, and placental function.

Origins of adult-onset disease

That events in utero affect pregnancy outcome is a fact. Preterm birth and IUGR are the most obvious, and possibly the most significant, examples of events in utero leading to post natal morbidity and mortality. What is new is the evidence that birth outcomes heretofore considered successful might lead to poor health outcomes in adult life. Epidemiologic studies have indicated that the effects of birth size on latter disease extend into the normal birth weight range, and thus are not restricted to the serious effects of IUGR or premature birth (Barker, 1991; Barker *et al.*, 1993; Curhan *et al.*, 1996a, b).

   This realization has led to a concerted search for mechanisms. Much of this search has centered on excessive or inappropriate activation of the HPA axis, both maternal and fetal. Activation of the fetal hypothalamic–pituitary–adrenal (HPA) axis is a common characteristic across species that results in increased output of fetal glucocorticoids, which contribute to mechanisms associated with the onset

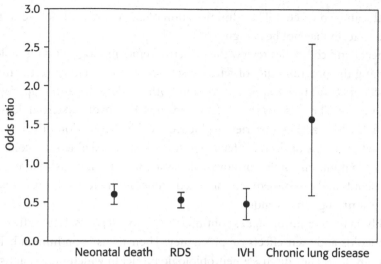

Figure I.5   A single course of antenatal steroids significantly decreases the risk of neonatal death, RDS, and IVH, but does not decrease the incidence of chronic lung disease. Data (means and 95% confidence intervals) are from Dudley *et al.* (2003)

of parturition and to the normal maturation of fetal organ systems. The fetus responds to an adverse intrauterine environment with precocious HPA activation, and premature upregulation of critical genes at each level along the axis. Thus in compromised pregnancies the fetus may be exposed inappropriately to sustained elevations of glucocorticoids.

An important theme in the chapters by Debra Sloboda and colleagues (Chapter 4) and Jonathon Seckl and colleagues (Chapter 5) is that glucocorticoids are potent steroids that have organizing effects on fetal organs. Key targets for in utero programming of physiology include glucocorticoid receptor gene expression and the CRH system. Sloboda and colleagues review data from animal models concerning the effects of exogenous glucocorticoids on pregnancy and fetal development.

The use of glucocorticoids to mature fetal lung tissue prior to preterm birth has had a significant positive effect on neonatal morbidity and mortality. A single course of antenatal corticosteroids significantly reduces the risk of respiratory distress syndrome (RDS), intraventricular hemorrhage (IVH), and neonatal mortality, although it does not reduce the overall incidence of chronic lung disease (Dudley *et al.*, 2003; Figure I.5). However, animal studies, such as the one described in Chapters 4 and 5, have demonstrated that glucocorticoid administration in late gestation can result in IUGR and significant alterations in metabolic and HPA axis function and regulation. This raises cautionary warnings concerning both the use of multiple doses of glucocorticoids to mature fetal lung tissue in pregnancies at risk for preterm birth, and the accuracy with which pregnancies at risk for preterm birth can be predicted. The administration of glucocorticoids to a fetus that is carried to term may not be benign.

Seckl and colleagues review the evidence (epidemiologic and physiologic) concerning the programming of fetal physiology in utero. They present the case that glucocorticoids play important roles in both appropriate and inappropriate programming. They discuss the placental enzyme 11β-hydroxysteroid dehydrogenase type 2, which acts as a barrier to glucocorticoids. Regulation of this enzyme may serve to increase or decrease fetal exposure to maternal glucocorticoids. They discuss programming of the cardiovascular system, liver, pancreas, and brain by glucocorticoids and the subsequent increased vulnerability to adult onset diseases such programming can engender.

Elysia Davis and colleagues continue the theme of stress, HPA activation, glucocorticoids and their effects on pregnancy. Their focus is on human behavior and human data. They discuss a neurobiologic model in which maternal psychosocial stress influences developmental outcomes that are mediated, in part, via maternal–placental–fetal neuroendocrine mechanisms. They present data on the consequences of stress during pregnancy on neuroendocrine processes and fetal and infant development. They also note the uniqueness of placental CRH in anthropoid primates, and that placental CRH and cortisol may contribute to the organization of the fetal central nervous system (Sandman *et al.*, 1997; Florio and Petraglia, 2001).

Feed-forward regulation of CRH by glucocorticoids

Until recently, it was the received view that glucocorticoids restrained CRH production. The model system was the HPA axis, wherein hypothalamic CRH stimulated pituitary adrenocorticotrophic hormone (ACTH) production, which in turn stimulated cortisol production by the adrenals. Cortisol crossed the blood–brain barrier and exerted negative feedback on CRH neurons in the hypothalamic paraventricular nucleus (PVN), restraining the system. It is a curious fact that independent groups of researchers, working on different CRH producing organs (the brain and the placenta) found at roughly the same time that glucocorticoids can also stimulate CRH production. Glucocorticoid added to cultured human placental tissue resulted in the upregulation of CRH gene expression (Robinson *et al.*, 1988; Jones *et al.*, 1989; Figure I.6). In several regions of the brain (e.g. amygdala and bed nucleus of the stria terminalis, and areas of the paraventricular region of the hypothalamus that project to the brainstem) CRH messenger ribonucleic acid (mRNA) expression similarly is upregulated by glucocorticoids (Swanson and Simmons, 1989; Makino *et al.*, 1994; Watts and Sanchez-Watts, 1995; Figure I.7).

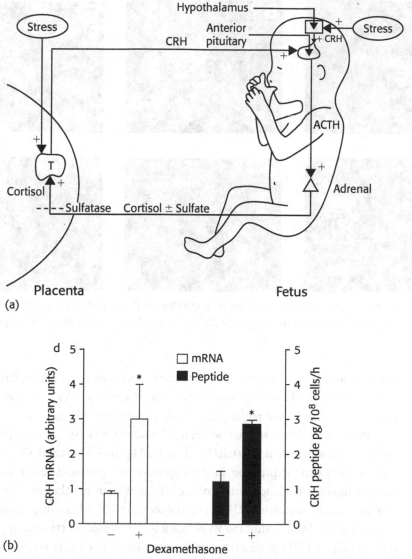

Figure I.6   (a) A positive feedback loop is established between the fetus and the placenta, where cortisol (either maternal or from the fetal) adrenal upregulates placental CRH messenger ribonucleic acid (mRNA) expression and CRH peptide content. Placental CRH stimulates the fetal HPA axis to produce more cortisol. (b) Dexamethasone increases CRH mRNA and CRH peptide concentration in cultured placental cells. From Robinson *et al.* (1988), with permission

The majority of CRH neurons within the PVN are clustered in the parvicellular division. Other regions with predominant CRH-containing neurons are the lateral bed nucleus of the stria terminalis and the central region of the central nucleus of the amygdala (CeA). To a smaller degree, there are CRH cells in the lateral

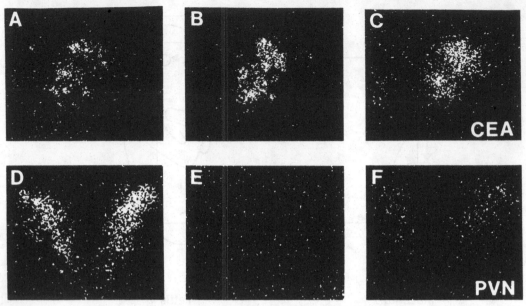

Figure I.7   Corticosterone decreases CRH expression in the rat PVN but increases CRH expression in rat central nucleus of the amygdala (CeA). From Makino *et al.* (1994), with permission

hypothalamus, prefrontal and cingulate cortex. In brainstem regions, CRH cells are clustered near the locus coeruleus (Barringtons' nucleus) (Valentino *et al.*, 1995), parabrachial region and regions of the solitary nucleus (Figure I.8).

In this volume, Watts reviews neural regulation of CRH axons. He emphasizes that there is cell specificity in how CRH and the CRH gene is regulated. Glucocorticoids repress CRH gene expression in the hypothalamic paraventricular nucleus (the familiar negative feedback system of the HPA axis), but in other regions (e.g. CeA) glucocorticoids stimulate CRH gene expression, and in others glucocorticoids have no effect at all. Even within the PVN, basal levels of glucocorticoids appear necessary to sustain CRH gene expression. Adrenalectomized rats show a suppressed CRH response in the PVN to hypovolemia rather than an exaggerated response (Tanimura and Watts, 2000). It turns out that the 'usual' negative restraint of CRH by glucocorticoids has actually only been seen in one (admittedly important) set of CRH expressing neurons. Thus the increase in human placental CRH mRNA expression when exposed to glucocorticoids does not appear to represent an unusual circumstance. The current state of knowledge supports the idea that glucocorticoids have variable effects on CRH regulation depending on cell type, and intracellular and extracellular factors. The original idea of glucocorticoids functioning as a negative feedback response molecule has been expanded to a more flexible, context-oriented understanding of regulation.

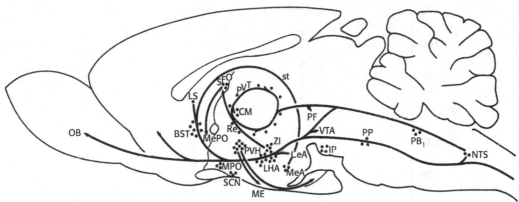

Figure I.8   The localization of CRH neurons in rat brain (from Swanson *et al.*, 1983). A partial list of the abbreviations that are relevant to this book: BST = bed nucleus of the stria terminalis; CeA = central nucleus of the amygdala; LHA = lateral hypothalamus; MeA = medial nucleus of the amygdala; PVH = paraventricular hypothalamic nuclei.

Glucocorticoids have both permissive, suppressive and stimulatory effects on diverse end-organ systems (Sapolsky, 2000), and are part of both positive and negative feedback systems regulating CRH expression. Jay Schulkin and colleagues review some of the evidence that surrounds the positive regulation of CRH gene expression in the placenta and the brain by glucocorticoids, and the possible roles of CRH and glucocorticoids in the regulation of human pregnancy and of behavior.

Glucocorticoids play important functional roles in facilitating gene expression of CRH in both the placenta and the brain. The placental production of CRH may in part function for the fetus, reminiscent of neural function, as both a sensory and effector system in providing important sources of adaptation to environmental demands (Wadhwa *et al.*, 2001). Pre-eclampsia, IUGR, preterm labor and birth, even multiple gestations are all associated with increased maternal serum CRH. Multiple gestations are not a pathology, but they produce increased strain on maternal physiology, and are associated with significantly higher fetal death rates (Kahn *et al.*, 2003). Exaggerated expression of CRH in the placenta may reflect states of adversity and an increased vulnerability to preterm delivery of the neonate (Majzoub *et al.*, 1999). Elevated placental production of CRH appears to be a marker of metabolic disorder or disruption of pregnancy in humans.

Rat and nonhuman primate studies suggest that prenatal and early life adversity can have lifelong consequences on stress responses and, potentially, on vulnerability to physical and psychiatric disorders (Heim and Nemeroff, 2002). Rat pups deprived of maternal closeness for 3 hours a day for a 2-week period were found to have higher levels of CRH mRNA expression in the PVN, CeA and the lateral bed nucleus of the stria terminalis as adults (Plotsky, 1996; Levine, 2000). Infant

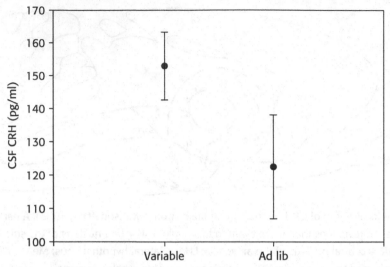

Figure I.9   Five-year old rhesus macaques whose mother experienced variable foraging conditions had higher CRH in their cerebral spinal fluid (CSF) than did monkeys whose mother experienced predictable foraging conditions. Data (mean and sem) from Coplan *et al.* (2001)

monkeys reared by mothers experiencing unpredictable foraging conditions had higher CRH in cerebrospinal fluid in adulthood than infant monkeys reared by mothers that had either a predictable overabundance or a scarcity of food. The studies show that unpredictability in early life, and not just chronic hardship, led to persistently higher CRH levels in the cerebrospinal fluid in adulthood, up to 5 years later (Coplan *et al.*, 2001; Figure I.9).

Glucocorticoids readily cross from the peripheral systemic circuitry into the brain. In extra-hypothalamic sites in the brain, the upregulation of CRH by glucocorticoids is linked to conditions of adversity or stress. It can result in fearful and anxious behaviors. Physiologic effects of the prenatal environment include changes in programming of the CeA, and a vulnerability in the infant toward perceiving events as fearful (Welberg and Seckl, 2001).

REFERENCES

Barker, D. J. P. (1991). *Fetal and Infant Origins of Adult Disease*. London: BMJ.

Barker, D. J. P., Gluckman, P. D., Godfrey, K. M. *et al.* (1993). Fetal nutrition and cardiovascular disease in adult life. *Lancet*, **341**, 938–41.

Bowman, M. E., Lopata, A. *et al.* (2001). Corticotropin-releasing hormone-binding protein in primates. *Am. J. Primatol.*, **53**(3), 123–30.

Campbell, E. A., Linton, E. A., Wolfe, C. D. *et al.* (1987). Plasma corticotropin-releasing hormone concentrations during pregnancy and parturition. *J. Clin. Endocrinol. Metab.*, **64**, 1054–9.

Coplan, J. D., Smith, E. L. P., Altemus, M. *et al.* (2001). Variable foraging demand rearing: sustained elevations in cisternal cerebrospinal fluid corticotropin-releasing factor concentrations in adult primates. *Biol. Psychiat.*, **50**, 200–4.

Curhan, G. C., Chertow, G. M., Willett, W. C. *et al.* (1996a). Birth-weight and adult hypertension and obesity in women. *Circulation*, **94**, 1310–15.

Curhan, G. C., Willett, W. C., Rimm, E. B. *et al.* (1996b). Birth weight and adult hypertension, diabetes mellitus, and obesity in US men. *Circulation*, **94**, 3246–50.

da Fonseca, E. B., Bittar, R. E., Carvalho, M. H. and Zugaib, M. (2003). Prophylactic administration of progesterone by vaginal suppository to reduce the incidence of spontaneous preterm birth in women at increased risk: a randomized placebo-controlled double-blind study. *Am. J. Obstet. Gynecol.*, **188**, 419–24.

Dudley, D. J., Waters, T. P. and Nathanielsz, P. W. (2003). Current status of single-course antenatal steroid therapy. *Clin. Obstet. Gynecol.*, **46**, 132–49.

Ellis, M. J., Livesey, J. H., Inder, W. J., Prickett, T. C. R. and Reid, R. (2002). Plasma corticotropin-releasing hormone and unconjugated estriol in human pregnancy: gestational patterns and ability to predict preterm labor. *Am. J. Obstet. Gynecol.*, **189**, 94–9.

Florio, P. and Petraglia, F. (2001). Human placental corticotropin releasing factor (CRF) in the adaptive response to pregnancy. *Stress*, **4**, 247–61.

Gluckman, P. D. and Pinal, C. S. (2002). Maternal–placental–fetal interactions in the endocrine regulation of fetal growth. *Endocrine*, **19**, 81–9.

Gluckman, P. D. and Pinal, C. S. (2003). Regulation of fetal growth by the somatotrophic axis. *J. Nutr.*, **133**, 1741S–6S.

Goland, R. S., Wardlaw, S. L. *et al.* (1986). High levels of corticotropin-releasing hormone immunoactivity in maternal and fetal plasma during pregnancy. *J. Clin. Endocrinol. Metab.*, **63**(5), 1199–203.

Goldenberg, R. L., Iams, J. D., Mercer, B. M. *et al.* (2003). What we have learned about the predictors of preterm birth. *Semin. Perinatol.*, **27**, 185–93.

Grino, M., Chrousos, G. P. and Margioris, A. N. (1987). The corticotropin-releasing hormone gene is expressed in human placenta. *Biochem. Biophys. Res. Commun.*, **148**, 1208–14.

Heim, C. and Nemeroff, C. B. (2002). Neurobiology of early life stress: clinical studies. *Semin. Clin. Neuropsychiat.*, **7**(2), 147–59.

Hobel, C. J., Dunkel-Schetter, C., Roesch, S. C., Castro, L. C. and Arora, C. P. (1999). Maternal plasma corticotropin-releasing hormone associated with stress at 20 weeks' gestation in pregnancies ending in preterm delivery. *Am. J. Obstet. Gynecol.*, **180**, S257–63.

Inder, W. J., Prickett, T. C. R., Ellis, M. J. *et al.* (2001). The utility of plasma CRH as a predictor of preterm delivery. *J. Clin. Endocrinol. Metab.*, **86**, 5706–10.

Jones, S. A., Brooks, A. N. and Challis, J. R. G. (1989). Steroids modulate corticotropin-releasing hormone production in human fetal membranes and placenta. *Clin. Endocrinol. Metabol.*, **68**, 825–30.

Kahn, B., Lumey, L. H., Zybert, P. A. *et al.* (2003). Prospective risk of fetal death in singleton, twin, and triplet gestations: implications for practice. *Obste. Gynecol.*, **102**, 685–92.

Laatikainen, T., Virtanen, T., Raisanen, I. and Salminen, K. (1987). Immunoreactive corticotropin-releasing factor and corticotropin during pregnancy and puerperium. *Neuropeptides*, **10**, 343–53.

Laatikainen, T., Virtanen, T., Kaaja, R. and Salminen-Lappalainen, K. (1991). Corticotropin-releasing hormone in maternal and cord plasma in pre-eclampsia. *Eur. J. Obstet. Gynecol. Reprod. Biol.*, **39**, 19–24.

Lacroix, M.-C., Guibourdenche, J., Frendo, J.-L., Pidoux, G. and Evain-Brion, D. (2002). Placental growth hormones. *Endocrine*, **19**, 73–9.

Leung, T. N., Chung, T. K. H., Madsen, G. *et al.* (2001). Rate of rise in maternal plasma corticotropin-releasing hormone and its relation to gestational length. *Br. J. Obstet. Gynaecol.*, **108**, 527–32.

Levine, S. (2000). Modulation of CRF gene expression by early experience. Neuropsychopharmacology, **23**, S77.

Majzoub, J. A., McGregor, J. A. *et al.* (1999). A central theory of preterm and term labor: putative role for corticotropin-releasing hormone. *Am. J. Obstet. Gynecol.*, **180**(1 Pt 3), S232–41.

Makino, S., Gold, P. W. and Schulkin, J. (1994). Corticosterone effects on corticotrophin-relasing hormone mRNA in the central nucleus of the amygdala and the parvocellular region of the paraventricular nucleus of the hypothalamus. *Brain Res.*, **640**, 105–12.

McKeown, K. J. and Challis, J. R. G. (2003). Regulation of 15-hydroxy prostaglandin dehydrogenase by corticotropin-releasing hormone through a calcium-dependent pathway in human chorion trophoblast cells. *J. Clin. Endocrinol. Metab.*, **88**, 1737–41.

McLean, M., Bistis, A., Davies, J. J. *et al.* (1995). A placental clock controlling the length of human pregnancy. *Nat. Med.*, **1**, 460–3.

McLean, M., Bisits, A., Davies, J. *et al.* (1999). Predicting risk of preterm delivery by second-trimester measurement of maternal plasma corticotropin-releasing hormone and alpha-fetoprotein concentrations. *Am. J. Obstet. Gynecol.*, **181**, 207–15.

Meis, P. J., Klebanoff, M., Thom, E. *et al.* (2003). Prevention of recurrent preterm delivery by 17 alpha-hydroxyprogesterone caproate. *N. Eng. J. Med.*, **348**, 2379–85.

Petraglia, F., Volpe, A., Genazzani., A. R. *et al.* (1990). Neuroendocrinology of the human placenta. *Front. Neuroendocrinlp.*, **11**, 6–37.

Plotsky, P. M. (1996). Early environmental regulation of forebrain glucocorticoid receptor gene expression: implications for adrenocortical responses to stress. *Dev. Neurosci.*, **18**, 49–72.

Regev, R. H., Lusky, A., Dolfin, T. *et al.* Israel Neonatal Network. (2003). Excess mortality and morbidity among small-for-gestational-age premature infants: a population-based study. *J Pediatr.*, **143**, 186–91.

Robinson, B. G., Emanuel, R. L. *et al.* (1988). Glucocorticoid stimulates expression of corticotropin-releasing hormone gene in human placenta. *Proc. Natl. Acad. Sci. USA.*, **85**(14), 5244–8.

Robinson, B. G., Arbiser, J. L., Emanuel, R. L. and Majzoub, J. A. (1989). Species-specific placental corticotropin releasing hormone messenger RNA and peptide expression. *Mol. Cell. Endocrinol.*, **62**, 337–41.

Sandman, C. A., Wadhwa, P. D., Chicz-DeMet, A., Dunkel-Schetter, C. and Porto, M. (1997). Maternal stress, HPA activity, and fetal/infant outcome. *Ann. NY Acad. Sci. USA*, **814**, 266–75.

Sapolsky, R. M. (2000). Glucocorticoids and hippocampal atrophy in neuropsychiatric disorders. *Arch. Gen. Psychiat.*, **57**, 925–35.

Sasaki, A., Liotta, A. S., Luckey, M. M. *et al.* (1984). Immunoreactive corticotropin-releasing factor is present in human maternal serum during the third trimester of pregnancy. *J. Clin. Endocrinol. Metab.*, **59**, 812–14.

Sasaki, A., Shinkawa, O., Margioris, A. N. *et al.* (1987). Immunoreactive corticotropin-releasing hormone in human plasma during pregnancy, labor and delivery. *J. Clin. Endocrinol. Metab.*, **64**, 224–9.

Swanson, L. W., Sawchenko, P. E., Rivier, J. and Vale, W. W. (1983). Organization of ovine corticotropin-releasing factor immunoreactive cells and fibers in the rat brain: an immunohistochemical study. *Neuroendocrinology*, **36**, 165–86.

Swanson, L. W. and Simmons, D. M. (1989). Differential steroid hormone and neural influences on peptide mRNA levels in CRH cells of the paraventricular nucleus: a hybridization histochemical study in the rat. *J. Comp. Neurol.*, **285**, 413–35.

Tanimura, S. M. and Watts, A. G. (2000). Adrenalectomy dramatically modifies the dynamics of neuropeptide and c-*fos* gene responses to stress in the hypothalamic paraventricular nucleus. *J. Neuroendocrinol.*, **12**, 715–22.

Vale, W., Spiess, J., Rivier, C. and Rivier, J. (1981). Characterization of a 41-residue ovine hypothalamic peptide that stimulates secretion of corticotropin and β-endorphin. *Science*, **78**, 1394–7.

Valentino, R. J., Pavcovich, L. A. and Hirata, H. (1995). Evidence for corticotropin-releasing hormone projections from Barrington's nucleus to the periaqueductal gray and dorsal motor nucleus of the vagus in the rat. *J. Comp. Neurol.*, **363**, 402–22.

Wadhwa, P. D., Sandman, C. A. *et al.* (2001). The neurobiology of stress in human pregnancy: implications for prematurity and development of the fetal central nervous system. *Prog. Brain. Res.*, **133**, 131–42.

Warren, W. B., Goland, R. S., Wardlaw, S. L. *et al.* (1990). Elevated maternal plasma corticotropin releasing hormone levels in twin gestation. *J. Perinat. Med.*, **18**, 39–44.

Warren, W. B., Patrick, S. L. and Goland, R. S. (1992). Elevated maternal plasma corticotropin-releasing hormone levels in pregnancies complicated by preterm labor. *Am. J. Obstet. Gynecol.*, **166**(4), 1198–204.

Watts, A. G. and Sanchez-Watts, G. (1995). Region-specific regulation of neuropeptide mRNAs in rat limbic forebrain neurones by aldosterone and corticosterone. *J. Physiol.*, **484**(Pt 3), 721–36.

Welberg, L. A. and Seckl, J. R. (2001). Prenatal stress, glucocorticoids and the programming of the brain. *J. Neuroendocrinol.*, **13**, 113–28.

1

Placental expression of neurohormones and other neuroactive molecules in human pregnancy

Felice Petraglia[1], Pasquale Florio[1] and Wylie W. Vale[2]

[1] Department of Pediatrics, Obstetrics and Reproductive Medicine, University of Siena, Siena School of Medicine, Siena, Italy
[2] Peptide Biology Laboratory, Salk Institute, La Jolla, CA, USA

Introduction

The human placenta and its accessory membranes (amnion and chorion) actually undertake the role of intermediary barriers and source(s) of active messengers in the maternal–fetal dialog. In the past decades, an accelerated progress in the understanding of physiological roles and of pathological influences of the placenta and other gestational intrauterine tissues (fetal membranes and deciduae) has occurred. These organs and tissues produce brain, pituitary, gonadal and adrenocortical hormones (Petraglia *et al.*, 1990b; 1996d; Petraglia, 1991; Reis *et al.*, 2001; 2002), chemically identical and as biologically active as their hypothalamic/gonadal counterparts and, when added to placental cell cultures, they modulate the release of both pituitary-like peptide hormones and gonadal/adrenal cortex-like steroid hormones. Thus, the intraplacental mechanism of control of hormone secretion resembles in many aspects the organization of hypothalamus–pituitary–target organ axes. Under this perspective, the human placenta may be considered as a neuroendocrine organ, since its secretion of substances analogous to neurohormones, neuropeptides, neurosteroids and monoamines (Table 1.1) have endocrine, paracrine and autocrine function (Petraglia *et al.*, 1996d).

Physiological functions of these placental secretions include:

(1) to maintain an equilibrium between the fetus and the mother;
(2) to provide a favorable uterine environment at implantation;
(3) to regulate fetal growth during pregnancy;
(4) to direct the appropriate signals for the timing of parturition.

Table 1.1 Neuropeptides, neurosteroids and monoamines produced by the human placenta

Brain peptides	Pituitary-like peptides and proteins	Neurosteroids	Monoamines and adrenal-like peptides
Corticotrophin-releasing factor	ACTH	Progesterone	Epinephrine
TRH	TSH	Allopregnanolone	Norepinephrine
GHRH	Growth hormone	Pregnenolone sulfate	Dopamine
Gonadotrophin-releasing hormone	hPL	5α-dihydro progesterone	Serotonin
Melatonin	Human chorionic gonadotropin		Adrenomedullin
Colecistokinin	Luteinizing hormone		
Methionine enkephalin	Follicle stimulating hormone		
Dynorphin	β-endorphin		
Neurotensin	Prolactin		
Vasointestinal peptide	Oxytocin		
Galanin	Leptin		
Somatostatin	Activin		
Calcitonin gene-related peptide	Follistatin		
Neuropeptide Y	Inhibin		
Substance P			
Endothelin			
ANP			
Renin			
Angiotensin			
Urocortin			

In other words, both maternal and fetal physiology during pregnancy are influenced by placental secretion of neurohormones and other regulatory molecules (Figure 1.1). Human placenta decisively contributes to all phases of gestation, and placental neurohormones are critical in providing a favorable uterine environment. When maternal or fetal acute or chronic hostile events occur, placental secretions may protect the feto-placental unit, and/or trigger parturition, thus helping the fetus to escape from a hostile environment.

The present chapter will review the experimental and clinical studies on the possible role of placental neurohormones and related molecules in physiological and pathological conditions occurring throughout gestation.

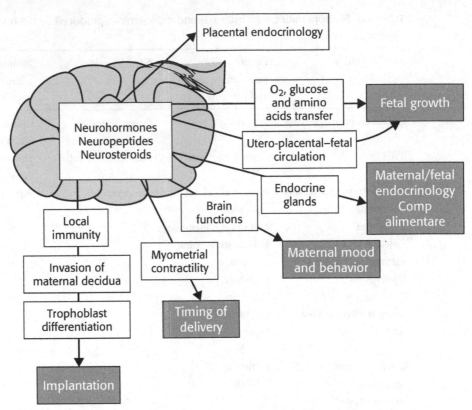

Figure 1.1   The putative role of human placenta throughout pregnancy. The secretion of neurohormones, neuropeptides and neurosteroids is able to affect several maternal and fetal functions through endocrine mechanisms, but at the same time is also able to affect several placental functions in autocrine/paracrine ways

Neurosteroids and monoamines

Neurosteroid is a generic denomination applied to the steroid hormones which are synthesized within the nervous system, either de novo from cholesterol, or by the metabolism of precursors obtained from an outside source. The placenta is a source of several neurosteroids comprising progesterone itself, its derivates 5α-pregnan-3a-ol-20-one (allopregnanolone) and 5α-dihydroprogesterone (5α-DHP), and its precursor pregnenolone sulfate (Dombroski *et al.*, 1997; Le Goascogne *et al.*, 2000). The levels of allopregnanolone in maternal serum increase progressively during gestation and, diversely from progesterone, are augmented in hypertensive complications of pregnancy (Luisi *et al.*, 2000). Apart from progesterone, the role of placental neurosteroids in the physiology of pregnancy is largely unknown. These hormones may contribute to the neurochemical and behavioral changes of pregnancy and puerperium, since they interfere with gabaergic circuits and have anxyolitic effects (Dombroski *et al.*, 1997). Placental neurosteroids may also contribute to myometrial quiescence, as suggested by their ability to reduce the contraction frequency of human myometrial strips in vitro (Lofgren *et al.*, 1992).

The placenta is a source and target for epinephrine, norepinephrine, dopamine and 5-hydroxitryptamin (serotonin). The enzymes involved in monoamine synthesis and metabolism as well as monoamine transporters and receptors have been identified in the placenta (Falkay and Kovacs, 1994; Bzoskie *et al.*, 1997; Vaillancourt *et al.*, 1998; Kenney *et al.*, 1999; Nguyen *et al.*, 1999). Several studies have suggested that local monoamines participate in the regulation of placental function. The placental metabolism and transport of these neurohormones has an important role in determining the availability and bioactivity of biogenic amines to both mother and fetus. In preeclampsia (PE) there is an increased activity of tyrosine hydroxylase in placental tissue and this is likely to contribute to the higher levels of catecholamines in maternal circulation (Manyonda *et al.*, 1998). It has been shown that placental norepinephrine transporter mRNA expression is reduced in some gestational diseases, resulting in increased norepinephrine levels in fetal circulation (Bzoskie *et al.*, 1997). The activity of serotonin transporter in placental cells is suppressed by agonistic stimulation of cannabinoid receptors, indicating that placental clearance of serotonin may account for adverse effects of cannabinoid use during pregnancy (Kenney *et al.*, 1999).

Peptide signaling and placental endocrinology

Human placenta plays a fundamental role in the physiology of pregnancy. Its most relevant role is to maintain an equilibrium between the fetus and the mother, regulating the body functions of both organisms in a complementary way. Initiation, maintenance and termination of pregnancy are related to placental functions. Under this interpretation, the capacity of hormonal production in placental cells is critical in providing a favorable uterine environment at implantation, in regulating fetal growth during pregnancy and in directing the appropriate signals for the timing of parturition.

Increasing evidence indicates that maternal or fetal physiological and pathological stress conditions influence placental secretion of neurohormones, so that endogenous or exogenous stress stimuli stimulate the placenta to take an active role in responding to these adverse conditions.

A major role for the various peptides produced by the placenta, fetal membranes and decidua is the control of local placental hormonogenesis. The various neurohormones act on local hormone secretion through paracrine and/or autocrine mechanisms, as their actions may occur in the same tissue where they originate as well as in the contiguous tissues.

CRH, CRH-BP and urocortin

Immunoreactive corticotropin-releasing hormone (CRH; Box 1.1) was first detected in extracts of human placenta obtained at full term from spontaneous delivery (Shibasaki *et al.*, 1982) and was found to be as bioactive as rat hypothalamic CRH or synthetic ovine CRH on the release of immunoreactive adrenocorticotrophic hormone (ACTH) and β-endorphin (β-END) from cultures of rat

Box 1.1 Corticotropin-releasing hormone

The CRH is a 41 amino acid peptide released from the medial eminence of the hypothalamus, acting at the corticotroph cells in the anterior pituitary to stimulate the release of ACTH and related peptides in response to stress events, and modulating behavioral, vascular and immune response to stress (Vale *et al.*, 1993). Human placenta, decidua, chorion and amnion also produce CRH (Petraglia *et al.*, 1992a; Warren and Silverman, 1995).

Expression and localization
Placental villi at term immunostained for CRH show the presence of the neurohormone in some cytotrophoblast cells (Saijonmaa *et al.*, 1988), as well as in syncytiotrophoblast cells (Warren and Silverman, 1995). Cytotrophoblast cells are transformed to syncytial cells, which release CRH factor when maintained in culture (Petraglia *et al.*, 1987c; Frim *et al.*, 1988; Jones *et al.*, 1989; Riley and Challis, 1991).

Other than from placental cells, CRH is also released from cultured amnion, chorion and decidual cells at term (Robinson *et al.*, 1988; Jones *et al.*, 1989; Riley and Challis, 1991) with an output similar to that by the placental cells (Jones *et al.*, 1989). Immunohistochemical localization of CRH in fetal membranes showed that CRH is distributed in the epithelial cells, in some cells of the subepithelial layer of amnion, and in cells of the reticular layer of chorion (Saijonmaa *et al.*, 1988; Warren and Silverman, 1995). Immunoreactive CRH is present in decidual cells (Petraglia *et al.*, 1992a) as well as in endometrial cells treated hormonally to achieve in vitro decidualization (Ferrari *et al.*, 1995).

Receptors
The CRH (and urocortin) interact with two distinct receptors (Valdenaire *et al.*, 1997): R1 (classified in R1a, R1b, R1c, and R1d subtypes) and R2 (R2a, R2b and R2g subtypes) (Petraglia *et al.*, 1990c; Leung and Peng, 1996). Fluorescent *in situ* hybridization and immunofluorescence demonstrated that syncytiotrophoblast

cells and amniotic epithelium are the cell types expressing CRH-R1a, -Rc (Karteris *et al.*, 1998) and -R2beta mRNA (Florio *et al.*, 2000).

The CRH receptors (mRNA and protein) have also been described in human myometrium (Grammatopoulos *et al.*, 1998). In particular, recent findings show the presence in pregnant myometrium of subtypes 1a, 1b, 2a and 2b, and the variant -Rc, whereas only the 1a, 1b and 2b receptors are detectable in non-pregnant myometrium (Hillhouse and Grammatopoulos, 2002). Urocortin binds to CRH receptors types 1 and 2, with a particularly high affinity for type 2 receptor (Vaughan *et al.*, 1995).

Levels in biological fluids

From intrauterine tissues, CRH is reversed into the maternal and umbilical cord plasma, as well as the amniotic fluid. Plasma CRH levels are low in non-pregnant women (<10 pg/ml) and become higher during the first trimester of pregnancy, rising steadily until term (Petraglia *et al.*, 1996d; Reis *et al.*, 1999; Reis and Petraglia, 2001; Florio *et al.*, 2002d). The CRH is also measurable in fetal circulation, and a linear correlation exists between maternal and fetal plasma CRH levels, despite umbilical cord plasma CRH levels are 20–30-fold lower than in maternal circulation (Economides *et al.*, 1987). In addition, CRH concentrations in umbilical venous plasma are higher than in the umbilical artery, supporting placenta as a major source of fetal plasma CRH (Goland *et al.*, 1988). The significant correlation between the amniotic fluid and maternal plasma CRH levels obtained simultaneously (Laatikainen *et al.*, 1988) suggests a placental source for amniotic CRH: amniotic fluid levels are similar to those circulating in cord plasma (Reis *et al.*, 1999).

anterior pituitary cells (Sasaki *et al.*, 1988). The structure of placental CRH mRNA is similar to that predicted for hypothalamic CRH mRNA (Florio *et al.*, 2002d). The content of immunoreactive CRH is higher in extracts of placenta obtained at term than in tissue obtained at 10 weeks of gestation (Schulte and Healy, 1987; Frim *et al.*, 1988) and a progressive increase of placental CRH content increase has been described during normal pregnancy, paralleling a similar time course of placental CRH mRNA expression, which starts from early gestation (7–8 weeks) (Grino *et al.*, 1987; Frim *et al.*, 1988).

Some mechanisms stimulating CRH release from medial hypothalamic eminence in the brain (Vale *et al.*, 1993) are identical to those operating in the human placenta (Figure 1.2). In fact, prostaglandins (PGs), neurotransmitters and peptides stimulates the release of CRH from cultured placental cells. Both prostaglandin F2 (PGF2) and E2 (PGE2) increases the CRH concentration in the culture medium

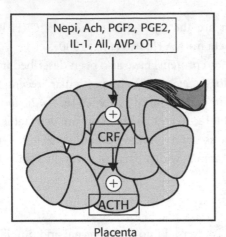 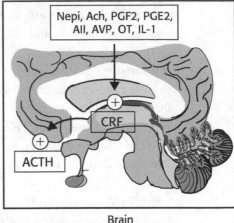

| Placenta | Brain |

Figure 1.2   The mechanisms stimulating CRF release from medial basal hypothalamus are in part chemically identical to those operating in the human placenta. PGF2 and PGE2, norepinephrine (Nepi), acetylcholine (Ach), angiotensin II (AII), arginine vasopressin (AVP), stimulate CRF in hypothalamus, as well as in placental cells. On the contrary, the effect of OT on CRF and HPA hormones in human placenta, is different being stimulatory. In turn, placental CRF stimulates ACTH secretion from cultured human placental cells

with a dose-dependent effect (Petraglia *et al.*, 1987c). Norepinephrine and acetylcholine are the most active neurotransmitters in increasing CRH release. In particular, the norepinephrine effect is reversed by prazosin, an α1-adrenergic antagonist, or yohimbine, an α2-adrenergic receptor antagonist. The involvement of both adrenergic receptor subtypes is further supported by the evidence that methoxamine or clonidine, α1- and α2-adrenergic receptor agonists, respectively, stimulate CRH release from placental cells (Petraglia *et al.*, 1989c). Acetylcholine acts via a muscarinic receptor: atropine or hexamethonium, specific muscarinic receptor antagonists, reverse the effect of acetylcholine on CRH release. In addition, the human placenta synthesizes acetylcholine and contains acetylcholine concentrations higher than in mammalian brain tissue (Petraglia, 1991; Petraglia *et al.*, 1996d; Reis *et al.*, 2001). Interestingly, the positive effect of norepinephrine and acetylcholine on placental immunoreactive CRH release agrees with the observation that these neurotransmitters stimulate CRH release from rat hypothalamic tissue in vitro and increase CRH levels in the hypophysial portal circulation (Plotsky *et al.*, 1989), suggesting a close correlation between hypothalamic and placental regulation of CRH release (Figure 1.2).

In agreement with the hypothalamic mechanisms of secretion, some neuropeptides also modulate placental CRH release. Angiotensin II and arginine vasopressin increase the release of placental CRH from cultured trophoblasts (Petraglia *et al.*, 1989c). On the contrary, oxytocin (OT) has different effects, being inhibitory to

CRH/hypothalamus–pituitary–adrenal (HPA) axis (Plotsky *et al.*, 1993), while stimulatory on CRH and ACTH secretion from cultured placental cells (Petraglia *et al.*, 1987c).

The CRH and both groups of neurotransmitters (norepinephrine and acetylcholine) and neuropeptides (angiotensin II, arginine vasopressin and OT) are involved in the stress-induced responses of the neuroendocrine system (Plotsky *et al.*, 1989). The release of CRH from cultured placental cells during the incubation with norepinephrine, acetylcholine, angiotensin II and arginine vasopressin, or OT suggests a possible in vivo interaction among these substances. In agreement with the regulation of the hypothalamic CRH, although interleukin (IL)-1 stimulates the release of CRH from cultured placental cells, on the contrary IL-2 has no effect (Petraglia *et al.*, 1989c). Since indomethacin prevents the CRH release induced by IL-1, it has been suggested that the action of IL-1 is mediated by PGs (Petraglia *et al.*, 1987a) (Figure 1.2).

The CRH-binding protein (CRH-BP) is a 37-kDa protein of 322 amino acids, mainly produced by the human brain and the liver (Petraglia *et al.*, 1996b) that is able to bind circulating CRH and urocortin, thus modulating their actions on pituitary gland (Potter *et al.*, 1992). Further, sources of CRH-BP during pregnancy are placental trophoblast, decidua and fetal membranes (Petraglia *et al.*, 1993a; 1996b). In detail, the syncytial layer of placental villi at term intensely expresses CRH-BP mRNA and immunoreactivity, whereas rare positively hybridized cells are observed within the cytotrophoblasts and mesenchymal cells. Large decidual cells, amniotic epithelial cells and chorionic cytotrophoblasts stained positively for CRH-BP mRNA and protein.

The CRH-BP is measurable in maternal plasma, and levels remain stable in nonpregnant women and during gestation until the third trimester of pregnancy (Petraglia *et al.*, 1996a, b; Reis *et al.*, 1999; Florio *et al.*, 2002d). At this time, maternal plasma CRH-BP concentrations significantly and rapidly decrease in the last 4–6 weeks before labor (Linton *et al.*, 1993; Petraglia *et al.*, 1996a, b; Reis *et al.*, 1999; Florio *et al.*, 2002d), returning to approximately non-pregnant levels during the first 24 h postpartum. Thus, opposite changes in concentrations of CRH (higher) and CRH-BP (lower) in maternal plasma occur at term, so that the availability of bioactive CRH increases during the activation of labor. Cord blood CRH-BP levels are higher (Petraglia *et al.*, 1997a), while amniotic fluid levels are lower than in maternal plasma and have a similar trend, decreasing until term pregnancy (Florio *et al.*, 1997).

Recently, another component of the CRH family, urocortin, has been described. Its sequence is similar to fish urotensin (63%) and human CRH (45%) (Vaughan *et al.*, 1995). Placental and decidual cells collected at 8–11 weeks or 38–40 weeks of gestation express urocortin mRNA and immunohistochemistry localized urocortin staining in syncytial cells of trophoblast as well as in amnion, chorion and decidua of fetal membranes (Petraglia *et al.*, 1996c; Florio *et al.*, 1999b). In detail, immunoreactive urocortin was then localized in syncytiotrophoblast cells and in some extent in cytotrophoblast cells of placental villi at term, as well as in fetal membranes and maternal decidua.

Urocortin levels are undetectable during pregnancy, with no rise with increasing gestational age as is seen for CRH (Glynn *et al.*, 1998). This lack of urocortin rise throughout pregnancy is further supported by an absence of gestational age-related changes in placental urocortin mRNA expression (Florio *et al.*, 1999b). Urocortin levels were higher at labor than those previously reported during pregnancy, but they did not change significantly at the different stages of labor when evaluated longitudinally. Some patients displayed a trend towards increasing levels, whilst others had variable concentrations (Florio *et al.*, 2002b).

Placental control of ACTH secretion

Placental ACTH, also called chorionic corticotropin (hCC) is a product of the proopiomelanocortin (POMC) gene and has the same structure and immuno-genic and biologic activity as pituitary ACTH (Waddell and Burton, 1993). Placental ACTH is localized to the cytotrophoblast in the first trimester and to the syncitiotrophoblast in the second and third trimesters (Cooper *et al.*, 1996). There is a significant increase of POMC gene expression in the placenta with the advance of gestation, which is manifested by increasing levels of POMC mRNA as well as immunoreactive ACTH (Cooper *et al.*, 1996). Among the possible local effects of placental ACTH are the stimulation of placental steroidogenesis (Barnea *et al.*, 1986) and reduction of vascular resistance (Clifton *et al.*, 1996).

The addition of CRH to primary trophoblast cell cultures stimulates ACTH secretion in a dose-dependent manner (Petraglia *et al.*, 1987c; 1999a). Moreover, the addition of a CRH antagonist is able to block the CRH-induced ACTH release from placental cells (Petraglia *et al.*, 1987c; 1999a). The concentration of CRH required for 50% of maximal stimulation of ACTH secretion is higher than the concentration necessary to release ACTH from cultured anterior pituitary cells (Petraglia *et al.*, 1987c). CRH-induced ACTH secretion is mediated by cyclic adenosine monophosphate (cAMP) as second messenger and evidence that this intracellular mechanism operates in placenta comes from the observation that dibutyryl cAMP and forskolin, a diterpene that stimulates adenylate cyclase activity, stimulate ACTH release from cultured trophoblast cells with the same intensity of corticotropin-releasing factor (CRF) without potentiating the effect of CRH (Petraglia *et al.*, 1987c).

The CRH-BP reverses the CRH-induced ACTH release from placental cells (Petraglia *et al.*, 1993a; 1996b), as in the pituitary (Potter *et al.*, 1992). These findings indicate a similarity between pituitary and placental CRH-induced ACTH release. However, in contrast to the corticosteroid negative feedback on pituitary ACTH secretion, glucocorticoids stimulate placental CRH secretion and mRNA expression (Petraglia *et al.*, 1987c; 1999a), and dexamethasone does not inhibit the effect of CRH on placental ACTH release (Petraglia *et al.*, 1987c; Robinson *et al.*, 1988).

In addition to CRH and urocortin, OT (Box 1.2) also is a potent stimulator of ACTH from cultured placental cells (Petraglia *et al.*, 1987c; 1989c; Margioris *et al.*, 1988). The effect resembles the neuroendocrine findings showing OT active on hypothalamic CRH and on pituitary POMC-related peptides, participating in the stress-induced events. The similarity between placental ACTH regulation and the brain CRH/ACTH system is also confirmed by the evidence that the addition of neuropeptide Y (NPY), IL-1, arginine vasopressin, angiotensin II, norepinephrine, or acetylcholine increase CRH release.

Box 1.2 Oxytocin

The OT is a neurophyseal hormone composed of nine amino acids, synthesized in the hypothalamus and stored in the neurohypophysis, where it acts as a neuro-transmitter involved in sexual and maternal behavior (Acher and Chauvet, 1995). The synthesis of OT has been demonstrated in peripheral sites including the ovary, decidua, chorion and placenta (Mitchell and Schmid, 2001) and, with respect to the biological actions, it acts in the breast and the intrauterine tissues to modulate lactation and parturition, respectively (Uvnas-Moberg and Eriksson, 1996; Challis *et al.*, 2000; Mitchell and Schmid, 2001).

Expression and localization

Northern blot analysis, ribonuclease protection assays and *in situ* hybridization analysis indicated local production of OT mRNA in trophoblast, amnion, chorion and decidua. The highest abundance was found in the decidua where the transcript appeared to be slightly smaller than that in the hypothalamus and ovary, considerably less in chorion and amnion and very low in trophoblast (Chibbar *et al.*, 1993). With respect to trophoblast localization a large quantity of OT-like substance exists in human placental tissue, mainly in the syncy-tiotrophoblast (Mitchell and Schmid, 2001).

By ribonuclease protection assays, a significantly higher amount of OT mRNA has been detected in tissue obtained after spontaneous labor compared with those obtained at term but before labor onset. This suggested that OT mRNA levels increase around the time of parturition either through increased transcription of the mRNA or increased stability of the mRNA, thus supporting a role for OT in the mechanism of labor onset. The OT peptide has been measured in human fetal membrane tissues with significantly higher concentrations in the decidua compared with the amnion or the chorion (Chibbar et al., 1993; Takemura et al., 1994; Mitchell and Schmid, 2001). The content of immunoreactive OT in total placenta extracts increases throughout gestation, in parallel to maternal blood levels (Chibbar et al., 1993; Mitchell and Schmid, 2001 Blanks and Thornton, 2003). Since placental content is approximately fivefold greater than in the posterior pituitary lobe, the main source of OT in pregnancy is the placenta (Reis et al., 2001). The OT is secreted from cultured placental cells (Florio et al., 1996), and in vitro studies showed an effect of OT in stimulating CRF (CRH) secretion from cultured placental cells (Petraglia et al., 1996d; Challis et al., 2000).

Receptors

The OT signaling is transduced to physiological actions via the OTR. The OTR is a 389 amino acid polypeptide with seven-transmembrane domains and belongs to the class I G-protein-coupled receptor (GPCR) family (Kimura et al., 1992). The OTR gene is present in single copy in the human genome and was mapped to the gene locus 3p25–3p26.2 (Inoue et al., 1994) and the human OTR mRNAs shows two different sizes, being of 3.6 Kb in breast and of 4.4 Kb in ovary, endometrium and myometrium (Mitchell and Schmid, 2001).

By in situ hybridization and immunohistochemistry OTR mRNA was detected in decidual cells and in the trophoblast of the chorion laeve, but not in the trophoblast into the placenta, suggesting differences in its expression in the trophoblast, depending on the localization. Indeed, the expression of OTR mRNA and protein in the amnion, the other fetally derived tissue at the feto-maternal interface, is much lower than that of trophoblasts in the chorion leave (Chibbar et al., 1993; Takemura et al., 1994; Mitchell and Schmid, 2001).

The promoter region of the human OTR gene contains several consensus sequences that have been reported to be affected by cytokines, such as TNF, IL-1 and IL-6 (Takemura et al., 1994). The concentrations of these cytokines in human amniotic fluid are increased at the time of parturition both in normal term or preterm labor in the absence of clinical evidence of infection (Reis et al., 2002). Thus, it is possible that the timing of human parturition is regulated to a large extent by the influence of the immune system on the OTR gene, not only in cases associated with intrauterine infection but also in the normal physiological process.

Levels in biological fluids

A number of technical difficulties have been found in measuring plasma OT in humans, due to the pulsatile OT secretion, the presence of oxytocinase, which metabolize OT (Tsujimoto *et al.*, 1992) and, to the antibodies used to measure OT. The OT is measurable in maternal plasma during pregnancy with a gradual rise of its levels with advancing gestation, but levels do not differ between early labor and late pregnancy (Fuchs *et al.*, 1981; 1991). It is secreted in discrete pulses and the frequency of these pulses is significantly higher during spontaneous labor than before the onset of labor (Fuchs *et al.*, 1991). After spontaneous VD, umbilical arterial plasma levels of OT are consistently higher than those in the umbilical vein, whilst the fetal arterio-venous difference is less pronounced at ECS section. At spontaneous VD, plasma levels from the umbilical cord artery are significantly higher than the maternal levels, and significantly higher than at elective abdominal delivery. Therefore, it is concluded that the human fetus can be an important source of OT (De Geest *et al.*, 1985) and this indirectly supports the hypothesis that locally produced OT may act without being reflected in maternal circulation.

CRH and pathologies of pregnancy

Several lines of evidence underlie the link between placental CRH and stress of parturition in humans. In fact, during spontaneous labor maternal plasma CRH levels progressively rise (Figure 1.3), reaching the maximum values at the most advanced stages of cervical dilation (Petraglia *et al.*, 1990a; Reis *et al.*, 1999; Florio *et al.*, 2002d). In addition, subjects who underwent elective Cesarean (ECS) delivery had plasma and amniotic fluid CRH levels significantly lower than patients after spontaneous vaginal delivery (VD) (Petraglia *et al.*, 1990a; Reis *et al.*, 1999; Florio *et al.*, 2002d). Moreover, the amount of CRH in placental extracts obtained at term after spontaneous VD is significantly greater than the amount of extracted from placentas obtained after Caesarean delivery (Petraglia *et al.*, 1990a). In addition, during spontaneous physiological labor a significant decrease in CRH-BP levels in maternal plasma (Linton *et al.*, 1993; McLean *et al.*, 1995), cord blood (Petraglia *et al.*, 1997a) and amniotic fluid (Florio *et al.*, 1997) has been observed.

Women with preterm labor have maternal plasma CRH levels significantly higher than those measured in the course of normal pregnancy (Korebrits *et al.*, 1998), but also in those who later develop preterm labor (McLean *et al.*, 1995) (Table 1.2). Taken together, this finding suggests that the increase in CRH levels in patients with preterm labor is not due to the process of labor itself, but indeed may be part of the mechanism controlling the onset of labor.

Maternal plasma CRH is higher in women with threatened preterm labor who give birth within 24 h from admission compared to those delivered after 24 h or with normal women at the same gestational age (Petraglia *et al.*, 1996a). However,

Table 1.2 Levels of placental neurohormones in gestational diseases

	Preterm labor	PIH	PE	IUGR
GnRH	+	− −	− −	− −
Activin A	+	+ +	+ + +	+ +
Inhibin A	n.e.	+ +	+ + +	+
CRF	+ +	+ +	+ + +	+ +
CRF-BP	−	− −	− − −	n.e.
NPY	+	n.e.	+ +	n.e.
CGRP	n.e.	n.e.	−	n.e.
PTHrP	n.e.	n.e.	n.e.	+ +
SST	+	+ +	n.e.	n.e.

+: increased; −: reduced; =: unchanged levels; n.e.: not evaluated.

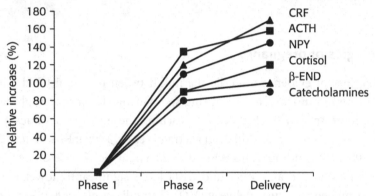

Figure 1.3   Stress hormones in maternal circulation at parturition. The sharp increase in the concentrations of CRF, cortisol and NPY around the time of labor reflects acute placental release. The placenta seems to participate in the stress response of human parturition

the continued elevation of CRH preceding clinical evidence of uterine contraction suggests that CRH secretion is not sufficient to induce initiation of labor, and other factors are required in this event (McLean *et al.*, 1995; Reis *et al.*, 1999; Florio *et al.*, 2002d). Maternal and fetal plasma CRH-BP levels are low in preterm labor (Berkowitz *et al.*, 1996; Petraglia *et al.*, 1997a) resembling the physiologic pattern observed at term. As CRH-BP modulates CRH actions on target organs, the precocious fall in CRH-BP levels has been suggested to be involved in the pathophysiology of preterm labor.

The PE, defined as hypertension associated with proteinuria, complicates 2–8% of pregnancies, and is an important cause of maternal and neonatal mortality (Roberts and Cooper, 2001). It is associated with abnormal placentation, due to the altered cytotrophoblast proliferation and invasion of endometrium, causing a reduced placental perfusion, the impairment of placental angiogenesis with the insufficiency and failure of spiral arteries remodeling (Roberts and Cooper, 2001). The reduced and/or low perfusion of placenta and the fetus is consequently the main cause of fetal growth restriction (FGR), a PE complication. Maternal concentrations of CRH are greatly increased in PE (Laatikainen *et al.*, 1991; Petraglia *et al.*, 1996a), in presence of plasma CRH-BP levels significantly lower than in healthy controls (Perkins *et al.*, 1995; Petraglia *et al.*, 1996a). In addition, also cord venous plasma CRH concentrations are significantly higher in patients with PE and higher than in cord arterial plasma, indicating the secretion of CRH from the placenta into the fetal circulation (Laatikainen *et al.*, 1991). In addition to CRH, also the remaining hormones with vasodilatory actions and involved in the stress response, such as ACTH and cortisol, are increased in the fetuses from PE pregnancies (Goland *et al.*, 1995) as well as in the FGR fetuses (Goland *et al.*, 1993).

Concentrations of CRH in the fetal circulation are significantly increased in pregnancies complicated by abnormal umbilical artery flow velocity waveforms, thus representing a stress-responsive compensatory mechanism in the human placenta (Giles *et al.*, 1996). It is not known whether this deranged secretion is part of the primary pathophysiology of these conditions or occurs as a secondary response to the increased vascular resistance in abnormal pregnancies. The concentration of CRH in the fetal circulation is significantly increased in pregnancies complicated by abnormal umbilical artery flow velocity waveforms, thus representing a stress-responsive compensatory mechanism in the human placenta.

Peptide signaling and fetal/maternal endocrinology

Neurohormones produced by human placenta, decidua and fetal membranes are secreted into maternal and fetal circulation, and amniotic fluid. In these compartments, levels may increase from early to term pregnancy, or just at term. However, the role of these changes in the regulation of maternal and fetal endocrinology may be of some relevance (Reis and Petraglia, 2001), as well as the putative role of the placenta as the central organ in this bidirectional system. A typical example is the modulation of the HPA axis activity and hormone secretion in pregnancy.

The activity of the maternal HPA axis is increased in pregnant women, and high levels of free and bound cortisol circulate in pregnant women (Challis *et al.*, 2000; Florio *et al.*, 2002d). Indeed, hypercortisolemia is characteristic of pregnancy, and the correlation between plasma CRH and salivary or urinary free cortisol levels would suggest that placental CRH is responsible for these alterations, even though other factors may act in modulating maternal HPA axis function in pregnancy (Goland *et al.*, 1994; Challis *et al.*, 2000). However, some discrepancies occur between CRH and ACTH. In fact, although plasma ACTH levels increase throughout pregnancy, they remain within the normal range of non-pregnant women (Barbieri, 1994). This is probably because CRH-BP counteracts the secretory action of CRH on both maternal pituitary and placental ACTH (Potter *et al.*, 1992; Petraglia *et al.*, 1993a; 1996b). Furthermore, injecting pregnant women with exogenous CRH does not induce an increase of circulating ACTH, suggesting that high cortisol levels may desensitize maternal pituitary corticotrophs (Schulte and Healy, 1987; Sasaki *et al.*, 1989; Schulte *et al.*, 1990).

Thus, some discrepancies exist in the HPA axis regulation between pregnant and non-pregnant women. In fact, the administration of exogenous glucocorticoid to pregnant women may increase maternal plasma and placental levels of immunoreactive CRH (Marinoni *et al.*, 1998), decreasing cortisol (Tropper *et al.*, 1987; Marinoni *et al.*, 1998) and ACTH levels (Marinoni *et al.*, 1998). To date, it is unclear whether maternal plasma ACTH originates from the maternal pituitary, placenta, or both. The diurnal rhythm for plasma ACTH, cortisol and β-END is maintained in pregnant women; however, CRH does not have a circadian rhythm (Chan *et al.*, 1993; Petraglia *et al.*, 1994a). These findings and the fact that the changes of plasma CRH do not correlate with those of ACTH or cortisol throughout normal pregnancy or out of the time of labor (Chan *et al.*, 1993; Florio *et al.*, 2002d) underlie the differences in HPA regulation in pregnancy and support the following statements:

(1) pituitary ACTH release is regulated centrally;
(2) placental CRH is not the only regulator of maternal ACTH and cortisol levels (Florio *et al.*, 2002d).

Placental CRH secreted into the fetal circulation may stimulate the production of pituitary ACTH as well as of adrenal hormones (Figure 1.4). The effect of CRH on fetal pituitary ACTH release is potentiated by arginine vasopressin and possibly mediated by cAMP, and may be antagonized by dexamethasone (Vale *et al.*, 1993). Recent studies revealed a direct effect of CRH on dehydroepiandrosterone sulfate (DHEA-S) release from cultured fetal adrenal cells (Smith *et al.*, 1998). Expression of mRNA encoding type 1 CRH receptor was identified in mid-gestation human fetal adrenals (Smith *et al.*, 1998) suggesting that the fetal adrenal cortex may be directly responsive to CRH (Figure 1.4). Placenta of humans and higher primates uses DHEA-S supplied by the fetal adrenals as the main substrate for estrogen synthesis, and estrogens produced by the placenta play a pivotal role in the endocrine control of pregnancy and induce many of the key changes involved at parturition (Challis *et al.*, 2000).

Human CRH increased DHEA-S production by cultured human fetal adrenal cortical cells in a dose-dependent fashion, being as effective as ACTH at stimulating

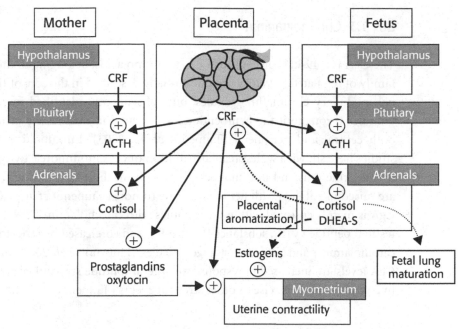

Figure 1.4   In vitro evidences for a role of CRF on placental, maternal and fetal endocrinology. Placental CRF at the end of pregnancy stimulates fetal pituitary ACTH secretion, which in turn stimulates fetal adrenal cortisol and DHEA-S production. The increasing concentrations of cortisol, in addition to maturating enzymes in organs critical for postnatal existence, further stimulate production of placental CRF by a feed-forward mechanism. The increasing production of DHEA-S provides additional substrate for placental aromatization to estrogen, which triggers the cascade leading to labor and delivery. In addition, CRF modulates directly the myometrial contractility, and indirectly by stimulating the release of uterotonic substances (prostaglandins, oxytocin)

DHEA-S production, although it was considerably less potent than ACTH in stimulating cortisol synthesis (Smith *et al.*, 1998). CRH did not alter cell number, indicating that it is not mitogenic for fetal adrenal cortical cells. Therefore, placental CRH production, which rises exponentially during human pregnancy, may play a key role in promoting DHEA-S production by the fetal adrenals, which could lead to an increase in placental estrogen synthesis (Smith *et al.*, 1998; Challis *et al.*, 2000; Florio *et al.*, 2002d).

With respect to neurohormones and fetal adrenal, several findings suggest a role for chromogranin A (CgA; Box 1.3). In fact, during pregnancy, the highest CgA levels found in the umbilical cord blood and mainly at parturition, are most probably of fetal adrenal origin and may have a role in preparing the fetus for the extra-uterine life (Florio *et al.*, 2002c). In fact, CgA is costored and coreleased with catecholamine (Taupenot *et al.*, 2003), and both increase significantly in cord blood during the

Box 1.3 Chromogranin A

The CgA is a 49-kDa glycoprotein of 439 amino acids, belonging to the granin family of regulated secretory proteins initially described in the core of the adrenal medullary chromaffin granules, but subsequently identified in secretory granules throughout the neuroendocrine system and in a variety of neurons, both central and peripheral (Taupenot *et al.*, 2003). Immunohistochemical studies have shown a widespread distribution of CgA immunoreactivity in neuroendocrine cells and in tumors originating from these cells and serum levels are raised in patients with neuroendocrine tumors (Taupenot *et al.*, 2003). The CgA is mainly costored within the granules with catecholamines, ENK, vasointestinal peptide (VIP), substance P and NPY, and coreleased by exocytosis with catecholamines and NPY from storage vesicules (Taupenot *et al.*, 2003). In plasma, CgA levels are increased in response to large-amplitude stressful events, that is hypoxia, physical exercise or other stressful events (Taupenot *et al.*, 2003).

Expression and localization

Syversen *et al.* (1992) showed the presence of CgA mRNA and peptide in intrauterine tissues as placental trophoblast, decidua and fetal membranes. The CgA immunoreactivity was demonstrated by immunofluorescence studies of isolated trophoblasts and decidual cells from term placentas. Double immunofluorescence of isolated trophoblasts showed colocalization of CgA with hPL and hCG. Since syncytiotrophoblasts are the placental source of hPL, that indicates that this cell is one site of CgA production. By Northern blotting, a distinct band corresponding to CgA mRNA was demonstrated in the human placental cell line (TPA-30-1), whereas in placental homogenates an mRNA band of a slightly larger size was found (Syversen *et al.*, 1992).

Biological fluids

CgA is measurable in maternal and fetal plasma, in umbilical cord blood and in amniotic fluid (Syversen *et al.*, 1992; Moftaquir-Handaj *et al.*, 1995; Florio *et al.*, 2002c). No significant differences were found in maternal CgA levels during pregnancy compared with levels out of pregnancy, even if median CgA level in maternal sera at term tended to be higher than at 6–11 weeks or in sera from non-pregnant women (Syversen *et al.*, 1992). In umbilical cord sera median CgA level was significantly higher than in term sera, whilst in amniotic fluid median CgA value was significantly higher at term than in second trimester (Syversen *et al.*, 1992).

With respect to labor, umbilical cord plasma and amniotic fluid levels of CgA were higher in women who had spontaneous VD than in those delivered by ECS (Moftaquir-Handaj *et al.*, 1995; Florio *et al.*, 2002c), suggesting a fetal origin, whilst no change was detected in maternal circulation (Florio *et al.*, 2002c).

stress of delivery (Padbury and Martinez, 1988; Moftaquir-Handaj *et al.*, 1995). The sympathoadrenergic system is activated to withstand the stress of birth, and several other neuropeptides, other than CgA, are secreted by the adrenal medulla into cord blood at the time of delivery, including catecholamines, enkephalins (ENK) and NPY (Poyner *et al.*, 2002; Taupenot *et al.*, 2003). The ability of the sympathoadrenal system to develop a response is essential for fetal life (during which the fetus grows under a state of relatively low oxygen tension), as well as for survival during parturition, when compression of the umbilical cord and the placental circulation occurs because of uterine contractions that intermittently deprive the infant of oxygen (Padbury and Martinez, 1988). The CgA levels in the fetal circulation at birth are associated with high levels of NPY (Lundberg *et al.*, 1986) and catecholamines (Wang *et al.*, 1999) so that CgA could inhibit the excessive catecholamine release to counteract the vasoconstrictive effects of catecholamines and NPY (Poyner *et al.*, 2002; Taupenot *et al.*, 2003). As CgA also possesses some function related to vasodilation (Poyner *et al.*, 2002; Taupenot *et al.*, 2003), umbilical cord CgA release could help to regulate and prevent the vascular constrictive effects of catecholamines and NPY when they are secreted in excess.

Peptide signaling and the control of myometrial contractility

For parturition to occur, the cervical connective tissue and smooth muscle must be capable of dilation to allow the passage of the fetus from the uterus, but the uterus itself must be converted from a quiescent structure with dysynchronous contractions to an active coordinately contracting organ. On this regard, the entire pregnancy may be viewed as the result of the constraint equilibrium between factors activating and others inhibiting myometrial contractility, so that the term or preterm labor is the consequence of shift-forward activating (uterotonic) factors, with the decrease of the role of quiescence (inhibitors) neurohormones (Figure 1.5).

(A) Role of OT

The major uterotonic factors triggering uterine contractility are OT and PGs (Petraglia *et al.*, 1996d; Challis *et al.*, 2000). Historically, OT was assumed to be the initiating factor of parturition because clinical administration initiates labor which is indistinguishable from spontaneous labor. After this 'proof of concept' experiment, the role of OT was extensively investigated in many animal species.

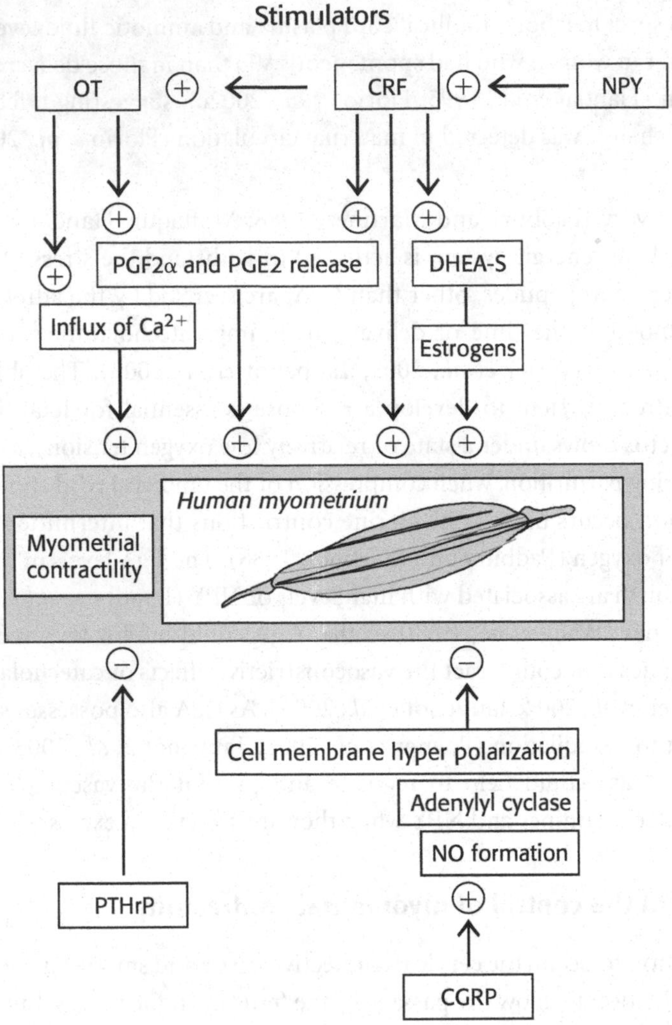

Figure 1.5   Human pregnancy may be viewed as the result of a constant equilibrium between activators and inhibitors of myometrial contractility. In particular, OT, PGs, CRF and NPY are able to stimulate, whilst CGRP and PTHrP inhibit the activity of the prenant myometrium activing on the uterine contractile machine

The initiation of term labor has been related to an increased myometrial responsiveness to OT near or at the time of parturition and, a variety of mechanisms have been invoked to initiate parturition. However, the involvement of the local OT production and secretion within the uterus is the final pathway of the mechanism leading to parturition linked to local PG release (Challis *et al.*, 2000) and an immediate influx of Ca^{2+} into the cytoplasm of myometrial cells from both extracellular and intracellular sites (Challis *et al.*, 2000). In fact, OT is not only a neurohormone but also a locally produced substance (Chibbar *et al.*, 1993; Petraglia *et al.*, 1996d; Challis *et al.*, 2000) with possible paracrine actions, able to stimulate PG production (Petraglia *et al.*, 1996d; Challis *et al.*, 2000). The PGs themselves may be uterotonic, and drive the arachidonic acid metabolism toward cyclo-oxygenase products rather than the less active lipoxygenase metabolites (Ticconi *et al.*, 1998). In explant culture of human choriodecidua, OT markedly increases the production of PGF2α, PGE2 and leukotrienes in contrast to amnion where PGE2 is the primary PG product (Pasetto *et al.*, 1992). Therefore, OT might have a dual role in fetal membranes: it could directly enhance PG production and also indirectly stimulate the synthesis and release of cytokines involved in the regulation of PG output by tissue (Zicari *et al.*, 2002).

At the end of pregnancy in the human and in the rat, there is a large increase in content of decidual mRNA encoding OT. The concentration of OT peptide for these two species in the decidua is not greater than that in the circulation and it would, if released, probably act on the endometrium rather than on the myometrium. Indeed, in cyclic ruminants, PG production by the endometrium in response to OT is the signal precipitating luteolysis, unless a blastocyst is present to block OT receptor (OTR) expression (Challis *et al.*, 2000). It is generally thought that changing secretion of estrogen and progesterone towards the end of pregnancy is important in the regulation of OT peptide and receptor gene expression. The content of OT mRNA in human decidua increases in vitro in response to estrogen, with no effect of progesterone, while in the rat endometrium in vivo the reported stimulatory action of estrogen is enhanced by progesterone (Chibbar *et al.*, 1995). Although there appears to be no change in OT metabolism around the time of parturition, OTR gene expression is upregulated (Takemura *et al.*, 1994), so that the onset of labor coincides with an increase in the paracrine rather than systemic release of OT. This local OT production seems to be regulated by other paracrine factors, such as CRH, activin A and PGs (Florio *et al.*, 1996) (Figure 1.5).

(B) Role of CRH

Labor and delivery are the main physiological stress conditions and among the neuroendocrine factors which play a role in the maintenance of uterine quiescence and involved in the onset of parturition, CRH has been one of the more investigated in the last decade. In vitro data support a role for CRH at labor (Figure 1.5). In fact, CRH and ACTH stimulate the release of PGF2α and PGE2 from cultured amnion, chorion, decidual and placental tissues (Jones *et al.*, 1989; Benedetto *et al.*, 1994; Petraglia *et al.*, 1995b; 1999a). These effects are inhibited in presence of antisera to CRH and to ACTH. Moreover, in placenta but not in amnion or decidua, the stimulatory effect of CRH on PGF2α and PGE2 output is attenuated in presence of an antibody to ACTH, thus supporting the possibility of paracrine stimulation by

CRH and ACTH of PG production in intrauterine tissues (Jones and Challis, 1990). The CRH markedly stimulates the release of immunoreactive OT from cultured placental cells in a dose-dependent fashion (Florio *et al.*, 1996). Moreover, the addition of CRH, but not of arginine vasopressin or NPY, increase the release of immunoreactive OT three- to fourfold from placental cells.

Recent data indicated a role played by CRH directly on myometrial contractility, due to the fact that CRH mediates its actions in the human myometrium via activation of two distinct classes of CRH receptors, R1 and R2 (Hillhouse and Grammatopoulos, 2002). Contrasting data exists on the net role played by CRH, some suggesting CRH as an important uterotonic, others as the main uterine quiescence factor (Challis *et al.*, 2000; Florio *et al.*, 2002d; Hillhouse and Grammatopoulos, 2002). It seems that different myometrial CRH receptors are recruited at labor, and that this recruitment may be dynamically and differentially modulated by the great hormonal changes occurring at term pregnancy, so that CRH actions in vivo may differ from actions reported in vitro, according to different myometrial CRH receptor expression and the induced affinity state.

For many years, investigators questioned whether there are fundamental differences between ovine pregnancy, in which the fetal adrenal gland plays a pivotal role in the process of parturition, and human pregnancy, in which the role of the fetal adrenal gland in this process is less clear (Challis *et al.*, 2000). Human placental CRH may directly and preferentially stimulate the fetal adrenocortical production of DHEA-S to as great an extent as ACTH, while stimulation of cortisol by CRH occurs to a much lesser degree than stimulation by ACTH (Smith *et al.*, 1998) (Figure 1.4). Further, placental CRH can stimulate production of proopimelanocortin and some of its derivatives in the placenta, including ACTH, α-MSH and β-END in syncitiotrophoblast cells in vitro (Reis *et al.*, 1999; Challis *et al.*, 2000; Florio *et al.*, 2002d; Hillhouse and Grammatopoulos, 2002). Placental CRH could, however, like fetal CRH, also stimulate fetal pituitary ACTH. Placental CRH may stimulate fetal pituitary ACTH, which then stimulates fetal adrenal DHEA-S, which is used by the placenta for conversion to estrogen by the process of aromatization (Challis *et al.*, 2000; Florio *et al.*, 2002d). This increase in estrogen then could serve as a trigger for the cascade of events leading to labor and parturition. In fact, estrogens increase uterine contractility by increasing myometrial excitability, myometrial responsivity to OT and other uterotonic agents, as well as stimulate the synthesis and the release of PGs by fetal membranes (Challis *et al.*, 2000; Florio *et al.*, 2002d). Further, estrogens stimulate proteolytic enzymes in the cervix, such as collagenase, which break down the extracellular matrix permitting the cervix to dilate.

Thus, consistent with the observation that CRH preferentially stimulates fetal adrenal DHEA-S directly, was the observation that CRH increased the abundance of mRNAs encoding the enzymes for the conversion of androgen to estrogen

(Smith *et al.*, 1998). Thus, it was hypothesized that the rapid rise in placental CRH which occurs at the end of gestation at the time when CRH-BP decreases, serves as the inciting event leading to placental aromatization (Reis *et al.*, 1999; Challis *et al.*, 2000; Florio *et al.*, 2002d; Hillhouse and Grammatopoulos, 2002). The increasing estrogen, then, would initiate the chain of events terminating in labor and delivery (Challis *et al.*, 2000; Florio *et al.*, 2002d). Thus, there may be a feto-placental unit which involves fetal glucocorticoids and placental CRH as well as that involving fetal DHEA-S and placental estrogen.

Thus, among the possible processes governing the initiation of human parturition are the following:

(1) The rise in placental CRH at the end of pregnancy stimulates fetal pituitary ACTH, which in turn stimulates increased fetal adrenal cortisol and DHEA-S production. The increasing concentrations of cortisol, in addition to maturating enzymes in organs critical for postnatal existence, further stimulate production of placental CRH by a feed-forward mechanism. The increasing production of DHEA-S provides additional substrate for placental aromatization to estrogen, which triggers the cascade leading to labor and delivery.

(2) The increasing production of placental CRH directly and preferentially stimulate fetal adrenal DHEA-S, which is then converted by placental aromatization to estrogens which trigger the cascade leading to parturition.

(3) CRH exerts direct effect on the myometrium and fetal membranes to increase myometrial contractility.

(C) Role of opioids

Opioids (Box 1.4) could play a role in the initiation of parturition. As parturition approaches, a central opioid inhibitory mechanism is activated that restrains the excitation of OT cells by brainstem inputs. In fact, OT secretion from the posterior pituitary gland is increased during parturition, stimulated by the uterine contractions that forcefully expel the fetuses. Opioid is the predominant damper of OT cells before and during parturition, limiting stimulation by extraneous stimuli, and perhaps facilitating optimal spacing of births and economical use of the store of OT accumulated during pregnancy (Russell *et al.*, 2003). In fact, β-END levels are elevated, approximately twofold higher than circulating plasma levels, in the colostrum and transitional milk of mothers who were vaginally delivered. Therefore, it was hypothesized that β-END may contribute to postnatal fetal adaptation, to overcoming birth stress of natural labor and delivery, and at the same time to the postnatal development of several related biologic functions of breast-fed infants (Zanardo *et al.*, 2001). The β-END appears to be related with glucocorticoid release, energy balance and the stimulation of lipolysis (Petraglia, 1991; Ahmed *et al.*, 1992;

Box 1.4 Opioid peptides

Opioid peptides have a morphine-like activity. Three families are recognized: END, ENK and DYN. They derive from three precursors of similar molecular size and sequence homology. The POMC is the precursor of ACTH, α-melanocyte-stimulating hormone (α-MSH), β-END and lipotropin. Proenkefalin (P-ENK) is the precursor of ENK and prodynorphin (P-DYN) of DYN, rimorphin, leu-morphin and neo-endorphins (Kieffer and Evans, 2002).

Expression and localization

The β-END, methionine enkephalin (M-ENK) and DYN 1–8 and 1–13 are the main opioid peptides identified in placental extracts. The DYN 1–8 seem to be the predominant opioid peptide present in placental villus tissue (Agbas *et al.*, 1995).

The β-END was the first detected endogenous opioid peptide in the human placenta (Ahmed *et al.*, 1992). Immunohistochemical staining of placental tissue for β-END immunoreactivity is positive in the syncytiotrophoblast in both early and term pregnancy (Odagiri *et al.*, 1979). Cultures of human placenta cells collected at term, release β-END (Liotta and Krieger, 1980) and it is measurable in homogenates of human amnion, chorion and decidua collected throughout gestation (Facchinetti *et al.*, 1990).

The M-ENK is the major representative of the other family of opioid peptides, the ENK. Syncytial and cytotrophoblast cells contain immunoreactive M-ENK, and its de novo syntesis in culture villi at term has been shown (Sastry *et al.*, 1980).

The third family of opioids is represented by DYN, and human placenta is also the source of the multiple forms of DYN despite dynorphins A(1–8) is the major opioid present in the placental extracts (Agbas *et al.*, 1995).

Receptors

Mu, kappa and delta are the main opioid receptor types. Each opioid exhibits distinct binding activity towards each type of opioid receptor. The mu-receptor has high affinity for M-ENK and β-END (as well as morphine and dynorphin A); the delta-receptor for leu-enkephalin; the kappa-receptor is the main target for the DYN (Kieffer and Evans, 2002).

Receptor subtypes for the various endogenous opioid peptides are present on placental cell membranes (Porthe *et al.*, 1981; 1982), but kappa receptors is the more important type present in the placenta, in fact the order of potency in cells in vitro from term trophoblast tissue was kappa $>>>$ mu $>$ delta (Cemerikic *et al.*, 1992). Placental content of kappa receptors increases with gestational age and term placental content of kappa receptors correlates with route of delivery (Ahmed *et al.*, 1992).

Levels in biological fluids

Placenta and membranes contribute to the secretion of β-END in the different fluid compartments. Concentration of β-END in maternal plasma during pregnancy have been reported as unchanged (Cemerikic *et al.*, 1992), decreased (Goebelsmann *et al.*, 1984), or progressively increasing (Newnham *et al.*, 1983; Panerai *et al.*, 1983; Facchinetti *et al.*, 1990), so that the question of a possible placental contribution to the circulating pool remains unsolved. However, the findings that β-END concentrations are higher in the placental tissue than in the maternal or cord plasma (Petraglia, 1991; Petraglia *et al.*, 1996d; Reis *et al.*, 2001); that immunoreactive β-END in placental homogenates in the first is significantly higher than in the second trimester; that at delivery the β-END content is greater than in the second trimester and that, in tissues collected at term, in the absence of labor, β-END levels are higher in tissues collected after VD (Facchinetti *et al.*, 1990) suggest that gestational tissues are important sources and that stress of delivery greatly stimulates the placental secretion (Figure 1.5). On the contrary, amniotic fluid β-END concentrations have a completely different gestational pattern, with no changes at parturition (Genazzani *et al.*, 1984; Kofinas *et al.*, 1987; Mauri *et al.*, 1990), suggesting a different source in this compartment.

Moreover, β-END is elevated, approximately twofold higher than circulating plasma levels, in the colostrum and transitional milk of mothers who were vaginally delivered. Therefore, it was hypothesized that β-END may contribute to postnatal fetal adaptation, to overcoming birth stress of natural labor and delivery, and at the same time to the postnatal development of several related biologic functions of breast-fed infants (Zanardo *et al.*, 2001).

Maternal plasma levels of M-ENK are not significantly different from those of non-pregnant women and do not change throughout pregnancy (Sastry *et al.*, 1980), supporting a local role of the peptide. DYN was measured in maternal blood, umbilical vein and amniotic fluid. No significant change was observed in the plasma level of DYN in the first and second trimester of pregnancy as compared with plasma obtained from non-pregnant women. However, a 2.2-fold increase in DYN plasmatic levels was observed during the third trimester as well as at delivery. High levels of DYN were also found in the amniotic fluid and the umbilical vein plasma. Levels of DYN in the maternal plasma at the third trimester of pregnancy and at delivery increase, therefore, a placental contribution to this phenomenon has been speculated (Valette *et al.*, 1986). High DYN levels are also detectable in amniotic fluid and in umbilical vein plasma (Valette *et al.*, 1986).

Petraglia *et al.*, 1996d; Reis *et al.*, 2001; Russell *et al.*, 2003). Another function attributed to β-END is the inhibition of painful sensations in women during childbirth (Russell *et al.*, 2003). Stress during delivery has been associated with elevated umbilical cord plasma β-END levels. Multiple regression modeling showed that forceps delivery, maternal β-END concentration, bradycardia, VD, and birth weight each made independent contributions to elevated cord β-END. Level of cord β-END independent of delivery stress exerted the primary influence upon child motor development and higher levels of stress-independent β-END may play a direct role in motor development (Rothenberg *et al.*, 1996).

(D) Role of NPY and CGRP

The NPY (Box 1.5) synthesis by cytotrophoblastic cells, amnion, chorion and decidua has been suggested to be involved in the mechanism leading to parturition. NPY stimulates the placental release of CRH (Petraglia *et al.*, 1989a) and, it is also able to modulate myometrial contractility (Stjernquist and Owman, 1987; Tenmoku *et al.*, 1988) (Figure 1.5). On the contrary, calcitonin gene-related peptide (CGRP; Box 1.6) may have a role in maintaining uterine quiescence during pregnancy, from early to term gestation (Samuelson *et al.*, 1985), as it is a potent

Box 1.5 Neuropeptide Y

Human NPY is a peptide of 36 amino acid residues (Grove and Smith, 2003) belonging to a family of regulatory peptides that also includes peptide tyrosine (PYY). By fluorescence *in situ* hybridization the NPY gene has been mapped to chromosome 7p15.1 and exists in single copy (Grove and Smith, 2003). The NPY expression is abundant and widespread in the central and peripheral nervous systems, in particular in brain, in sympathetic neurons innervating cardiovascular and respiratory systems, gastrointestinal and genitourinary tracts (Grove and Smith, 2003). Physiological effects attributed to NPY include the stimulation of food intake and inhibition of anxiety in the central nervous system (CNS) (Grove and Smith, 2003; Pedrazzini *et al.*, 2003); presynaptic inhibition of neurotransmitter release in the CNS and the periphery; vasoconstriction (Michel and Rascher, 1995); inhibition of insulin release; regulation of gut motility; gastrointestinal and renal epithelial secretion (Grove and Smith, 2003; Pedrazzini *et al.*, 2003). Moreover, there is evidence that NPY is involved in the regulation of anterior pituitary hormone secretion: in particular, NPY plays a critical role in stimulating the basal pattern of luteinizing hormone (LH) release (Grove and Smith, 2003; Pedrazzini *et al.*, 2003).

Expression and localization

With respect to gestational tissues, NPY is produced by human placenta, maternal decidua and fetal membranes. Acidic extracts of human placental tissue collected at term pregnancy contained high immunoreactive NPY (ir-NPY) concentrations. The extracted ir-NPY eluted from high-pressure liquid chromatography (HPLC) with the same retention time as synthetic NPY. Its presence in placental cells was confirmed by immunohistochemical findings showing an intense NPY in the cytoplasm of the epithelial amnion cells and of the cytotrophoblast cells, and intermediate trophoblast of the chorion. To further support the local production of NPY, primary cultures of human placental cells released ir-NPY into the culture medium and the addition of high K+ concentrations increased the release of the peptide (Petraglia *et al.*, 1989a; 1993b).

Receptors

Binding sites for NPY are present in all peripheral cells of placental terminal villi (Petraglia *et al.*, 1989a; Robidoux *et al.*, 1998). All NPY receptors mediate their responses through pertussis toxin sensitive G-proteins of the Gi/0 family, resulting in inhibition of adenylate cyclase activity, but they are also able to increase intracellular Ca^{2+} levels (Balasubramaniam, 2003). A variety of receptor subtypes for NPY exists, that is Y1, Y2, Y3, Y4, Y5, Y6 receptor, and NPGPR (Balasubramaniam, 2003). The Y1 (Wharton *et al.*, 1993) and Y3 receptor (Robidoux *et al.*, 1998) and NPGPR (Cikos *et al.*, 1999) have been identified also within placenta. The NPY1R and NPY3R are located on brush-border membranes of syncytiotrophoblastic cells of placental villi (Robidoux *et al.*, 1998).

Biological fluids

During pregnancy, NPY is secreted from human placental tissues in maternal and fetal circulation and, in amniotic fluid, NPY levels are higher than in non-pregnant women, without significant changes throughout gestation. Maternal plasma levels increased threefold during labor, thus suggesting that the peptide may play a role in the stress response of parturition. In fact, during labor maternal plasma NPY levels progressively increased, matching the highest levels at the most advanced stages of cervical dilation and at the time of VD (Petraglia *et al.*, 1989b) (Figure 1.5). Moreover, plasma NPY values fall immediately after delivery, supporting the placental origin of the circulating NPY during pregnancy. The NPY is also measurable in amniotic fluid and umbilical cord serum, and levels are comparable to those found in maternal circulation, being highest at term and mainly during the early or late stages of labor (Petraglia *et al.*, 1989b).

A recent study by the use of radioimmunoassay showed that maternal plasma NPY levels in pregnant women with eclampsia and preeclampsia are significantly elevated with respect to that in normotensive pregnant women (Table 1.2). At 6 days after delivery the concentration of plasma NPY was significantly decreased in women with eclampsia and preeclampsia, and in women with normotension, compared with the value measured on admission. Probably, elevated plasma NPY levels may play a key role in the development of eclampsia and preeclampsia (Khatun *et al.*, 2000).

Box 1.6 Calcitonin-gene-related peptide

The CGRP is a 37 amino acid neuropeptide produced by tissue-specific alternative splicing of the primary transcript of the calcitonin gene (Poyner *et al.*, 2002). A second gene encoding a similar peptide (β-CGRP) has also been identified in rat and human (Poyner *et al.*, 2002), and various tissues, including the CNS, the heart and kidney, are able to express the peptide.

The distribution of CGRP-producing cells and pathways in the brain and other tissues suggests functions for CGRP in nociception, ingestive behavior, and modulation of the autonomic and endocrine systems. Moreover, CGRP also shows potent vasodilator actions and probably is an important regulator of vascular tone and blood flow (Poyner *et al.*, 2002).

Expression and localization

The CGRP mRNA is expressed by human placenta, but mainly by decidual cells (Graf *et al.*, 1996; Knerr *et al.*, 2002; Tsatsaris *et al.*, 2002; Yallampalli *et al.*, 2002). The mRNAs levels measured in the human placenta by RT-PCR in normal and preeclamptic women were significantly reduced in PE compared with controls, in chorionic plate but not in villi specimens. In general, CGRP gene expression indicated by mRNA amounts was slightly higher in chorionic plate tissue than in placental villi (Knerr *et al.*, 2002). Moreover, in placentae of preeclamptic and HELLP syndrome women, a reduction of CGRP mRNAs has been shown in contrast to unchanged mRNA levels of their receptors (Knerr *et al.*, 2002).

With respect to decidual cells, they are an important source of a CGRP-like substance within the placenta that may regulate vasodilation and influence placental hormone secretion (Graf *et al.*, 1996). Moreover, decidual cells express both CGRP mRNA and protein, that is secreted by decidual cells in vitro (Tsatsaris *et al.*, 2002).

Receptors

Two classes of CGRP receptors exist: one is sensitive to hCGRP(8–37) C-terminal fragment, while the other is insensitive to this fragment. The CGRP acts at the cellular level by binding to a seven-transmembrane domain GPCR, and receptors are linked to the activation of adenilate cyclase in several systems and in intracellular calcium level modulation (Born *et al.*, 2002). In human placentae there are specific binding sites for CGRP, able to bind α- and β-CGRP in a dose-dependent and saturable manner consistent with a single binding site of high affinity, with a low affinity for calcitotin (Foord and Craig, 1987).

The CGRP receptors are localized on human syncytiotrophoblast brush-border membrane (facing the mother) and in basal plasma membrane (facing the fetus), and are able to bind CGRP in a specific, rapid, time dependent and of high-affinity manner (Lafond *et al.*, 1997). The expression of CGRP receptors has been also detected by Southern blot hybridization and RT-PCR in decidual cells and extravillous trophoblast cells (Tsatsaris *et al.*, 2002). In addition to placental and decidual sites, CGRP receptors are also expressed by human myometrium (Casey *et al.*, 1997; Dong *et al.*, 1999) and, the myometrial expression is increased during pregnancy and significantly downregulated after labor (Dong *et al.*, 1999). Indeed, CGRP receptors are abundant in myometrial cells of pregnant women who are not in labor and, are minimal in uterine specimens from women in labor and in the non-pregnant state (Dong *et al.*, 1999). Finally, the sensitivity of myometrial tissues to CGRP significantly decreases at term labor (Chan *et al.*, 1997).

Levels in biological fluids

The CGRP is secreted in maternal and fetal circulation in increasing amounts from early to term gestation (Yallampalli *et al.*, 2002). Pregnant women at term have higher plasma CGRP levels than non-pregnant women and spontaneous labor does not alter maternal CGRP levels, as levels do not differ between VD and ECS section, and do not correlate with cervical ripening throughout labor (Florio *et al.*, 2001b).

There is a controversial report about maternal plasma CGRP concentrations in PE. In fact, no differences were found between severe PE and normal pregnancy, as levels were similar to those in non-pregnant women (Schiff *et al.*, 1995). Also fetal plasma CGRP do not change and levels in the supernatants of placental extracts do not differ between preeclamptic and normal pregnancies (Schiff *et al.*, 1995). On the contrary, recently maternal circulating CGRP concentrations were reported significantly lower in women with PE, thus contributing to the development and maintenance of hypertension during pregnancy (Halhali *et al.*, 2001) (Table 1.2).

relaxant of a variety of smooth muscle tissues (Brain *et al.*, 1985). In fact, CGRP can induce dose-dependent relaxation in spontaneously contracting pregnant myometrium, via activation of adenylyl cyclase (Casey *et al.*, 1997), and this relaxing effect of CGRP is lower in myometrium obtained from women after labor and in non-pregnant women (Chan *et al.*, 1997; Dong *et al.*, 1999). The inhibitory action of CGRP on myometrial contractions may be also dependent on nitric oxide (NO) formation (Shew *et al.*, 1993), but also involves the hyper polarization of cell membrane potentials via activation of membrane potassium channels (Chan *et al.*, 1997). The CGRP relaxation induced in uterus collected after spontaneous or OT-induced labor was 60 times less effective than in tissues from pregnant women not in labor (Chan *et al.*, 1997).

(E) Role of PTHrP

Recent evidence from sheep suggest that parathyroid hormone-related peptide (PTHrP; Box 1.7) may be an important modulator of placental calcium transport.

Box 1.7 Parathyroid hormone-related peptide

The PTHrP is a 141 amino acids protein involved in endochondral bone development and epithelial–mesenchymal interactions during the formation of the mammary glands and teeth (Strewler, 2000). Eight of the first 13 amino acids in the mature PTHrP peptide are identical to those of PTH but the sequence diverges completely after amino acid 13, and the subsequent region accounts for the distinctive biological actions of the two peptides (Strewler, 2000). The PTHrP regulates local tissue functions, in contrast to the systemic hormonal function of PTH. However, PTHrP functions as a poly-hormone that gives rise to several biologically active peptides, each of which presumably has it own receptor (Strewler, 2000). PTHrP is produced by many tissues, binds to the same receptor as PTH and has major effects on development (Fiaschi-Taesch and Stewart, 2003).

Expression and localization

The placenta and the mammary glands are the main sources of PTHrP (Ardawi *et al.*, 1997). In fact, its mRNA has been identified in placenta, myometrium, decidua and fetal membranes (Ferguson *et al.*, 1992; Bowden *et al.*, 1994; Emly *et al.*, 1994; Curtis *et al.*, 1997) and the peptide is localized in both syncytiotrophoblast and cytotrophoblast cells (Clemens *et al.*, 2001). With respect to mRNA levels, the expression is higher in placental amnion than in reflected amnion (Ferguson *et al.*, 1992). By using immunohistochemistry, a differential localization of immunoreactive PTHrP (ir-PTHrP)(1–34) and ir-PTHrP(67–86) in the human placenta and fetal membranes was found (Ramirez *et al.*, 1995), with PTHrP(1–34) localized strongly to the syncytiotrophoblast of the placenta, while PTHrP(67–86) was present predominantly in the endothelial cells of capillaries in the placental villi. Moreover, the staining for ir-PTHrP(1–34) was less in placenta and membranes obtained from women at the time of labor than at ECS section in the absence of labor, whereas ir-PTHrP(67–86) staining did not differ significantly (Ramirez *et al.*, 1995).

Receptors

The PTH/PTHrP receptor is a seven-transmembrane domain, G-protein-linked receptor which signals via both adenilate cyclase and phospholipase C (Strewler, 2000). Using real-time protein-coupled receptor (RT-PCR), PTH/PTHrP receptor mRNA was expressed in the myometrium and in preterm and term samples of placenta, amnion over placenta, reflected amnion and choriodecidua (Curtis *et al.*, 1998). In details, PTHrP receptor has been found in human trophoblast in proximity to sites of PTHrP expression (Ferguson *et al.*, 1998), thus suggesting possible autocrine and paracrine functions of PTHrP in all preterm and term tissues, including amnion, chorodecidua, placenta and myometrium (Curtis *et al.*, 1998; Ferguson *et al.*, 1998).

Levels in biological fluids

Plasma levels of PTHrP increase throughout pregnancy with higher levels at term (Hirota *et al.*, 1997) and PTHrP produced in either the feto-placental unit or the breast, or both, can reach the circulation of pregnant women in the third trimester and at 1 month postpartum in women with breast- and mixed-feeding (Hirota *et al.*, 1997).

The PTHrP is detectable in fetal blood and concentrations are lower in maternal blood (Bucht *et al.*, 1995; Papantoniou *et al.*, 1996). Moreover, PTHrP levels were higher in fetal than maternal circulation (Bucht *et al.*, 1995) and, concentrations in the umbilical artery are higher than in the vein, thus suggesting that the fetus is the main source of PTHrP in the cord blood circulation (Papantoniou *et al.*, 1996). The concentrations in umbilical cord plasma were increased in intrauterine growth restriction (IUGR), but unaltered in diabetes (Strid *et al.*, 2003) (Table 1.2). In preeclamptic women, the PTHrP expression in placenta and amnion was not increased in association with maternal hypertension, placental insufficiency and vasoconstriction. The PTHrP mRNA expression was decreased in choriodecidua in association with term but not preterm PE, thus suggesting that PTHrP is not involved in the placental pathophysiology of PE in late gestation (Curtis *et al.*, 1998; Clemens *et al.*, 2001).

It has been demonstrated that partially purified fetal parathyroid extracts of PTHrP increased placental calcium transport (Rodda *et al.*, 1988; Care *et al.*, 1990), and that parathyroid hormones (PTH) and PTHrP(1–34) regulate the calcium transport across the fetal facing, but not the maternal facing, of the syncytiotrophoblast (Farrugia *et al.*, 2000). Moreover, acting through the PTH/PTHrP receptor, the two molecules may contribute to the overall maintenance of calcium transfer across placenta (Rodda *et al.*, 1988; Care *et al.*, 1990).

Calcium is a factor that is also related to the physiology of the myometrium and calcium channel blockers effectively inhibit undesired uterine activity (Challis *et al.*, 2000). The PTH/PTHrP regulates calcium homeostasis in various target tissue, and hyperparathyroidism complicating pregnancy involves an increased incidence of premature birth but no statistically significant differences were observed in the levels of calcium and other minerals salts, between preterm labor, preterm non-labor, term labor and term non-labor (Lurie *et al.*, 1997). However, in rats PTH/PTHrP(1–34) acts on myometrial smooth muscle to cause relaxation (Shew *et al.*, 1984; Williams *et al.*, 1994), and inhibits OT-induced rat uterine contractions in vitro (Dalle *et al.*, 1992). Moreover, PTHrP may facilitate the myometrial quiescence characteristic of the first 95% of normal pregnancy (Figure 1.5).

Peptide signaling and the control of fetal–placental blood flow

The control of fetal–placental blood flow is very important throughout pregnancy, as the nutrients and oxygen to the fetus come from the mother and have to pass the placental barrier. In fact, the fetal vessels of the human placenta are not innervated, so that the control of blood flow in this vascular bed is partly dependant on locally produced and circulating vasoactive factors (Boura *et al.*, 1994). The tight regulation of the blood flow through the uterine arteries (from the mother to the placenta) and the umbilical cord (from the placenta to the fetus) is critical for the growth and differentiation of the embryo/fetal tissues (Reis *et al.*, 2002). In healthy pregnant women an increase in the uterine blood flow and a decrease in uterine vascular resistance are typical features. The mechanism causing this decreased vascular resistance is poorly understood. It is probably the result of multiple factors, including a loss of smooth muscle in myometrial resistance vessels (spiral arteries and terminations of radial arteries), an increased angiogenesis, as well as an augmented local uterine artery vasodilation probably related to an increased role of endogenous vasodilators (Kuo *et al.*, 1990; Poston *et al.*, 1995).

Pregnancy is associated with various cardiovascular changes such as increased blood volume and cardiac output, and decreased blood pressure and peripheral vascular resistance. The decrease in peripheral vascular resistance occurring in pregnancy (Poston *et al.*, 1995) has been attributed to increased production of vasorelaxant, which acts on the vascular endothelium to cause the release of several relaxant factors (Moncada and Vane, 1979; Furchgott, 1993), as well as directly on vascular smooth muscle causing relaxation (Brayden and Nelson, 1992). CRH, NPY, CGRP and PTHrP play a major role in regulating locally the tone of blood vessels.

(A) Effects of CRH and NPY

Several in vitro evidences demonstrated that CRH has vasodilatory effects in a number of species (Ramirez *et al.*, 1995). In fact, CRH caused dilation of the mesenteric arteries in vivo (MacCannell *et al.*, 1984) and both in rat and human i.v. administration of CRH lowers arterial pressure due to peripheral vasodilation caused by a direct action on vascular smooth muscle (Hermus *et al.*, 1987; Kiang and Wei, 1987; Corder *et al.*, 1992). However, in most animals and in non-pregnant humans, peripheral concentrations of CRH are low (Vale *et al.*, 1993), which suggests that CRH may play a minimal role in the control of vascular tone. In contrast, in the pregnant human, plasma CRH concentrations rise exponentially, peaking at term (Ramirez *et al.*, 1995; Challis *et al.*, 2000; Hillhouse and Grammatopoulos, 2002).

The CRH, when administered chronically in pregnant rats, causes a decrease in blood pressure (Jain *et al.*, 1998), and it is also a potent relaxant of the uterine artery of pregnant rats, acting both on the endothelium (mediated by NO–cGMP system) and the vascular smooth muscle (Jain *et al.*, 1999). Animal studies revealed that reduced uterine blood flow and consequent hypoxia induce an increased expression and secretion of CRH, and consequently of ACTH and cortisol (Sue-Tang *et al.*, 1992). As CRH acts as vasodilator in placental circulation, increased CRH could act systemically or be released locally in the placenta as a compensatory mechanisms to reduce uterine resistance to blood flow (Gagnon *et al.*, 1997). In humans, an impaired placental CRH secretion has been associated with the lack of uterine artery dilation and the decrease of the utero-placental blood flow through uterine arteries, supporting the concept that at mid-gestation placental CRH is involved in the control of the uterine artery tone (Florio *et al.*, 2003b).

Recent investigations have shown that CRH is a potent dilatator of the human fetal–placental circulation (Clifton *et al.*, 1994; 1995; 1996), acting at concentrations comparable to plasma CRH levels in maternal and fetal circulation. Placental CRH may, therefore, have a significant physiological role as a regulator of feto-placental vascular tone. This effect is due to endothelial-independent pathways (Kiang and Wei, 1987; Corder *et al.*, 1992), but in some species CRH may also operate via endothelium-dependant mechanism, acting on specific receptors expressed by endothelium, as in the case of human umbilical vein endothelial cells (HUVEC) (Simoncini *et al.*, 1999).

In the human fetal–placental circulation CRH causes vasodilation via a NO- and cGMP-mediated pathway, as the addition of a blocker of NO formation and

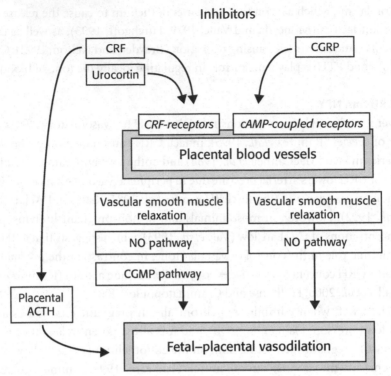

Figure 1.6   Placental CRF, urocortin, NPY, CGRP and PTHrP are involved in the fine control of the fetal–placental blood flow

inhibitors of cGMP formation respectively cause marked attenuation of CRH–stimulated vasodilation. The addition of CRH to preconstricted placental vessels is able to attenuate all constrictor mechanisms without variation in CRH potency as a vasodilator agent. The CRH-induced vasodilation appears to be mediated by a CRH receptor, as the vasodilatory response to CRH is antagonized in the presence of a CRH receptor antagonists (Clifton *et al.*, 1994; 1995). The CRH-induced vasodilation occurred at concentrations comparable to plasma CRH levels found in the maternal and fetal circulations (Challis *et al.*, 2000; Florio *et al.*, 2002d, Hillhouse and Grammatopoulos, 2002; Reis *et al.*, 1999), and CRH is approximatately 50 times more potent than prostacyclin (Clifton *et al.*, 1995) (Figure 1.6).

Urocortin has the same effects of CRH: administered i.v. in rats it is more potent than CRH in causing hypotension (Vaughan *et al.*, 1995; Torpy *et al.*, 1999) and, with respect to placental circulation, it causes vasodilation, reducing fetal–placental vascular resistance via CRH type 2 receptors, and being more potent that CRH (Leitch *et al.*, 1998) (Figure 1.6).

As syncytiotrophoblast is the main source of CRH during pregnancy (Petraglia *et al.*, 1990b; 1996d; Petraglia, 1991; Reis *et al.*, 1999; 2001; 2002; Florio *et al.*,

2002d; Hillhouse and Grammatopoulos, 2002), placental CRH may access the fetal–placental circulation to cause dilation by paracrine or endocrine mechanisms. It may be released locally to affect the vascular smooth muscle and endothelium, or it may be secreted into the feto-placental circulation and travel to its site of action through the placental vascular system. Finally, CRH may maximize the release of products such as POMC peptides (Florio et al., 2002d; Petraglia et al., 1987c; 1999a) or PGs (Challis et al., 2000) in vivo, by causing vasodilation of placental vascular tissue (Clifton et al., 1996) (Figure 1.6).

The NPY is involved in regulation of the local uterine blood flow (Fried et al., 1986; Fallgren et al., 1989; Ekesbo et al., 1991; Fried and Samuelson, 1991). Since level of NPY in plasma is increased in women with eclampsia, preeclampsia and hypertension (Fried et al., 1986), perhaps elevated plasma NPY values may play a key role in the development of these pathologies.

(B) Effect of CGRP

The CGRP is a potent vasodilator in a variety of animal and human systems (Poyner et al., 2002; Yallampalli et al., 2002) and, the mode of action of CGRP is still under investigation, as in some tissues it appears to act independently on endothelium, apparently by interacting directly with coupled cAMP receptors on smooth muscle (Fiscus et al., 1992), or via mechanisms mediated by the release of vasodilator NO (Fiscus et al., 1991). On the basis of these evidences, it has been suggested that CGRP may play a role in the control of vasoactivity of the human fetal–placental circulation (Mandsager et al., 1994) (Figure 1.6) and, of preconstricted human chorionic plate vessels in vitro through two classes of receptors and also independently of NO pathway (Firth and Pipkin, 1989). The CGRP participates in regulation of the vascular adaptations occurring during normal pregnancy, and it appears to be involved in the pathophysiology of preeclampsia (Kraayenbrink et al., 1993; Schiff et al., 1995). In fact, in rats the coadministration of L-NAME (a drug that increases blood pressure) and CGRP prevented the gestational (not the postpartum) L-NAME hypertension and decreased pup mortality to 6.4% but did not reverse the decreased fetal weight (Yallampalli et al., 1996; Gangula et al., 1997; Parida et al., 1998). The same phenomenon was evident in the presence of adequate levels of progesterone in the postpartum period, as if CGRP regulates vascular adaptations during pregnancy and these effects may be progesterone dependent (Figure 1.6).

Sex steroid hormones are raised during pregnancy, and the increase of plasma CGRP levels might be related to steroid hormone levels as levels are higher in women than in men, and mainly in women taking contraceptive pills (Valdermarsson et al., 1990). Taken together, we could hypothesize that the relaxant effect of CGRP on the non-pregnant and pregnant uterus, as well as its vasodilatory actions are, at least in part, under progesterone control. In fact, progesterone treatment of ovariectomized mice resulted in a significant increase in the responsiveness of the myometrium to CGRP (Naghashpour and Dahl, 2000) and, recent studies in female rats indicate that the vasodilator effects of CGRP are sex steroid hormone dependent, as chronic CGRP administration to pregnant rats increased systolic blood pressure, indicating a role for CGRP in maintaining a normotensive state during pregnancy (Gangula *et al.*, 2002). Furthermore, sex hormones increase both the synthesis of CGRP (Gangula *et al.*, 2000) and the responsiveness to synthetic CGRP in the vasculature (Gangula *et al.*, 2001).

(C) Effect of PTHrP

The PTHrP is a potent vasodilator (Winquist *et al.*, 1987; Nickols *et al.*, 1990) through the activation of myometrial cells of adenylyl cyclase and its expression in vascular smooth muscle cells increases in response to hypertension, vasoconstrictor agents, increased flow, shear stress and stretch. The PTHrP has vasodilator effect in the human fetal–placental circulation (Macgill *et al.*, 1997), and is 100 times more potent than PTH (Mandsager *et al.*, 1994). The expression of PTHrP in utero may be stimulated by hormones including estradiol, prolactin and placental lactogen (Dvir *et al.*, 1995), by cytokines and growth factors (Casey *et al.*, 1992; Dvir *et al.*, 1995) and mechanical stimuli (Daifotis *et al.*, 1992).

Inhibin-related peptides

Inhibins and activins (Box 1.8) are growth factors belonging to the transforming growth factor-β (TGF-β) superfamily, and composed by two subunits. Inhibins are heterodimers of a α subunit with a β subunit (inhibin A = $\alpha\beta$A; inhibin B = $\alpha\beta$B) while activins are omodimer of β subunit (activin A = βAβA; activin B = βBβB; and activin AB = βAβB) (Vale *et al.*, 1988). They were originally identified from gonads as factors acting antagonistically in the endocrine regulation of pituitary follicle-stimulating hormone (FSH) production, but successive descriptions of their expression in numerous cells types and tissues outside the hypothalamic–pituitary–gonadal axis indicate different functions, particularly as modulators of cell growth, differentiation and apoptosis (Luisi *et al.*, 2001). The βA subunit is also expressed from the first trimester of gestation, with the highest value at term, while the βB-subunit, present in the outer syncytial layer, is detected only at term (Petraglia *et al.*, 1991; 1992b). The βA-subunit is localized in the external syncytial layer of placental villi, in some structure of the stroma, in maternal decidual cells and in some amnion and chorionic cells (Petraglia *et al.*, 1990d; 1991; 1993c; 1994c) but, in term trophoblasts, also in endothelial cells within the placental villi (Schneider-Kolsky *et al.*, 2002).

Box 1.8 Inhibin-related peptides

Inhibins and activins are growth factors belonging to the TGF-β superfamily, and composed by two subunits. Inhibins are heterodimers of a α subunit with a β subunit (inhibin A = αβA; inhibin B = αβB) while activins are omodimers of β subunit (activin A = βAβA; activin B = βBβB; activin AB = βAβB) (Vale *et al.*, 1988).

Expression and localization
Human placenta synthesizes inhibins and activins (Petraglia, 1997; Florio *et al.*, 2001a). The α subunit mRNA in the human trophoblast is expressed from the first trimester of gestation, with the highest values at term (Petraglia *et al.*, 1991), and it is localized within the structure of placental villi (cyto- and intermediate trophoblast, mesenchymal cells) (Petraglia *et al.*, 1987b; 1991; 1992b), maternal decidua (Petraglia *et al.*, 1990d), amnion and chorionic cells (Petraglia *et al.*, 1993c).

Receptors and binding proteins
Activins signal through a heteromeric complex of receptor serine kinases which include at least two type I (IA and IB) and two type II (IIA and IIB) receptors. These receptors are all transmembrane proteins, composed of a ligand-binding extracellular domain, a transmembrane domain and a cytoplasmic domain with predicted serine/threonine specificity (Gray *et al.*, 2002).

Levels in biological fluids
During the first trimester of pregnancy, maternal serum levels of inhibin A and activin A are higher than in non-pregnancy (Florio *et al.*, 2001a), while inhibin B (Petraglia *et al.*, 1997b) does not significantly differ from levels detected during the menstrual cycle. At this gestational period, coelomatic fluid activin A and inhibin B levels are higher than in maternal serum and amniotic fluid (Luisi *et al.*, 1998). In amniotic fluid, inhibin A is not detectable (Riley *et al.*, 1996). In this trimester of pregnancy, the feto-placental unit is the main source of circulating activin A and inhibin A (Muttukrishna *et al.*, 1997). During the second trimester of pregnancy, inhibin A and activin A further increase in maternal serum and amniotic fluid, whilst inhibin B increases only in amniotic fluid (Petraglia *et al.*, 1995a, c; 1999b; Muttukrishna *et al.*, 1996; Wallace *et al.*, 1997; Muttukrishna *et al.*, 2000). At term, maternal serum levels of inhibin A (Florio *et al.*, 1999a; Muttukrishna *et al.*, 2000), inhibin B (Petraglia *et al.*, 1997b) and

activin A (Petraglia *et al.*, 1994a; Florio *et al.*, 1999a; Muttukrishna *et al.*, 2000) and those in amniotic fluid (Wallace *et al.*, 1997) are at their highest. Inhibins A and B and activin A are also measurable in umbilical cord blood (Wallace *et al.*, 1997; Florio *et al.*, 1999a).

Inhibin and activin secretion from cultured placental cells is controlled by both positive and negative regulatory mechanisms involving hormones and growth factors (Petraglia *et al.*, 1996d). The FSH, human chorionic gonadotropin (hCG), PGs, epidermal growth factor (EGF) and TGF-α are potent stimulators, while TGF-β and activin A are suppressors for inhibin production in cultured trophoblast cells (Petraglia *et al.*, 1996d; 1987b). Furthermore, it was found that the addition of gonadotropin-releasing hormone (GnRH) and glucocorticoids induces an increases in the release of the inhibin in cultured human trophoblast cells (Keelan *et al.*, 1994). With respect to activin A, GnRH, inhibin, TGF-β, dexamethasone, cAMP and IL-1α have no effect on its production in cultured trophoblast cells, while its production can be stimulated by phorbol ester (Rabinovici *et al.*, 1992; Keelan *et al.*, 1994), tumor necrosis factor (TNF)-α, IL-1β and granulocyte and monocyte colony stimulating factor (GMCSF) (Keelan *et al.*, 1998; Mohan *et al.*, 2001) (Figure 1.7).

First and second trimester placentae express the various receptor proteins in the syncytium, whereas at term the distribution is confined to vascular endothelial cells of villous blood vessels. In the fetal membranes they are localized to some epithelial cells, mesenchime and chorionic trophoblast (Schneider-Kolsky *et al.*, 2002).

The activity of activin A is tightly regulated by follistatin, a structurally unrelated protein, that binds with high affinity to activin and neutralizes its activity (Luisi *et al.*, 2001). This affinity is similar to that for activin receptors, thus it plays a major role in regulating activin bioavailability on target tissues and functions. Recently, a new binding protein of 70 amino acids for activin A has been identified, namely follistatin-related gene (FLRG), closely related to follistatin (Hayette *et al.*, 1998), that interacts physically with activin A and, preventing the binding on ActRs, regulates activin A functions (Hayette *et al.*, 1998; Tsuchida *et al.*, 2001). Follistatin and FLRG are both present in trophoblast, decidua and fetal membranes amnion and chorion), but FLRG protein immunolocalization differs from that shown for follistatin. FLRG is predominantly present in the walls of decidual and placental blood vessels (Ciarmela *et al.*, 2003), whilst follistatin is more localized in cyto- and syncytiotrophoblast cells (Petraglia *et al.*, 1994c).

The measurement of inhibin-related proteins during pregnancy may have important clinical implications. In fact, at first/second trimester serum inhibin A

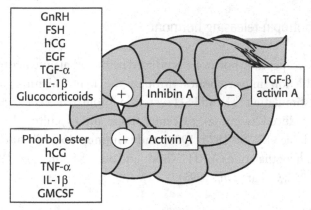

Figure 1.7   Factors regulating the release of activin and inhibin from human placental cells in culture

and activin A assay may be of value in diagnosis and short-term follow-up of molar pregnancy, as levels are highest in molar pregnancies (Florio *et al.*, 2002e); also of early pregnancy viability (Luisi *et al.*, 2003), fetal demise (Petraglia *et al.*, 1999b), pregnancy-induced hypertension (Muttukrishna *et al.*, 2000) and PE (Petraglia *et al.*, 1999b; Florio *et al.*, 2002a; 2003a) (Table 1.2). In particular, the measurement of inhibin A and activin A may offer important prognostic informa- tion in predicting early the onset of PE several months before the onset of symptoms (Florio *et al.*, 2003a; Lambert-Messerlian *et al.*, 2000; Silver *et al.*, 2002). Although placental mRNA expression of the α and βA-subunits is increased in PE (Florio *et al.*, 2003a; Silver *et al.*, 2002), the increased levels of activin A appear to be more specifically a reflection of increased placental production than do the increased levels of inhibin A (Silver *et al.*, 2002).

Placental control of hCG secretion

Placental GnRH (Box 1.9) stimulates secretion of hCG in vitro (Khodr and Siler- Khodr, 1980), in agreement with the neuroendocrine action of the hypothalamic counterpart (Figure 1.8). In addition, since several factors regulating the release of GnRH from hypothalamus also regulate the secretion of placental GnRH, they may also have a local role in modulating indirectly the placental hCG release. Indeed, activin A stimulates, whilst inhibin A inhibits, the placental secretion of hCG, 17β-estradiol and progesterone (Petraglia *et al.*, 1989d; Keelan *et al.*, 1994). In details, the effects of activin A and inhibin A on placental hCG release is com- parable to pituitary/FSH regulation. In addition, the cellular colocalization of activin A, inhibin A and GnRH suggests the occurrence of autocrine events in the regulation of hCG release (Petraglia *et al.*, 1992b). The addition of an inhibin anti- serum increases the placental hCG release (Petraglia *et al.*, 1987b; 1989d), whilst

Box 1.9 Gonadotropin-releasing hormone

The GnRH is a decapeptidic hormone produced by hypothalamic neurons that controls reproduction in vertebrates through the hypothalamic–pituitary–gonadal axis by stimulating LH and FSH secretion (Stojilkovic *et al.*, 1994). The GnRH is also produced by human placental tissue and by cultured placental cells (Khodr and Siler-Khodr, 1978; 1980) and is immunologically and chemically identical to hypothalamic GnRH (Khodr and Siler-Khodr, 1978; 1980; Tan and Rousseau, 1982; Gohar *et al.*, 1996).

Expression and localization
Placental GnRH message has been found in human placenta, from the first trimester to term, by *in situ* reverse transcription-polymerase chain reaction and immunocytochemistry, with abundant signals both in the cyto- and syncytiotrophoblast (Wolfahrt *et al.*, 1998). The GnRH staining is reported to be intense in cytotrophoblast and in the villous stroma from early placentae (8 weeks of pregnancy) (Miyake *et al.*, 1982), but GnRH immunoreacivity has been also demonstrated in the syncytiotrophoblast of the normal human placenta from the first half of pregnancy, in syncytiotrophoblast cells of hydatidiform mole and choriocarcinoma (Seppala *et al.*, 1980). The total placental concentration of immunoreactive GnRH, as measured by RIA, progressively increases during the first 24 weeks of gestation and remains relatively constant in the third trimester (Siler-Khodr and Khodr, 1978) whilst, on the contrary, the mRNA expression remains constant throughout gestation (Kelly *et al.*, 1991).

Receptors
The human placenta contains specific binding sites for GnRH that interact with GnRH agonists and antagonists (Leung and Peng, 1996). By *in situ* hybridization, GnRH receptor (GnRHR) mRNAs were detected in the human placenta and localized to the cytotrophoblast and syncytiotrophoblast cell layers (Lin *et al.*, 1995). Using primers specific to the human GnRHR, the predicted PCR product was obtained from human placenta cells (Boyle *et al.*, 1998; Wolfahrt *et al.*, 1998) and choriocarcinoma cell line (JAR and JEG-3) (Lamharzi *et al.*, 1998; Yin *et al.*, 1998) and the receptor expressed in the placenta is identical to the counterpart of pituitary (Cheng *et al.*, 2000). The placental GnRHR is coupled to the protein kinase C (PKC) and cAMP/protein kinase A (PKA) pathways (Cheng *et al.*, 2000). Moreover, there is evidence that GnRH induces activation of the mitogen-activated protein kinase (MAPK) signaling pathway in normal and carcinoma cells of the human ovary and placenta (Kang *et al.*, 2000).

The contemporary presence of GnRH and GnRHR in identical cells strongly suggests an autocrine/paracrine regulation by GnRH in human placenta. On this regard, two classes of placental GnRH-binding sites have been described to date: high affinity (Kd = $10-8$ mol/l) and low affinity (Kd = $10-5$ mol/l) (Cheng *et al.*, 2000; Kang *et al.*, 2000). From first trimester to term, the human placenta contains low-affinity GnRH-binding sites that interact with GnRH agonist or antagonist (Bramley *et al.*, 1992; 1994; Cheng *et al.*, 2000; Kang *et al.*, 2000). The GnRHR levels decrease observed between 10 and 20 weeks of gestation is probably due to a decreased expression/synthesis (or increased catabolism) of placental GnRHR, or increased occupancy (or downregulation) of placental GnRHR by an endogenous GnRH-like ligand (Bramley *et al.*, 1992; 1994). The mRNA of the high-affinity GnRH-binding site is expressed in human cytotrophoblast and syncytiotrophoblast cell layers (Lin *et al.*, 1995). The GnRH administration to pregnant women increases serum levels of hCG in the first trimester, but not in the third trimester (Iwashita *et al.*, 1993), probably due to the decreased number of GnRHRs in the term placenta (Lin *et al.*, 1995).

Levels in biological fluids

The GnRH is measurable in the maternal circulation, and levels are significantly higher during pregnancy than in non-pregnant cycling women, in particular in the first half of pregnancy (Siler-Khodr *et al.*, 1984). Pulsatile changes of maternal GnRH values have been shown, with highest amplitude in the first trimester and lowest at term (Petraglia *et al.*, 1994a) and, maternal levels at 25–35 weeks of gestation are higher in women who later had post-term pregnancies (Gohar *et al.*, 1996).

the addition of recombinant inhibin inhibits it secretion (Petraglia *et al.*, 1987b; 1989d). These effects are mediated at least in part by GnRH, as preincubation with a GnRH antagonist partially reduced the increase of hCG after immunoneutralization of inhibin (Petraglia *et al.*, 1987b). Activin A increases hCG and GnRH-induced hCG release from cultured human placental cells collected at first trimester and at term (Petraglia *et al.*, 1987b; 1994c). The effect of activin A on GnRH release is potentiated by estradiol or estriol, reduced by progesterone and antagonized by tamoxifen or RU486. In addition, progesterone reverses the effect of estriol, thus suggesting that estrogens and progesterone have opposite effects on placental hCG release. Finally, follistatin inhibits activin A-induced hCG release, as it binds and inactivates activin A (Petraglia *et al.*, 1994c) (Figure 1.8).

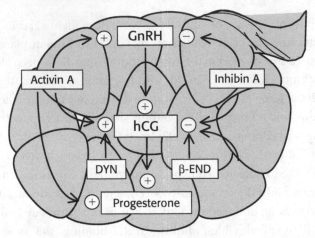

Figure 1.8   Paracrine control of hCG release by the placental syncytiotrophoblasts. The stimulatory effects of GnRH and activin, and the inhibitory effects of inhibin resemble the control of pituitary FSH release

Opioid peptides (β-END and dynorphins (DYN)) play a role in regulating secretion of hPL (Newnham *et al.*, 1983; Petraglia *et al.*, 1990b; 1996a; Petraglia, 1991; Ahmed *et al.*, 1992; Reis *et al.*, 2001) and hCG release from trophoblast tissue (Cemerikic *et al.*, 1992). Indeed, DYN has a significant stimulatory effect upon pulsatile hCG secretion in the first trimester placenta cell cultures (Barnea *et al.*, 1991a), whilst β-END in vitro inhibits hCG secretion (Barnea *et al.*, 1991b) (Figure 1.8).

Conclusions

The physiological maternal and fetal adaptations during human gestation are regulated by human placenta through the secretion of several neurohormones. Thus, fluid balance, blood pressure, digestion, respiration, fuel and mineral metabolism, immune response, and several behavioral functions are reprogrammed during pregnancy and occur under the modulation of hormonal changes, from very early gestation till after the fetal delivery. The excessive/reduced release of some placental neurohormones in association with gestational diseases may be part of an adaptive response of placenta and fetal membranes to adverse environmental conditions, such as hypertension, hypoxia and infection, or to malformations of the fetus and placenta. In a scenery of maternal and/or fetal stress elicited by a number of pathological conditions, the neurohormones produced and secreted by the human placenta appear to play a role in coordinating the adaptive changes in uterine perfusion, maternal metabolism, fluid balance and possibly uterine contractility.

REFERENCES

Acher, R. and Chauvet, J. (1995). The neurohypophysial endocrine regulatory cascade: precursors, mediators, receptors, and effectors. *Front. Neuroendocrinol.*, **16**, 237–89.

Agbas, A., Ahmed, M. S., Millington, W. *et al.* (1995). Dynorphin A(1–8) in human placenta: amino acid sequence determined by tandem mass spectrometry. *Peptides*, **16**, 623–27.

Ahmed, M. S., Cemerikic, B. and Agbas, A. (1992). Properties and functions of human placental opioid system. *Life Sci.*, **50**, 83–97.

Ardawi, M. S., Nasrat, H. A. and BA'Aqueel, H. S. (1997). Calcium-regulating hormones and parathyroid hormone-related peptide in normal human pregnancy and postpartum: a longitudinal study. *Eur. J. Endocrinol.*, **137**, 402–9.

Balasubramaniam, A. (2003). Neuropeptide Y (NPY) family of hormones: progress in the development of receptor selective agonists and antagonists. *Curr. Pharm. Des.*, **9**, 1165–75.

Barbieri, R. L. (1994). The maternal adenohypophysis. In D. Tulchinsky and A. B. Little, eds., *Maternal–Fetal Endocrinology*, 2nd edn., Philadelphia: WB Saunders Co.

Barnea, E. R., Lavy, G., Fakih, H. and Decherney, A. H. (1986). The role of ACTH in placental steroidogenesis. *Placenta*, **7**, 307–13.

Barnea, E. R., Ashkenazy, R. and Sarne, Y. (1991a). The effect of dynorphin on placental pulsatile human chorionic gonadotropin secretion in vitro. *J. Clin. Endocrinol. Metab.*, **73**, 1093–8.

Barnea, E. R., Ashkenazy, R., Tal, Y., Kol, S. and Sarne, Y. (1991b). Effect of beta-endorphin on human chorionic gonadotrophin secretion by placental explants. *Hum. Reprod.*, **6**, 1327–31.

Benedetto, C., Petraglia, F., Marozio, L. *et al.* (1994). Corticotropin-releasing hormone increases prostaglandin F2 alpha activity on human myometrium in vitro. *Am. J. Obstet. Gynecol.*, **171**, 126–31.

Berkowitz, G. S., Lapinski, R. H., Lockwood, C. J. *et al.* (1996). Corticotropin-releasing factor and its binding protein: maternal serum levels in term and preterm deliveries. *Am. J. Obstet. Gynecol.*, **174**, 1477–83.

Blanks, A. M. and Thornton, S. (2003). The role of oxytocin in parturition. *BJOG*, **110**, 46–51.

Born, W., Fischer, J. A. and Muff, R. (2002). Receptors for calcitonin gene-related peptide, adrenomedullin, and amylin: the contributions of novel receptor-activity-modifying proteins. *Receptor. Channel.*, **8**, 201–9.

Boura, A. L., Walters, W. A., Read, M. A. and Leitch, I. M. (1994). Autacoids and control of human placental blood flow. *Clin. Exp. Pharmacol. Physiol.*, **21**, 737–48.

Bowden, S. J., Emly, J. F., Hughes, S. V. *et al.* (1994). Parathyroid hormone-related protein in human term placenta and membranes. *J. Endocrinol.*, **142**, 217–24.

Boyle, T. A., Belt-Davis, D. I. and Duello, T. M. (1998). Nucleotide sequence analyses predict that human pituitary and human placental gonadotropin-releasing hormone receptors have identical primary structures. *Endocrine*, **9**, 281–7.

Brain, S. D., Williams, T. J., Tippins, J. R., Morris, H. R. and MacIntyre, I. (1985). Calcitonin gene-related peptide is a potent vasodilator. *Nature*, **313**, 54–6.

Bramley, T. A., McPhie, C. A. and Menzies, G. S. (1992). Human placental gonadotrophin-releasing hormone (GnRH) binding sites: I. Characterization, properties and ligand specificity. *Placenta*, **13**, 555–81.

Bramley, T. A., McPhie, C. A. and Menzies, G. S. (1994). Human placental gonadotrophin-releasing hormone (GnRH) binding sites: III. Changes in GnRH binding levels with stage of gestation. *Placenta*, **15**, 733–45.

Brayden, J. E. and Nelson, M. T. (1992). Regulation of arterial tone by activation of calcium-dependent potassium channels. *Science*, **256**, 532–5.

Bucht, E., Rong, H., Bremme, K. *et al.* (1995). Midmolecular parathyroid hormone-related peptide in serum during pregnancy, lactation and in umbilical cord blood. *Eur. J. Endocrinol.*, **132**, 438–43.

Bzoskie, L., Yen, J., Tseng, Y. T. *et al.* (1997). Human placental norepinephrine transporter mRNA: expression and correlation with fetal condition at birth. *Placenta*, **18**, 205–10.

Care, A. D., Abbas, S. K., Pickard, D. W. *et al.* (1990). Stimulation of ovine placental transport of calcium and magnesium by mid-molecule fragments of human parathyroid hormone-related protein. *Exp. Physiol.*, **75**, 605–8.

Casey, M. L., Mibe, M., Erk, A. and MacDonald, P. C. (1992). Transforming growth factor-beta 1 stimulation of parathyroid hormone-related protein expression in human uterine cells in culture: mRNA levels and protein secretion. *J. Clin. Endocrinol. Metab.*, **74**, 950–2.

Casey, M. L., Smith, J., Alsabrook, G. and MacDonald, P. C. (1997). Activation of adenylyl cyclase in human myometrial smooth muscle cells by neuropeptides. *J. Clin. Endocrinol. Metab.*, **82**, 3087–92.

Cemerikic, B., Schabbing, R. and Ahmed, M. S. (1992). Selectivity and potency of opioid peptides in regulating human chorionic gonadotropin release from term trophoblast tissue. *Peptides*, **13**, 897–903.

Challis, J. R. G., Matthews, S. G., Gibb, W. and Lye, S. J. (2000). Endocrine and paracrine regulation of birth at term and preterm. *Endocr. Rev.*, **21**, 514–50.

Chan, E. C., Smith, R., Lewin, T. *et al.* (1993). Plasma corticotropin releasing hormone, β-endorphin and cortisol inter-relationship during human pregnancy. *Acta Endocrinol.*, **128**, 339–44.

Chan, K. K., Robinson, G. and Pipkin, F. B. (1997). Differential sensitivity of human nonpregnant and pregnant myometrium to calcitonin gene-related peptide. *J. Soc. Gynecol. Invest.*, **4**, 15–21.

Cheng, K. W., Nathwani, P. S. and Leung, P. C. (2000). Regulation of human gonadotropin-releasing hormone receptor gene expression in placental cells. *Endocrinology*, **141**, 2340–9.

Chibbar, R., Miller, F. D. and Mitchell, B. F. (1993). Synthesis of oxytocin in amnion, chorion, and decidua may influence the timing of human parturition. *J. Clin. Invest.*, **91**, 185–92.

Chibbar, R., Wong, S., Miller, F. D. and Mitchell, B. F. (1995). Estrogen stimulates oxytocin gene expression in human chorio-decidua. *J. Clin. Endocrinol. Metab.*, **80**, 567–72.

Ciarmela, P., Florio, P., Toti, P. *et al.* (2003). Human placenta and fetal membranes express follistatin-related gene (FLRG) mRNA and protein. J. E. I. (in press).

Cikos, S., Gregor, P. and Koppel, J. (1999). Sequence and tissue distribution of a novel G-protein-coupled receptor expressed prominently in human placenta. *Biochem. Biophys. Res. Commun.*, **256**, 352–6.

Clemens, T. L., Cormier, S., Eichinger, A. *et al.* (2001). Parathyroid hormone-related protein and its receptors: nuclear functions and roles in the renal and cardiovascular systems, the placental trophoblasts and the pancreatic islets. *Br. J. Pharmacol.*, **134**, 1113–36.

Clifton, V. L., Read, M. A., Leitch, I. M. *et al.* (1994). Corticotropin-releasing hormone-induced vasodilatation in the human fetal placental circulation. *J. Clin. Endocrinol. Metab.*, **79**, 666–9.

Clifton, V. L., Read, M. A., Leitch, I. M. *et al.* (1995). Corticotropin-releasing hormone-induced vasodilatation in the human fetal–placental circulation: involvement of the nitric oxide-cyclic guanosine 3′,5′-monophosphate-mediated pathway. *J. Clin. Endocrinol. Metab.*, **80**, 2888–93.

Clifton, V. L., Read, M. A., Boura, A. L., Robinson, P. J. and Smith, R. (1996). Adrenocorticotropin causes vasodilatation in the human fetal–placental circulation. *J. Clin. Endocrinol. Metab.*, **81**, 1406–10.

Cooper, E. S., Greer, I. A. and Brooks, A. N. (1996). Placental proopiomelanocortin gene expression, adrenocorticotropin tissue concentrations, and immunostaining increase throughout gestation and are unaffected by prostaglandins, antiprogestins, or labor. *J. Clin. Endocrinol. Metab.*, **81**, 4462–9.

Corder, R., Turnill, D., Ling, N. and Gaillard, R. C. (1992). Attenuation of corticotropin releasing factor-induced hypotension in anesthetized rats with the CRF antagonist, alpha-helical CRF9–41; comparison with effect on ACTH release. *Peptides*, **13**, 1–6.

Curtis, N. E., Ho, P. W., King, R. G. *et al.* (1997). The expression of parathyroid hormone-related protein mRNA and immunoreactive protein in human amnion and choriodecidua is increased at term compared with preterm gestation. *J. Endocrinol.*, **154**, 103–12.

Curtis, N. E., King, R. G., Moseley, J. M. *et al.* (1998). Intrauterine expression of parathyroid hormone-related protein in normal and pre-eclamptic pregnancies. *Placenta*, **19**, 595–601.

Daifotis, A. G., Weir, E. C., Dreyer, B. E. and Broadus, A. E. (1992). Stretch-induced parathyroid hormone-related peptide gene expression in the rat uterus. *J. Biol. Chem.*, **267**, 23455–8.

Dalle, M., Dauprat-Dalle, P. and Barlet, J. P. (1992). Parathyroid hormone-related peptide inhibits oxytocin-induced rat uterine contractions in vitro. *Arch. Int. Physiol. Biochim. Biophys.*, **100**, 251–4.

De Geest, K., Thiery, M., Piron-Possuyt, G. and Vanden Driessche, R. (1985). Plasma oxytocin in human pregnancy and parturition. *J. Perinat. Med.*, **13**, 3–13.

Dombroski, R. A., Casey, M. L. and MacDonald, P. C. (1997). 5-alpha-dihydroprogesterone formation in human placenta from 5alpha-pregnan-3beta/alpha-ol-20-ones and 5-pregnan-3beta-yl-20-one sulfate. *J. Steroid Biochem. Mol. Biol.*, **63**, 155–63.

Dong, Y. L., Fang, L., Kondapaka, S. *et al.* (1999). Involvement of calcitonin gene-related peptide in the modulation of human myometrial contractility during pregnancy. *J. Clin. Invest.*, **104**, 559–65.

Dvir, R., Golander, A., Jaccard, N. *et al.* (1995). Amniotic fluid and plasma levels of parathyroid hormone-related protein and hormonal modulation of its secretion by amniotic fluid cells. *Eur. J. Endocrinol.*, **133**, 277–82.

Economides, D., Linton, E., Nicolaides, K. *et al.* (1987). Relationship between maternal and fetal corticotrophin-releasing hormone-41 and ACTH levels in human mid-trimester pregnancy. *J. Endocrinol.*, **114**, 497–501.

Ekesbo, R., Alm, P., Ekstrom, P., Lundberg, L. M. and Akerlund, M. (1991). Innervation of the human uterine artery and contractile responses to neuropeptides. *Gynecol. Obstet. Invest.*, **31**, 30–6.

Emly, J. F., Gregory, J., Bowden, S. J. *et al.* (1994). Immunohistochemical localization of parathyroid hormone-related protein (PTHrP) in human term placenta and membranes. *Placenta*, **15**, 653–60.

Facchinetti, F., Garuti, G., Petraglia, F., Mercantini, F. and Genazzani, A. R. (1990). Changes in beta-endorphin in fetal membranes and placenta in normal and pathological pregnancies. *Acta Obstet. Gynecol. Scand.*, **69**, 603–7.

Falkay, G. and Kovacs, L. (1994). Expression of two alpha 2-adrenergic receptor subtypes in human placenta: evidence from direct binding studies. *Placenta*, **15**, 661–8.

Fallgren, B., Edvinsson, L., Ekblad, E. and Ekman, R. (1989). Involvement of perivascular neuro-peptide Y nerve fibres in uterine arterial vasoconstriction in conjunction with pregnancy. *Regul. Pept.*, **24**, 119–30.

Farrugia, W., de Gooyer, T., Rice, G. E., Moseley, J. M. and Wlodek, M. E. (2000). Parathyroid hormone(1–34) and parathyroid hormone-related protein(1–34) stimulate calcium release from human syncytiotrophoblast basal membranes via a common receptor. *J. Endocrinol.*, **166**, 689–95.

Ferguson II, J. E., Gorman, J. V., Bruns, D. E. *et al.* (1992). Abundant expression of parathyroid hormone-related protein in human amnion and its association with labor. *Proc. Natl. Acad. Sci. USA*, **89**, 8384–8.

Ferguson II, J. E., Seaner, R. M., Bruns, D. E., Iezzoni, J. C. and Bruns, M. E. (1998). Expression and specific immunolocalization of the human parathyroid hormone/parathyroid hormone-related protein receptor in the uteroplacental unit. *Am. J. Obstet. Gynecol.*, **179**, 321–9.

Ferrari, A., Petraglia, F. and Gurpide, E. (1995). Corticotropin releasing factor decidualizes human endometrial stromal cells in vitro. Interaction with progestin. *J. Steroid. Biochem. Mol. Biol.*, **54**, 251–5.

Fiaschi-Taesch, N. M. and Stewart, A. F. (2003). Minireview: parathyroid hormone-related protein as an intracrine factor – trafficking mechanisms and functional consequences. *Endocrinology*, **144**, 407–11.

Firth, K. F. and Pipkin, F. B. (1989). Human alpha- and beta-calcitonin gene-related peptides are vasodilators in human chorioic plate vasculature. *Am. J. Obstet. Gynecol.*, **161**, 1318–19.

Fiscus, R. R., Zhou, H. L., Wang, X. *et al.* (1991). Calcitonin gene-related peptide (CGRP)-induced cyclic AMP, cyclic GMP and vasorelaxant responses in rat thoracic aorta are antagonized by blockers of endothelium-derived relaxant factor (EDRF). *Neuropeptides*, **20**, 133–43.

Fiscus, R. R., Wang, X. and Hao, H. (1992). hCGRP8–37 antagonizes vasodilations and cAMP responses to rat CGRP in rat caudal artery. *Ann. New York Acad. Sci.*, **657**, 513–15.

Florio, P., Lombardo, M., Gallo, R. *et al.* (1996). Activin A, corticotropin-releasing factor and prostaglandin F2 alpha increase immunoreactive oxytocin release from cultured human placental cells. *Placenta*, **17**, 307–11.

Florio, P., Woods, R. J., Genazzani, A. R., Lowry, P. J. and Petraglia, F. (1997). Changes in amniotic fluid immunoreactive corticotropin-releasing factor (CRF) and CRF-binding protein levels in pregnant women at term and during labor. *J. Clin. Endocrinol. Metab.*, **82**, 835–8.

Florio, P., Benedetto, C., Luisi, S. *et al.* (1999a). Activin A, inhibin A, inhibin B and parturition: changes of maternal and cord serum levels according to the mode of delivery. *Br. J. Obstet. Gynaecol.*, **106**, 1061–5.

Florio, P., Rivest, S., Reis, F. M. *et al.* (1999b). Lack of gestational-related changes of urocortin gene expression in human placenta. *Prenat. Neonat. Med.*, **4**, 296–300.

Florio, P., Franchini, A., Reis, F. M. *et al.* (2000). Human placenta, chorion, amnion and decidua express different variants of corticotropin-releasing factor receptor messenger RNA. *Placenta*, **21**, 32–7.

Florio, P., Cobellis, L., Luisi, S. *et al.* (2001a). Changes in inhibins and activin secretion in healthy and pathological pregnancies. *Mol. Cell. Endocrinol.*, **180**, 123–30.

Florio, P., Margutti, A., Apa, R. *et al.* (2001b). Maternal plasma calcitonin gene-related peptide levels do not change during labour and are not influenced by delivery route. *J. Soc. Gynecol. Invest.*, **8**(3), 165–8.

Florio, P., Ciarmela, P., Luisi, S. *et al.* (2002a). Pre-eclampsia with fetal growth restriction: placental and serum activin A and inhibin A levels. *Gynecol. Endocrinol.*, **16**, 365–72.

Florio, P., Cobellis, L., Woodman, J. *et al.* (2002b). Levels of maternal plasma corticotropin-releasing factor and urocortin during labor. *J. Soc. Gynecol. Invest.*, **9**, 233–7.

Florio, P., Mezzesimi, A., Turchetti, V. *et al.* (2002c). High levels of human chromogranin A in umbilical cord plasma and amniotic fluid at parturition. *J. Soc. Gynecol. Invest.*, **9**, 32–6.

Florio, P., Severi, F. M., Ciarmela, P. *et al.* (2002d). Placental stress factors and maternal–fetal adaptive response: the corticotropin-releasing factor family. *Endocrine*, **19**, 91–102.

Florio, P., Severi, F. M., Cobellis, L. *et al.* (2002e). Serum activin A and inhibin A. New clinical markers for hydatidiform mole. *Cancer*, **94**, 2618–22.

Florio, P., Reis, F. M., Pezzani, I. *et al.* (2003a). The addition of activin A and inhibin A measurement to uterine artery Doppler velocimetry to improve the early prediction of pre-eclampsia. *Ultrasound Obstet. Gynecol.*, **21**, 165–9.

Florio, P., Severi, F. M., Fiore, G. *et al.* (2003b). Impaired uterine artery blood flow at mid gestation and low levels of maternal plasma corticotropin-releasing factor. *J. Soc. Gynecol. Invest.*, **10**, 294–7.

Foord, S. M. and Craig, R. K. (1987). Isolation and characterisation of a human calcitonin-gene-related-peptide receptor. *Eur. J. Biochem.*, **170**, 373–9.

Fried, G. and Samuelson, U. (1991). Endothelin and neuropeptide Y are vasoconstrictors in human uterine blood vessels. *Am. J. Obstet. Gynecol.*, **164**, 1330–6.

Fried, G., Hokfelt, T., Lundberg, J. M., Terenius, L. and Hamberger, L. (1986). Neuropeptide Y and noradrenaline in human uterus and myometrium during normal and pre-eclamptic pregnancy. *Hum. Reprod.*, **1**, 359–64.

Frim, D. M., Emanuel, R. L., Robinson, B. G. *et al.* (1988). Characterization and gestational regulation of corticotropin-releasing hormone messenger RNA in human placenta. *J. Clin. Invest.*, **82**, 287–92.

Fuchs, A. R., Husslein, P. and Fuchs, F. (1981). Oxytocin and the initiation of human parturition. II. Stimulation of prostaglandin production in human decidua by oxytocin. *Am. J. Obstet. Gynecol.*, **141**, 694–7.

Fuchs, A. R., Romero, R., Keefe, D. *et al.* (1991). Oxytocin secretion and human parturition: pulse frequency and duration increase during spontaneous labor in women. *Am. J. Obstet. Gynecol.*, **165**, 1515–23.

Furchgott, R. F. (1993). Introduction to EDRF research. *J. Cardiovasc. Pharmacol.*, **22**, S1–2.

Gagnon, R., Murotsuki, J., Challis, J. R., Fraher, L. and Richardson, B. S. (1997). Fetal sheep endocrine responses to sustained hypoxemic stress after chronic fetal placental embolization. *Am. J. Physiol.*, **272**, E817–23.

Gangula, P. R., Supowit, S. C., Wimalawansa, S. J. *et al.* (1997). Calcitonin gene-related peptide is a depressor in NG-nitro-L-arginine methyl ester-induced hypertension during pregnancy. *Hypertension*, **29**, 248–53.

Gangula, P. R., Wimalawansa, S. J. and Yallampalli, C. (2000). Pregnancy and sex steroid hormones enhance circulating calcitonin gene-related peptide concentrations in rats. *Hum. Reprod.*, **15**, 949–53.

Gangula, P. R., Zhao, H., Wimalawansa, S. J. *et al.* (2001). Pregnancy and steroid hormones enhance the systemic and regional hemodynamic effects of calcitonin gene-related peptide in rats. *Biol. Reprod.*, **64**, 1776–83.

Gangula, P. R., Dong, Y. L., Wimalawansa, S. J. and Yallampalli, C. (2002). Infusion of pregnant rats with calcitonin gene-related peptide (CGRP)(8–37), a CGRP receptor antagonist, increases blood pressure and fetal mortality and decreases fetal growth. *Biol. Reprod.*, **67**, 624–9.

Genazzani, A. R., Facchinetti, F. and Parrini, D. (1981). Beta-lipotrophin and beta-endorphin plasma levels during pregnancy. *Clin. Endocrinol. (Oxford)*, **14**, 409–18.

Genazzani, A. R., Petraglia, F., Parrini, D. *et al.* (1984). Lack of correlation between amniotic fluid and maternal plasma contents of beta-endorphin, beta-lipotropin, and adrenocorticotropic hormone in normal and pathologic pregnancies. *Am. J. Obstet. Gynecol.*, **148**, 198–203.

Giles, W. B., McLean, M., Davies, J. J. and Smith, R. (1996). Abnormal umbilical artery Doppler waveforms and cord blood corticotropin-releasing hormone. *Obstet. Gynecol.*, **87**, 107–11.

Glynn, B. P., Wolton, A., Rodriguez-Linares, B., Phaneuf, S. and Linton, E. A. (1998). Urocortin in pregnancy. *Am. J. Obstet. Gynecol.*, **179**, 533–9.

Goebelsmann, U., Abboud, T. K., Hoffman, D.I. and Hung, T. T. (1984). Beta-endorphin in pregnancy. *Eur. J. Obstet. Gynecol. Reprod. Biol.*, **17**, 77–89.

Gohar, J., Mazor, M. and Leiberman, J. R. (1996). GnRH in pregnancy. *Arch. Gynecol. Obstet.*, **259**, 1–6.

Goland, R. S., Wardlaw, S. L., Blum, M., Tropper, P. J. and Stark, R. I. (1988). Biologically active corticotropin-releasing hormone in maternal and fetal plasma during pregnancy. *Am. J. Obstet. Gynecol.*, **159**, 884–90.

Goland, R. S., Jozak, S., Warren, W. B. *et al.* (1993). Elevated levels of umbilical cord plasma corticotropin-releasing hormone in growth-retarded fetuses. *J. Clin. Endocrinol. Metab.*, **77**, 1174–9.

Goland, R. S., Jozak, S. and Conwell, I. (1994). Placental corticotropin-releasing hormone and the hypercorticolism of pregnancy. *Am. J. Obstet. Gynecol.*, **171**, 1287–91.

Goland, R. S., Tropper, P. J., Warren, W. B. *et al.* (1995). Concentrations of corticotrophin-releasing hormone in the umbilical-cord blood of pregnancies complicated by pre-eclampsia. *Reprod. Fertil. Dev.*, **7**, 1227–30.

Graf, A. H., Hutter, W., Hacker, G. W. *et al.* (1996). Localization and distribution of vasoactive neuropeptides in the human placenta. *Placenta*, **17**, 413–21.

Grammatopoulos, D., Dai, Y., Chen, J. *et al.* (1998). Human corticotropin-releasing hormone receptor: differences in subtype expression between pregnant and nonpregnant myometria. *J. Clin. Endocrinol. Metab.*, **83**(1998), 2539–44.

Gray, P. C., Bilezikjian, L. M. and Vale, W. (2002). Antagonism of activin by inhibin and inhibin receptors: a functional role for betaglycan. *Mol. Cell. Endocrinol.*, **188**, 254–60.

Grino, M., Chrousos, G. P. and Margioris, A. N. (1987). The corticotropin releasing hormone gene is expressed in human placenta. *Biochem. Biophys. Res. Commun.*, **148**, 1208–14.

Grove, K. L. and Smith, M. S. (2003). Ontogeny of the hypothalamic neuropeptide Y system. *Physiol. Behav.*, **79**, 47–63.

Halhali, A., Wimalawansa, S. J., Berentsen, V. *et al.* (2001). Calcitonin gene- and parathyroid hormone-related peptides in preeclampsia: effects of magnesium sulfate. *Obstet. Gynecol.*, **97**, 893–7.

Hayette, S., Gadoux, M., Martel, S. *et al.* (1998). FLRG (follistatin-related gene), a new target of chromosomal rearrangement in malignant blood disorders. *Oncogene*, **16**, 2949–54.

Hermus, A. R., Pieters, G. F., Willemsen, J. J. *et al.* (1987). Hypotensive effects of ovine and human corticotrophin-releasing factors in man. *Eur. J. Clin. Pharmacol.*, **31**, 531–4.

Hillhouse, E. W. and Grammatopoulos, D. K. (2002). Role of stress peptides during human pregnancy and labour. *Reproduction*, **124**, 323–9.

Hirota, Y., Anai, T. and Miyakawa, I. (1997). Parathyroid hormone-related protein levels in maternal and cord blood. *Am. J. Obstet. Gynecol.*, **177**, 702–6.

Inoue, T., Kimura, T., Azuma, C. *et al.* (1994). Structural organization of the human oxytocin receptor gene. *J. Biol. Chem.*, **269**, 32451–6.

Iwashita, M., Kudo, Y., Shinozaki, Y. and Takeda, Y. (1993). Gonadotropin-releasing hormone increases serum human chorionic gonadotropin in pregnant women. *Endocr. J.*, **40**, 539–44.

Jain, V., Shi, S. Q., Vedernikov, Y. P. *et al.* (1998). In vivo effects of corticotropin-releasing factor in pregnant rats. *Am. J. Obstet. Gynecol.*, **178**, 186–91.

Jain, V., Vedernikov, Y. P., Saade, G. R., Chwalisz, K. and Garfield, R. E. (1999). Endothelium-dependent- and independent mechanisms of vasorelaxation by corticotropin-releasing factor in pregnant rat uterine artery. *J. Pharmacol. Exp. Ther.*, **288**, 407–13.

Jones, S. A. and Challis, J. R. (1990). Effects of corticotropin-releasing hormone and adrenocorticotropin on prostaglandin output by human placenta and fetal membranes. *Gynecol. Obstet. Invest.*, **29**, 165–8.

Jones, S. A., Brooks, A. N. and Challis, J. R. (1989). Steroids modulate corticotropin-releasing hormone production in human fetal membranes and placenta. *J. Clin. Endocrinol. Metab.*, **68**, 825–30.

Kang, S. K., Tai, C. J., Cheng, K. W. and Leung, P. C. (2000). Gonadotropin-releasing hormone activates mitogen-activated protein kinase in human ovarian and placental cells. *Mol. Cell. Endocrinol.*, **170**, 143–51.

Karteris, E., Grammatopoulos, D., Dai, Y. *et al.* (1998). The human placenta and fetal membranes express the corticotropin-releasing hormone receptor 1alpha (CRH-1alpha) and the CRH-C variant receptor. *J. Clin. Endocrinol. Metab.*, **83**, 1376–9.

Keelan, J., Song, Y. and France, J. T. (1994). Comparative regulation of inhibin, activin and human chorionic gonadotropin production by placental trophoblast cells in culture. *Placenta*, **15**, 803–18.

Keelan, J. A., Groome, N. P. and Mitchell, M. D. (1998). Regulation of activin-A production by human amnion, decidua and placenta in vitro by pro-inflammatory cytokines. *Placenta*, **19**, 429–34.

Kelly, A. C., Rodgers, A., Dong, K. W. *et al.* (1991). Gonadotropin-releasing hormone and chorionic gonadotropin gene expression in human placental development. *DNA Cell. Biol.*, **10**, 411–21.

Kenney, S. P., Kekuda, R., Prasad, P. D. *et al.* (1999). Cannabinoid receptors and their role in the regulation of the serotonin transporter in human placenta. *Am. J. Obstet. Gynecol.*, **181**, 491–7.

Khatun, S., Kanayama, N., Belayet, H. M. *et al.* (2000). Increased concentrations of plasma neuropeptide Y in patients with eclampsia and preeclampsia. *Am. J. Obstet. Gynecol.*, **182**, 896–900.

Khodr, G. S. and Siler-Khodr, T. M. (1978). Localization of luteinizing hormone-releasing factor in the human placenta. *Fertil. Steril.*, **29**, 523–30.

Khodr, G. S. and Siler-Khodr, T. M. (1980). Placental luteinizing hormone-releasing and its synthesis. *Science*, **207**, 315–17.

Kiang, J. G. and Wei, E. T. (1987). Corticotropin-releasing factor inhibits thermal injury. *J. Pharmacol. Exp. Ther.*, **243**, 517–20.

Kieffer, B. L. and Evans, C. J. (2002). Opioid tolerance-in search of the holy grail. *Cell*, **108**, 587–90.

Kimura, T., Tanizawa, O., Mori, K., Brownstein, M. J. and Okayama, H. (1992). Structure and expression of a human oxytocin receptor. *Nature*, **356**, 526–9.

Knerr, I., Dachert, C., Beinder, E. *et al.* (2002). Adrenomedullin, calcitonin gene-related peptide and their receptors: evidence for a decreased placental mRNA content in preeclampsia and HELLP syndrome. *Eur. J. Obstet. Gynecol. Reprod. Biol.*, **101**, 47–53.

Kofinas, G. D., Kofinas, A. D., Pyrgerou, M. and Reyes, F. I. (1987). Amniotic fluid beta-endorphin levels and labor. *Obstet. Gynecol.*, **69**, 945–7.

Korebrits, C., Ramirez, M. M., Watson, L. *et al.* (1998). Maternal corticotropin-releasing hormone is increased with impending preterm birth. *J. Clin. Endocrinol. Metab.*, **83**, 1585–91.

Kraayenbrink, A. A., Dekker, G. A., van Kamp, G. J. and van Geijn, H. P. (1993). Endothelial vasoactive mediators in preeclampsia. *Am. J. Obstet. Gynecol.*, **169**, 160–5.

Kuo, L., Davis, M. J. and Chilian, W. M. (1990). Endothelium-dependent, flow-induced dilation of isolated coronary arterioles. *Am. J. Physiol.*, **259**, H1063–70.

Laatikainen, T. J., Raisanen, I. J. and Salminen, K. R. (1988). Corticotropin-releasing hormone in amniotic fluid during gestation and labor and in relation to fetal lung maturation. *Am. J. Obstet. Gynecol.*, **159**, 891–5.

Laatikainen, T., Virtanen, T., Kaaja, R. and Salminen-Lappalainen, K. (1991). Corticotropin-releasing hormone in maternal and cord plasma in pre-eclampsia. *Eur. J. Obstet. Gynecol. Reprod. Biol.*, **39**, 19–24.

Lafond, J., St-Pierre, S., Masse, A., Savard, R. and Simoneau, L. (1997). Calcitonin gene-related peptide receptor in human placental syncytiotrophoblast brush-border and basal plasma membranes. *Placenta*, **18**, 181–8.

Lambert-Messerlian, G. M., Silver, H. M., Petraglia, F. *et al.* (2000). Second-trimester levels of maternal serum human chorionic gonadotropin and inhibin a as predictors of preeclampsia in the third trimester of pregnancy. *J. Soc. Gynecol. Invest.*, **7**, 170–4.

Lamharzi, N., Halmos, G., Armatis, P. and Schally, A. V. (1998). Expression of mRNA for luteinizing hormone-releasing hormone receptors and epidermal growth factor receptors in human cancer cell lines. *Int. J. Oncol.*, **12**, 671–5.

Le Goascogne, C., Eychenne, B., Tonon, M. C. *et al.* (2000). Neurosteroid progesterone is up-regulated in the brain of jimpy and shiverer mice. *Glia*, **29**, 14–24.

Leitch, I. M., Boura, A. L., Botti, C. *et al.* (1998). Vasodilator actions of urocortin and related peptides in the human perfused placenta in vitro. *J. Clin. Endocrinol. Metab.*, **83**, 4510–13.

Leung, P. C. and Peng, C. (1996). Gonadotropin-releasing hormone receptor: gene structure, expression and regulation. *Biol. Signals*, **5**, 63–9.

Lin, L. S., Roberts, V. J. and Yen, S. S. (1995). Expression of human gonadotropin-releasing hormone receptor gene in the placenta and its functional relationship to human chorionic gonadotropin secretion. *J. Clin. Endocrinol. Metab.*, **80**, 580–5.

Linton, E. A., Perkins, A. V., Woods, R. J. *et al.* (1993). Corticotropin releasing hormone-binding protein (CRH-BP): plasma levels decrease during the third trimester of normal human pregnancy. *J. Clin. Endocrinol. Metab.*, **76**, 260–2.

Liotta, A. S. and Krieger, D. T. (1980). In vitro biosynthesis and comparative posttranslational processing of immunoreactive precursor corticotropin/beta-endorphin by human placental and pituitary cells. *Endocrinology*, **106**, 1504–11.

Lofgren, M., Holst, J. and Backstrom, T. (1992). Effects in vitro of progesterone and two 5 alpha-reduced progestins, 5 alpha-pregnane-3,20-dione and 5 alpha-pregnane-3 alpha-ol-20-one, on contracting human myometrium at term. *Acta Obstet. Gynecol. Scand.*, **71**, 28–33.

Luisi, S., Battaglia, C., Florio, P. *et al.* (1998). Activin A and inhibin B in extra-embryonic coelomic and amniotic fluids, and maternal serum in early pregnancy. *Placenta*, **19**, 435–8.

Luisi, S., Petraglia, F., Benedetto, C. *et al.* (2000). Serum allopregnanolone levels in pregnant women: changes during pregnancy, at delivery, and in hypertensive patients. *J. Clin. Endocrinol. Metab.*, **85**, 2429–33.

Luisi, S., Florio, P., Reis, F. M. and Petraglia, F. (2001). Expression and secretion of activin A: possible physiological and clinical implications. *Eur. J. Endocrinol.*, **145**, 225–36.

Luisi, S., Florio, P., D'Antona, D. *et al.* (2003). Maternal serum inhibin A levels are a marker of a viable trophoblast in incomplete and complete miscarriage. *Eur. J. Endocrinol.*, **148**, 233–6.

Lundberg, J. M., Hemsen, A., Fried, G., Theodorsson-Norheim, E. and Lagercrantz, H. (1986). Co-release of neuropeptide Y (NPY)-like immunoreactivity and catecholamines in newborn infants. *Acta Physiol. Scand.*, **126**, 471–3.

Lurie, S., Fink, A. and Hagay, Z. J. (1997). Parathyroid hormone levels in preterm and term labor. *J. Perinat. Med.*, **25**, 292–4.

MacCannell, K. L., Hamilton, P. L., Lederis, K., Newton, C. A. and Rivier, J. (1984). Corticotropin releasing factor-like peptides produce selective dilatation of the dog mesenteric circulation. *Gastroenterology*, **87**, 94–102.

Macgill, K., Moseley, J. M., Martin, T. J. *et al.* (1997). Vascular effects of PTHrP (1–34) and PTH (1–34) in the human fetal-placental circulation. *Placenta*, **18**, 587–92.

Mandsager, N. T., Brewer, A. S. and Myatt, L. (1994). Vasodilator effects of parathyroid hormone, parathyroid hormone-related protein, and calcitonin gene-related peptide in the human fetal–placental circulation. *J. Soc. Gynecol. Invest.*, **1**, 19–24.

Manyonda, I. T., Slater, D. M., Fenske, C. *et al.* (1998). A role for noradrenaline in pre-eclampsia: towards a unifying hypothesis for the pathophysiology. *Br. J. Obstet. Gynaecol.*, **105**, 641–8.

Margioris, A. N., Grino, M., Protos, P., Gold, P. W. and Chrousos, G. P. (1988). Corticotropin-releasing hormone and oxytocin stimulate the release of placental proopiomelanocortin peptides. *J. Clin. Endocrinol. Metab.*, **66**, 922–6.

Marinoni, E., Korebrits, C., Di Iorio, R., Cosmi, E. V. and Challis, J. R. (1998). Effect of betamethasone in vivo on placental corticotropinreleasing hormone in human pregnancy. *Am. J. Obstet. Gynecol.*, **178**, 770–8.

Mauri, A., Serri, F., Caminiti, F. *et al.* (1990). Correlation between amniotic levels of alpha-MSH, ACTH and beta-endorphin in late gestation and labour in normal and complicated pregnancies. *Acta Endocrinol. (Copenhagen)*, **123**, 637–42.

McLean, M., Bisit, A., Davies, J. J. *et al.* (1995). A placental clock controlling the length of human pregnancy. *Nat. Med.*, **1**, 460–3.

Michel, M. C. and Rascher W. (1995). Neuropeptide Y: a possible role in hypertension? *J. Hypertens.*, **13**, 385–95.

Mitchell, B. F. and Schmid, B. (2001). Oxytocin and its receptor in the process of parturition. *J. Soc. Gynecol. Invest.*, **8**, 122–33.

Miyake, A., Sakumoto, T., Aono, T. *et al.* (1982). Changes in luteinizing hormone-releasing hormone in human placenta throughout pregnancy. *Obstet. Gynecol.*, **60**, 444–9.

Moftaquir-Handaj, A., Barbe, F., Barbarino-Monnier, P., Aunis, D. and Boutroy, M. J. (1995). Circulating chromogranin A and catecholamines in human fetuses at uneventful birth. *Pediatr. Res.*, **37**, 101–5.

Mohan, A., Asselin, J., Sargent, I. L., Groome, N. P. and Muttukrishna, S. (2001). Effect of cytokines and growth factors on the secretion of inhibin A, activin A and follistatin by term placental villous trophoblasts in culture. *Eur. J. Endocrinol.*, **145**, 505–11.

Moncada, S. and Vane, J. R. (1979). Arachidonic acid metabolites and the interactions between platelets and blood-vessel walls. *New Engl. J. Med.*, **300**, 1142–7.

Muttukrishna, S., Fowler, P. A., George, L., Groome, N. P. and Knight, P. G. (1996). Changes in peripheral serum levels of total activin A during the human menstrual cycle and pregnancy. *Clin. Endocrinol. Metab.*, **81**, 3328–34.

Muttukrishna, S., Child, T. J., Groome, N. P. and Ledger, W. L. (1997). Source of circulating levels of inhibin A, pro alpha C-containing inhibins and activin A in early pregnancy. *Hum. Reprod.*, **12**, 1089–93.

Muttukrishna, S., North, R. A., Morris, J. *et al.* (2000). Serum inhibin A and activin A are elevated prior to the onset of pre-eclampsia. *Hum. Reprod.*, **15**, 1640–5.

Naghashpour, M. and Dahl, G. (2000). Sensitivity of myometrium to CGRP varies during mouse estrous cycle and in response to progesterone. *Am. J. Physiol. Cell. Physiol.*, **278**, C561–9.

Newnham, J. P., Tomlin, S., Ratter, S. J., Bourne, G. L. and Rees, L. H. (1983). Endogenous opioid peptides in pregnancy. *Br. J. Obstet. Gynaecol.*, **90**, 535–8.

Nguyen, T. T., Tseng, Y. T., McGonnigal, B. *et al.* (1999). Placental biogenic amine transporters: in vivo function, regulation and pathobiological significance. *Placenta*, **20**, 3–11.

Nickols, G. A., Nickols, M. A. and Helwig, J. J. (1990). Binding of parathyroid hormone and parathyroid hormone-related protein to vascular smooth muscle of rabbit renal microvessels. *Endocrinology*, **126**, 721–7.

Odagiri, E., Sherrell, B. J., Mount, C. D., Nicholson, W. E. and Orth, D. N. (1979). Human placental immunoreactive corticotropin, lipotropin, and beta-endorphin: evidence for a common precursor. *Proc. Natl. Acad. Sci. USA*, **76**, 2027–31.

Padbury, J. F. and Martinez, A. M. (1988). Sympathoadrenal system activity at birth: integration of postnatal adaptation. *Semin. Perinatol.*, **12**, 163–72.

Panerai, A. E., Martini, A., Di Giulio, A. M. *et al.* (1983). Plasma beta-endorphin, beta-lipotropin, and met-enkephalin concentrations during pregnancy in normal and drug-addicted women and their newborn. *J. Clin. Endocrinol. Metab.*, **57**, 537–43.

Papantoniou, N. E., Papapetrou, P. D., Antsaklis, A. J. *et al.* (1996). Circulating levels of immunoreactive parathyroid hormone-related protein and intact parathyroid hormone in human fetuses and newborns. *Eur. J. Endocrinol.*, **134**, 437–42.

Parida, S. K., Schneider, D. B., Stoss, T. D., Pauly, T. H. and McGillis, J. P. (1998). Elevated circulating calcitonin gene-related peptide in umbilical cord and infant blood associated with maternal and neonatal sepsis and shock. *Pediatr. Res.*, **43**, 276–82.

Pasetto, N., Zicari, A., Piccione, E. *et al.* (1992). Influence of labor and oxytocin on in vitro leukotriene release by human fetal membranes and uterine decidua at term gestation. *Am. J. Obstet. Gynecol.*, **166**, 1500–6.

Pedrazzini, T., Pralong, F. and Grouzmann, E. (2003). Neuropeptide Y: the universal soldier. *Cell Mol. Life Sci.*, **60**, 350–77.

Perkins, A. V., Linton, E. A., Eben, F. *et al.* (1995) Corticotrophin-releasing hormone and corticotrophin-releasing hormone binding protein in normal and pre-eclamptic human pregnancies. *Br. J. Obstet. Gynaecol.*, **102**, 118–22.

Petraglia, F. (1991). Placental neurohormones: secretion and physiological implications. *Mol. Cell. Endocrinol.*, **78**, C109–12.

Petraglia, F. (1997). Inhibin, activin and follistatin in the human placenta – a new family of regulatory proteins. *Placenta*, **18**, 3–8.

Petraglia, F., Lim, A. T. and Vale, W. (1987a). Adenosine 3′,5′-monophosphate, prostaglandins, and epinephrine stimulate the secretion of immunoreactive gonadotropin-releasing hormone from cultured human placental cells. *J. Clin. Endocrinol. Metab.*, **65**, 1020–5.

Petraglia, F., Sawchenko, P., Lim, A. T., Rivier, J. and Vale, W. (1987b). Localization, secretion, and action of inhibin in human placenta. *Science*, **237**, 187–9.

Petraglia, F., Sawchenko, P. E., Rivier, J. and Vale, W. (1987c). Evidence for local stimulation of ACTH secretion by corticotropin-releasing factor in human placenta. *Nature*, **328**, 717–9.

Petraglia, F., Calzà, L., Giardino, L. *et al.* (1989a). Identification of immunoreactive neuropeptide-gamma in human placenta: localization, secretion, and binding sites. *Endocrinology*, **124**, 2016–22.

Petraglia, F., Coukos, G., Battaglia, C. *et al.* (1989b). Plasma and amniotic fluid immunoreactive neuropeptide-Y level changes during pregnancy, labor, and at parturition. *J. Clin. Endocrinol. Metab.*, **69**, 324–8.

Petraglia, F., Sutton, S. and Vale, W. (1989c). Neurotransmitters and peptides modulate the release of immunoreactive corticotropin-releasing factor from cultured human placental cells. *Am. J. Obstet. Gynecol.*, **160**, 247–51.

Petraglia, F., Vaughan, J. and Vale, W. (1989d). Inhibin and activin modulate the release of gonadotropin-releasing hormone, human chorionic gonadotropin, and progesterone from cultured human placental cells. *Proc. Natl. Acad. Sci. USA*, **86**, 5114–17.

Petraglia, F., Calza, L., Garuti, G. C. *et al.* (1990a). Presence and synthesis of inhibin subunits in human decidua. *J. Clin. Endocrinol. Metab.*, **71**, 487–92.

Petraglia, F., Calza, L., Garuti, G. C. *et al.* (1990b). New aspects of placental endocrinology. *J. Endocrinol. Invest.*, **13**, 353–71.

Petraglia, F., Giardino, L., Coukos, G. *et al.* (1990c). Corticotropin-releasing factor and parturition: plasma and amniotic fluid levels and placental binding sites. *Obstet. Gynecol.*, **75**, 784–90.

Petraglia, F., Vaughan, J. and Vale, W. (1990d). Steroid hormones modulate the release of immunoreactive gonadotropin-releasing hormone from cultured human placental cells. *J. Clin. Endocrinol. Metab.*, **70**, 1173–8.

Petraglia, F., Garuti, G. C., Calza, L. *et al.* (1991). Inhibin subunits in human placenta: localization and messenger ribonucleic acid levels during pregnancy. *Am. J. Obstet. Gynecol.*, **165**, 750–8.

Petraglia, F., Tabanelli, S., Galassi, M. C. *et al.* (1992a). Human decidua and in vitro decidualized endometrial stromal cells at term contain immunoreactive corticotropin-releasing factor (CRF) and CRF messenger ribonucleic acid. *J. Clin. Endocrinol. Metab.*, **74**, 1427–31.

Petraglia, F., Woodruff, T. K., Botticelli, G. *et al.* (1992b). Gonadotropin-releasing hormone, inhibin, and activin in human placenta: evidence for a common cellular localization. *J. Clin. Endocrinol. Metab.*, **74**, 1184–8.

Petraglia, F., Anceschi, M. M., Calza, L. *et al.* (1993a). Inhibin and activin in human fetal membranes: evidence for a local effect on prostaglandin release. *J. Clin. Endocrinol. Metab.*, **77**, 542–8.

Petraglia, F., Calzà, L., Giardino, L. *et al.* (1993b). Maternal decidua and fetal membranes contain immunoreactive neuropeptide Y. *J. Endocrinol. Invest.*, **16**, 201–5.

Petraglia, F., Potter, E., Cameron, V. A. *et al.* (1993c). Corticotropin-releasing factor-binding protein is produced by human placenta and intrauterine tissues. *J. Clin. Endocrinol. Metab.*, **77**, 919–24.

Petraglia, F., Gallinelli, A., De Vita, D. *et al.* (1994a). Activin at parturition: changes of maternal serum levels and evidence for binding sites in placenta and fetal membranes. *Obstet. Gynecol.*, **84**, 278–82.

Petraglia, F., Gallinelli, A., Grande, A. *et al.* (1994b). Local production and action of follistatin in human placenta. *J. Clin. Endocrinol. Metab.*, **78**, 205–10.

Petraglia, F., Genazzani, A. D., Aguzzoli, L. *et al.* (1994c). Pulsatile fluctuations of plasma-gonadotropin-releasing hormone and corticotropin-releasing factor levels in healthy pregnant women. *Acta Obstet. Gynecol. Scand.*, **73**, 284–9.

Petraglia, F., Aguzzoli, L., Gallinelli, A. *et al.* (1995a). Hypertension in pregnancy: changes in activin A maternal serum concentration. *Placenta*, **16**, 447–54.

Petraglia, F., Benedetto, C., Florio, P. *et al.* (1995b). Effect of corticotropin-releasing factor-binding protein on prostaglandin release from cultured maternal decidua and on contractile activity of human myometrium in vitro. *J. Clin. Endocrinol. Metab.*, **80**, 3073–6.

Petraglia, F., De Vita, D., Gallinelli, A., *et al.* (1995c). Abnormal concentration of maternal serum activin-A in gestational diseases. *J. Clin. Endocrinol. Metab.*, **80**, 558–61.

Petraglia, F., Florio, P., Benedetto, C. *et al.* (1996a). High levels of corticotropin-releasing factor (CRF) are inversely correlated with low levels of maternal CRF-binding protein in pregnant women with pregnancy-induced hypertension. *J. Clin. Endocrinol. Metab.*, **81**, 852–6.

Petraglia, F., Florio, P., Gallo, R. et al. (1996b). Corticotropin-releasing factor-binding protein: origins and possible functions. *Horm. Res.*, **45**, 187–91.

Petraglia, F., Florio, P., Gallo, R. et al. (1996c). Human placenta and fetal membranes express human urocortin mRNA and peptide. *J. Clin. Endocrinol. Metab.*, **81**, 3807–10.

Petraglia, F., Florio, P., Nappi, C. and Genazzani, A. R. (1996d). Peptide signaling in human placenta and membranes: autocrine, paracrine, and endocrine mechanisms. *Endocr. Rev.*, **17**, 156–86.

Petraglia, F., Florio, P., Simoncini, T. et al. (1997a). Cord plasma corticotropin-releasing factor-binding protein (CRF-BP) in term and preterm labour. *Placenta*, **18**, 115–19.

Petraglia, F., Luisi, S., Benedetto, C. et al. (1997b). Changes of dimeric inhibin B levels in maternal serum throughout healthy gestation and in women with gestational diseases. *J. Clin. Endocrinol. Metab.*, **82**, 2991–5.

Petraglia, F., Santuz, M., Florio, P. et al. (1998). Paracrine regulation of human placenta: control of hormonogenesis. *J. Reprod. Immunol.*, **39**, 221–33.

Petraglia, F., Florio, P., Benedetto, C. et al. (1999a). Urocortin stimulates placental adrenocorticotropin and prostaglandin release and myometrial contractility in vitro. *J. Clin. Endocrinol. Metab.*, **84**, 1420–3.

Petraglia, F., Gomez, R., Luisi, S. et al. (1999b). Increased midtrimester amniotic fluid activin A: a risk factor for subsequent fetal death. *Am. J. Obstet. Gynecol.*, **180**, 194–7.

Plotsky, P. M., Cunningham Jr., E. T. and Widmaier, E. P. (1989). Catecholaminergic modulation of corticotropin-releasing factor and adrenocorticotropin secretion. *Endocr. Rev.*, **10**, 437–58.

Plotsky, P. M., Thrivikraman, K. V. and Meaney, M. J. (1993). Central and feedback regulation of hypothalamic corticotropin-releasing factor secretion. *Ciba Found. Symp.*, **172**, 59–75.

Porthe, G., Valette, A. and Cros, J. (1981). Kappa opiate binding sites in human placenta. *Biochem. Biophys. Res. Commun.*, **101**, 1–6.

Porthe, G., Valette, A., Moisand, A., Tafani, M. and Cros, J. (1982). Localization of human placental opiate binding sites on the syncytial brush border membrane. *Life Sci.*, **31**, 2647–54.

Poston, L., McCarthy, A. L. and Ritter, J. M. (1995). Control of vascular resistance in the maternal and feto-placental arterial beds. *Pharmacol. Ther.*, **65**, 215–39.

Potter, E., Behan, D. P., Linton, E. A. et al. (1992). The central distribution of a corticotropin-releasing factor (CRF)-binding protein predicts multiple sites and modes of interaction with CRF. *Proc. Natl. Acad. Sci. USA*, **89**, 4192–6.

Poyner, D. R., Sexton, P. M., Marshall, I. et al. (2002). International Union of Pharmacology. XXXII. The mammalian calcitonin gene-related peptides, adrenomedullin, amylin, and calcitonin receptors. *Pharmacol. Rev.*, **54**, 233–46.

Rabinovici, J., Goldsmith, P. C., Librach, C. L. and Jaffe, R. B. (1992). Localization and regulation of the activin-A dimer in human placental cells. *J. Clin. Endocrinol. Metab.*, **75**, 571–6.

Ramirez, M. M., Fraher, L. J., Goltzman D. et al. (1995). Immunoreactive parathyroid hormone-related protein: its association with preterm labor. *Eur. J. Obstet. Gynecol. Reprod. Biol.*, **63**, 21–6.

Reis, F. M. and Petraglia, F. (2001). The placenta as a neuroendocrine organ. *Front. Horm. Res.* **27**, 216–28.

Reis, F. M., Fadalti, M., Florio, P. and Petraglia, F. (1999). Putative role of placental corticotropin-releasing factor in the mechanisms of human parturition. *J. Soc. Gynecol. Invest.*, **6**, 109–19.

Reis, F. M., Florio, P., Cobellis, L. *et al.* (2001). Human placenta as a source of neuroendocrine factors. *Biol. Neonate.*, **79**, 150–6.

Reis, F. M., D'Antona, D. and Petraglia, F. (2002). Predictive value of hormone measurements in maternal and fetal complications of pregnancy. *Endocr. Rev.*, **23**, 230–57.

Riley, S. C. and Challis, J. R. (1991). Corticotropin-releasing hormone production by the placenta and fetal membranes. *Placenta*, **12**, 105–19.

Riley, S. C., Wathen, N. C., Chard, T., Groome, N. P. and Wallace, E. M. (1996). Inhibin in extra-embryonic coelomic and amniotic fluids and maternal serum in early pregnancy. *Hum. Reprod.*, **11**, 2772–6.

Roberts, J. M. and Cooper, D. W. (2001). Pathogenesis and genetics of pre-eclampsia. *Lancet*, **357**, 53–6.

Robidoux, J., Simoneau, L., St-Pierre, S. *et al.* (1998). Human syncytiotrophoblast NPY receptors are located on BBM and activate PLC-to-PKC axis. *Am. J. Physiol.*, **274**, E502–9.

Robinson, B. G., Emanuel, R. L., Frim, D. M. and Majzoub, J. A. (1988). Glucocorticoid stimulates expression of corticotropin-releasing hormone gene in human placenta. *Proc. Natl. Acad. Sci. USA*, **85**, 5244–8.

Rodda, C. P., Kubota, M., Heath, J. A. *et al.* (1988). Evidence for a novel parathyroid hormone-related protein in fetal lamb parathyroid glands and sheep placenta: comparisons with a similar protein implicated in humoral hypercalcaemia of malignancy. *J. Endocrinol.*, **117**, 261–71.

Rothenberg, S. J., Chicz-DeMet, A., Schnaas, L. *et al.* (1996). Umbilical cord beta-endorphin and early childhood motor development. *Early Hum. Dev.*, **46**, 83–95.

Russell, J. A., Leng, G. and Douglas, A. J. (2003). The magnocellular oxytocin system, the fount of maternity: adaptations in pregnancy. *Front. Neuroendocrinol.*, **24**, 27–61.

Saijonmaa, X., Laatikainen, T. and Walhstrom, T. (1988). Corticotropin releasing factor in human placenta: localization, concentration and release in vitro. *Placenta*, **9**, 373–85.

Samuelson, U. E., Dalsgaard, C. J., Lundberg, J. M. and Hokfelt, T. (1985). Calcitonin gene-related peptide inhibits spontaneous contractions in human uterus and fallopian tube. *Neurosci. Lett.*, **62**, 225–30.

Sasaki, A., Tempst, P., Lotta, A. S. *et al.* (1988). Isolation and characterization of a corticotropin-releasing hormone-like peptide from human placenta. *J. Clin. Endocrinol. Metab.*, **67**, 768–73.

Sasaki, A., Shinkawa, O. and Yoshinaga, K. (1989). Placental corticotropin-releasing hormone may be a stimulator of maternal pituitary adrenocorticotropic hormone secretion in humans. *J. Clin. Invest.*, **84**, 1997–01.

Sastry, B. V., Barnwell, S. L., Tayeb, O. S., Janson, V. E. and Owens, L. K. (1980). Occurrence of methionine enkephalin in human placental villus. *Biochem. Pharmacol.*, **29**, 475–8.

Schiff, E., Friedman, S. A., Sibai, B. M., Kao, L. and Schifter, S. (1995). Plasma and placental calcitonin gene-related peptide in pregnancies complicated by severe preeclampsia. *Am. J. Obstet. Gynecol.*, **173**, 1405–9.

Schneider-Kolsky, M. E., Manuelpillai, U., Waldron, K., Dole, A. and Wallace, E. M. (2002). The distribution of activin and activin receptors in gestational tissues across human pregnancy and during labour. *Placenta*, **23**, 294–302.

Schulte, H. M. and Healy, D. L. (1987). Corticotropin releasing hormone- and adreno-corticotropin-like immunoreactivity in human placenta, peripheral and uterine vein plasma. *Horm. Metab. Res.*, **16**, 44–6.

Schulte, H. M., Weisner, D. and Allolio, B. (1990). The corticotropin releasing hormone test in late pregnancy: lack of adrenocorticotrophin and cortisol response. *Clin. Endocrinol.*, **33**, 99–106.

Seppala, M., Wahlstrom, T., Lehtovirta, P., Lee, J. N. and Leppalouto, J. (1980). Immuno-histochemical demonstration of luteinizing hormone-releasing factor-like material in human syncytiotrophoblast and trophoblastic tumours. *Clin. Endocrinol. (Oxford)*, **12**, 441–51.

Shew, R. L., Yee, J. A. and Pang, P. K. (1984). Direct effect of parathyroid hormone on rat uterine contraction. *J. Pharmacol. Exp. Ther.*, **230**, 1–6.

Shew, R. L., Papka, R. E., McNeill, D. L. and Yee, J. A. (1993). NADPH-diaphorase-positive nerves and the role of nitric oxide in CGRP relaxation of uterine contraction. *Peptides*, **14**, 637–41.

Shibasaki, T., Odagiri, E., Shizume, K. and Ling, N. (1982). Corticotropin releasing factor-like activity in human placental extracts. *J. Clin. Endocrinol. Metab.*, **55**, 384–6.

Siler-Khodr, T. M. and Khodr, G. S. (1978). Content of luteinizing hormone-releasing factor in the human placenta. *Am. J. Obstet. Gynecol.*, **130**, 216–19.

Siler-Khodr, T. M., Khodr, G. S. and Valenzuela, G. (1984). Immunoreactive gonadotropin-releasing hormone level in maternal circulation throughout pregnancy. *Am. J. Obstet. Gynecol.*, **150**, 376–9.

Silver, H. M., Lambert-Messerlian, G. M., Reis, F. M. *et al.* (2002). Mechanism of increased maternal serum total activin a and inhibin a in preeclampsia. *J. Soc. Gynecol. Invest.*, **9**, 308–12.

Simoncini, T., Apa, R., Reis, F. M. *et al.* (1999). Human umbilical vein endothelial cells: a new source and potential target for corticotropin-releasing factor. *J. Clin. Endocrinol. Metab.*, **84**, 2802–6.

Smith, R., Mesiano, S., Chan, E. C., Brown, S. and Jaffe, R. B. (1998). Corticotropin-releasing hormone directly and preferentially stimulates dehydroepiandrosterone sulfate secretion by human fetal adrenal cortical cells. *J. Clin. Endocrinol. Metab.*, **83**, 2916–20.

Stjernquist, M. and Owman, C. (1987). Interaction of noradrenaline, NPY and VIP with the neurogenic cholinergic response of the rat uterine cervix in vitro. *Acta Physiol. Scand.*, **131**, 553–62.

Stojilkovic, S. S., Reinhart, J. and Catt, K. J. (1994). Gonadotropin-releasing hormone receptors: structure and signal transduction pathways. *Endocr. Rev.*, **15**, 462–99.

Strewler, G. J. (2000). The parathyroid hormone-related protein. *Endocrinol. Metab. Clin. North Am.*, **29**, 629–45.

Strid, H., Bucht, E., Jansson, T., Wennergren, M. and Powell, T. L. (2003). ATP dependent ca(2+) transport across basal membrane of human syncytiotrophoblast in pregnancies complicated by intrauterine growth restriction or diabetes. *Placenta*, **24**, 445–52.

Sue-Tang, A., Bocking, A. D., Brooks, A. N. *et al.* (1992). Effects of restricting uteroplacental blood flow on concentrations of corticotrophin-releasing hormone, adrenocorticotrophin, cortisol, and prostaglandin E2 in the sheep fetus during late pregnancy. *Can. J. Physiol. Pharmacol.*, **70**, 1396–402.

Syversen, U., Waldum, H. L., O'Connor, D. T. (1992). Rapid, high-yield isolation of human chromogranin A from chromaffin granules of pheochromocytomas. *Neuropeptides*, **22**, 235–40.

Takemura, M., Kimura, T., Nomura, S. *et al.* (1994). Expression and localization of human oxytocin receptor mRNA and its protein in chorion and decidua during parturition. *J. Clin. Invest.*, **93**, 2319–23.

Tan, L. and Rousseau, P. (1982). The chemical identity of the immunoreactive LHRH-like peptide biosynthesized in the human placenta. *Biochem. Biophys. Res. Commun.*, **109**, 1061–71.

Taupenot, L., Harper, K. L. and O'Connor, D. T. (2003). The chromogranin-secretogranin family. *New Engl. J. Med.*, **348**, 1134–49.

Tenmoku, S., Ottesen, B., O'Hare, M. M. *et al.* (1988). Interaction of NPY and VIP in regulation of myometrial blood flow and mechanical activity. *Peptides*, **9**, 269–75.

Ticconi, C., Mauri, A., Zicari, A. *et al.* (1998). Interrelationships between oxytocin and eicosanoids in human fetal membranes at term gestation: which role for leukotriene B4? *Gynecol. Endocrinol.*, **12**, 129–34.

Torpy, D. J., Webster, E. L., Zachman, E. K., Aguilera, G. and Chrousos, G. P. (1999). Urocortin and inflammation: confounding effects of hypotension on measures of inflammation. *Neuroimmunomodulation*, **6**, 182–6.

Tropper, P. J., Goland, R. S., Wardlaw, S. L., Fox, H. E. and Frantz, A. G. (1987). Effects of betamethasone on maternal plasma corticotropin releasing factor, ACTH and cortisol during pregnancy. *J. Perinat. Med.*, **15**, 221–5.

Tsatsaris, V., Tarrade, A., Merviel, P. *et al.* (2002). Calcitonin gene-related peptide (CGRP) and CGRP receptor expression at the human implantation site. *J. Clin. Endocrinol. Metab.*, **87**, 4383–90.

Tsuchida, K., Matsuzaki, T., Yamakawa, N., Liu, Z. and Sugino, H. (2001). Intracellular and extracellular control of activin function by novel regulatory molecules. *Mol. Cell. Endocrinol.*, **180**, 25–31.

Tsujimoto, M., Mizutani, S., Adachi, H. *et al.* (1992). Identification of human placental leucine aminopeptidase as oxytocinase. *Arch. Biochem. Biophys.*, **292**, 388–92.

Uvnas-Moberg, K. and Eriksson, M. (1996). Breastfeeding: physiological, endocrine and behavioural adaptations caused by oxytocin and local neurogenic activity in the nipple and mammary gland. *Acta Paediatr.*, **85**, 525–30.

Vaillancourt, C., Petit, A. and Belisle, S. (1998). Expression of human placental D2-dopamine receptor during normal and abnormal pregnancies. *Placenta*, **19**, 73–80.

Valdenaire, O., Giller, T., Breu, V., Gottiwik, J. and Kilpatric, G. (1997). A new functional isoform of the human CRF2 receptor for corticotropin-releasing factor. *Biochim. Biophys. Acta*, **135**, 129–32.

Valdermarsson, S., Edvinsson, L., Hedner, P. and Ekman, R. (1990). Hormonal influence on CGRP in man: effects of sex differences and contraceptive pills. *Scand. J. Clin. Lab. Invest.*, **18**, 385–8.

Vale, W., Rivier, C., Hsueh, A. *et al.* (1988). Chemical and biological characterization of the inhibin family of protein hormones. *Recent Prog. Horm. Res.*, **44**, 1–34.

Vale, W., Rivier, C., Brown, M. R. *et al.* (1993). Chemical and biological characterization of corticotropin releasing factor. *Recent Prog. Horm. Res.*, **39**, 245–70.

Valette, A., Desprat, R., Cros, J. *et al.* (1986). Immunoreactive dynorphine in maternal blood, umbilical vein and amniotic fluid. *Neuropeptides*, **7**, 145–51.

Vaughan, J., Donaldson, C., Bittencourt, J. *et al.* (1995). Urocortin, a mammalian neuropeptide related to fish urotensin I and to corticotropin-releasing factor. *Nature*, **378**, 287–92.

Waddell, B. J. and Burton, P. J. (1993). Release of bioactive ACTH by perifused human placenta at early and late gestation. *J. Endocrinol.*, **136**, 345–53.

Wallace, E. M., Riley, S. C., Crossley, J. A. *et al.* (1997). Dimeric inhibins in amniotic fluid, maternal serum, and fetal serum in human pregnancy. *J. Clin. Endocrinol. Metab.*, **82**, 218–22.

Wang, L., Zhang, W. and Zhao, Y. (1999). The study of maternal and fetal plasma catecholamines levels during pregnancy and delivery. *J. Perinat. Med.*, **27**, 195–8.

Warren, W. B. and Silverman, A. J. (1995). Cellular localization of corticotrophin releasing hormone in the human placenta, fetal membranes and decidua. *Placenta*, **16**, 147–56.

Wharton, J., Gordon, L., Byrne, J. *et al.* (1993). Expression of the human neuropeptide tyrosine Y1 receptor. *Proc. Natl. Acad. Sci. USA*, **90**, 687–91.

Williams, E. D., Leaver, D. D., Danks, J. A., Moseley, J. M. and Martin, T. J. (1994). Effect of parathyroid hormone-related protein (PTHrP) on the contractility of the myometrum and localization of PTHrP in the uterus of pregnant rats. *J. Reprod. Fertil.*, **102**, 209–14.

Winquist, R. J., Baskin, E. P. and Vlasuk, G. P. (1987). Synthetic tumor-derived human hypercalcemic factor exhibits parathyroid hormone-like vasorelaxation in renal arteries. *Biochem. Biophys. Res. Commun.*, **149**, 227–32.

Wolfahrt, S., Kleine, B. and Rossmanith, W. G. (1998). Detection of gonadotrophin releasing hormone and its receptor mRNA in human placental trophoblasts using in-situ reverse transcription-polymerase chain reaction. *Mol. Hum. Reprod.*, **4**, 999–1006.

Yallampalli, C., Dong, Y. L. and Wimalawansa, S. J. (1996). Calcitonin gene-related peptide reverses the hypertension and significantly decreases the fetal mortality in pre-eclampsia rats induced by N(G)-nitro-L-arginine methyl ester. *Hum. Reprod.*, **11**, 895–9.

Yallampalli, C., Chauhan, M., Thota, C. S., Kondapaka, S. and Wimalawansa, S. J. (2002). Calcitonin gene-related peptide in pregnancy and its emerging receptor heterogeneity. *Trend. Endocrinol. Metab.*, **13**, 263–9.

Yin, H., Cheng, K. W., Hwa, H. L. *et al.* (1998). Expression of the messenger RNA for gonadotropin-releasing hormone and its receptor in human cancer cell lines. *Life Sci.*, **62**, 2015–23.

Zanardo, V., Nicolussi, S., Carlo, G. *et al.* (2001). Beta endorphin concentrations in human milk. *J. Pediatr. Gastroenterol. Nutr.*, **33**, 160–4.

Zicari, A., Ticconi, C., Realacci, M. *et al.* (2002). Hormonal regulation of cytokine release by human fetal membranes at term gestation: effects of oxytocin, hydrocortisone and progesterone on tumour necrosis factor-alpha and transforming growth factor-beta 1 output. *J. Reprod. Immunol.*, **56**, 123–36.

2

The regulation of human parturition

Roger Smith, Sam Mesiano, Richard Nicholson, Vicki Clifton,
Tamas Zakar, Eng-Cheng Chan, Andrew Bisits and Warwick Giles

Mothers and Babies Research Centre, John Hunter Hospital, Newcastle, Australia

Preterm birth accounts for 70% of neonatal mortality and is a common cause for intellectual handicap among survivors. Approximately 50% of cases of cerebral palsy are associated with preterm birth, in turn preterm birth increases the risk of cerebral palsy by 40 times! (Goldenberg, 2002). Preterm labor thus afflicts individuals at the very beginning of their lives, depriving them of opportunities and increasing health and educational costs for families and society in general. Unfortunately the rates of preterm birth have not changed for over 30 years due to an inability to predict the event and lack of effective therapies.

This clinical problem has driven research into the mechanisms that regulate the timing of human birth and the disorders which cause preterm birth.

For reasons of ethics most research in the past has focused on animal work, especially in the sheep. Unfortunately studies have revealed substantial differences between parturition in humans and that in other animals. Thus animal studies provide us with clues as to how systems operate to regulate delivery in mammals but frustrate us with uncertainty as to whether particular mechanisms operate in the human. Experimental in vivo studies provide the strongest evidence for cause and effect, yet the closer we come to the human state in our near relatives the apes, the larger the ethical constraints on experimental studies become. This biological equivalent of Heisenberg's Uncertainty Principle difficulty continues to restrict opportunities for interventional, experimental studies of relevance to human parturition. Recent observational studies have started to clarify the mechanisms regulating the process and timing of human birth. Complemented by in vitro experimental studies using human tissue which can examine cause and effect relationships progress is occurring. Only when we have a good understanding of the normal physiology which determines the timing of human birth, can we hope to understand the disturbances that occur in pathology leading to preterm birth. With such an understanding we may be in a position to rationally identify predictors of preterm delivery, methods of preventing preterm delivery and, when these fail, methods of successfully intervening to generate a healthy newborn able to fully participate in our society. This chapter outlines the progress made over the last decade.

Clues from parturition in mammals

In the overwhelming majority of mammals parturition is associated with a fall in circulating progesterone concentrations and often a rise in circulating estrogens (see Figure 2.1). This is seen as a type of switch from the pro-pregnancy environment created by high concentrations of progesterone to the parturition inducing phenotype created by estrogen. Different mammals use different mechanisms to create the withdrawal of progesterone. In goats luteolysis initiated by endometrial-derived prostaglandin PGF2α plays a key role. In mice PGF2α also plays a key role in luteolysis and COX1 induction in the myometrium is present at labor; neither occurs in humans (Bethin et al., 2003). In sheep pioneering work by Mont Liggins indicated a fetal mechanism involving the fetal hypothalamic–pituitary–adrenal (HPA) axis (Liggins, 1973a, b; 1994). This model has contributed much to our understanding.

In the sheep, progesterone levels are high for the majority of pregnancy (Figure 2.1). The sheep placenta converts cholesterol to progesterone but is unable to produce estrogen because it lacks the 17α-hydroxylase, 17,20 lyase enzyme required for this conversion. Late in pregnancy, possibly stimulated by placentally derived

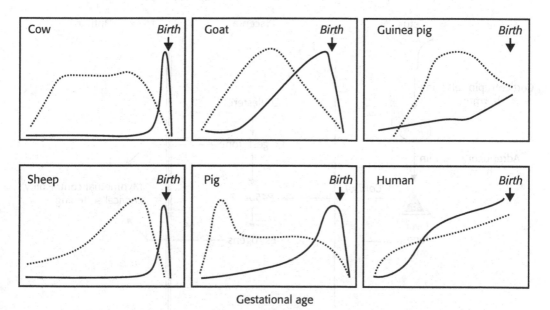

Gestational age

Figure 2.1   Variations in the pattern of estrogen and progesterone during pregnancy in different mammals; solid lines represent estrogen and dashed lines represent progesterone

prostaglandin E2 (Young *et al.*, 1996), the fetal hypothalamus releases increased amounts of the neuropeptide corticotropin-releasing hormone (CRH). The CRH stimulates fetal pituitary adrenocorticotropic hormone (ACTH) secretion which in turn drives fetal adrenal synthesis of cortisol. Rising concentrations of fetal cortisol induce placental expression of 17α-hydroxylase leading to conversion of progesterone into estrogen (see Figure 2.2). Maternal progesterone levels consequently fall while estrogen rises. Rising levels of estrogen initiate transcription of many contraction-associated genes in the myometrium, such as that coding for the oxytocin receptor. These changes lead to the onset of labor in the sheep. Damage to the sheep fetal hypothalamus, pituitary, or adrenal leads to a failure of parturition and the continuation of the pregnancy even to the extent of maternal death related to continued fetal growth and abdominal compression. Importantly, these events do not occur in human pregnancy. Clinical conditions occur where the fetal hypothalamus, pituitary, or adrenal fail to develop; yet labor occurs close to the normal time. Pregnant women do not remain pregnant indefinitely, regardless of the presence of pathology, while preterm delivery is common. The process in sheep cannot be extrapolated to the human. Why is this so?

Conflict as a source of evolutionary drive

The astonishing variety of processes observed in mammalian pregnancy has stimulated debate on the evolutionary pressures which have produced this situation.

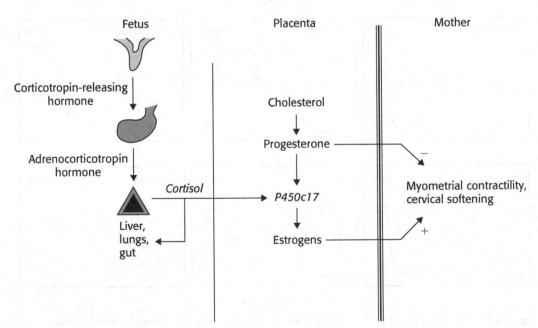

Figure 2.2   Mechanism of progesterone withdrawal at term in the sheep

David Haig from Harvard has cogently argued the Paternal–Maternal Conflict hypothesis to explain the rapid evolutionary divergence which has occurred in reproductive processes (Haig, 1993). Under this hypothesis paternal investment in any given pregnancy is restricted to that individual fetus to which he has contributed genetic material, any other pregnancy carried by that mother may not be his progeny. From the maternal point of view all of her offspring current and future are of equal value. The paternal genome acting through the fetus and placenta therefore has an interest in maximizing the maternal resources contributed to that particular fetus even at the expense of other potential offspring of that mother. The mother has a strong interest in the fetus but may wish to modify its demands to preserve resources for future offspring. This setting of paternal–maternal conflict produces rapid evolutionary change, as each participant seeks to push the seesaw in a different direction. For every metabolically advantageous mutation developed by the paternal genome, the mother will seek a modifying or restricting, contrary change. For these reasons extrapolation from experiments conducted in reproductive processes in one mammal to another are particularly hazardous.

The endocrinology of parturition in primates

If the sheep is not a particularly good model for the human, surely primates are better. It is clear that pregnancy among the different primates is more similar than between primates and other mammalian classes, nevertheless intriguing differences exist. The neuropeptide CRH is made in the placentas of all primates studied except the lemurs and not at all in non-primates (Robinson et al., 1989; Bowman et al., 2001). However the pattern of production of this peptide and its concentrations in maternal plasma vary considerably across the primates. Thus, while an exponential rise is seen across gestation in apes, baboons show a peak in mid-pregnancy and similar changes are seen in production of estradiol (Goland et al., 1992; Smith et al. 1993; 1999). Additionally while the human possesses a circulating binding protein for CRH many primates do not (Bowman et al., 2001). Apes provide a good model of human parturition based on present data, unfortunately experimental studies in apes are, if anything, harder to perform than those in humans due to ethical issues, availability of animals, expense and dangers related to human pathogens present in apes. Animal studies will continue to provide important clues for studies of human reproductive physiology but direct extrapolation is evidently not appropriate. Experimental studies in humans are not ethically possible, on some occasions nature's experiments, in the form of naturally occurring mutations, provide valuable insights into physiology but, in general, recent human research has progressed through observational studies.

CRH and the timing of birth in humans

Recent studies on the regulation of the timing of human birth have addressed two related but different questions: how is the duration of gestation determined and how are the events of labor precipitated? The questions have different clinical corollaries: how can we predict premature birth and how can we prevent preterm delivery? Effective methods to identify women at high-risk of preterm delivery are required in order to establish satisfactory trials of methods to prevent preterm delivery if women at low-risk of preterm delivery are to be saved from needless exposure to experimental pharmaceuticals.

While many biochemical markers have been examined for their ability to predict preterm delivery the most extensive studies have been conducted on CRH. CRH is synthesized in the placenta and released preferentially into the maternal compartment. Production and maternal plasma concentrations increase exponentially through gestation peaking at the time of delivery (Figure 2.3). Early studies determined that women in preterm labor had elevated maternal plasma concentrations compared to gestational-age matched control women (Goland *et al.*, 1986; Wolfe *et al.*, 1988). Subsequently, prospective longitudinal studies (McLean *et al.*, 1995; Prickett *et al.*, 2000) revealed that women destined to deliver preterm had more rapid exponential rises while women who would deliver late had slower rates of rise. A type of timing mechanism appears to exist in the human placenta which determined the length of gestation. Several important concepts arose from this work. Firstly, it

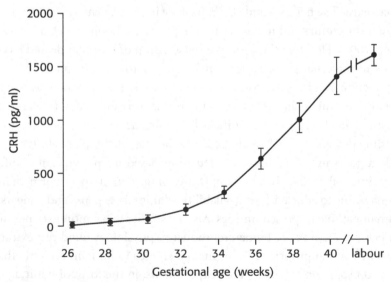

Figure 2.3   CRH increases exponentially in pregnant women's plasma. Adapted from Campbell *et al.* (1987)

established that, for at least a proportion of women, it is possible to predict the timing of delivery months in advance. This reveals the possibility of developing useful diagnostic tests to predict women at high-risk of preterm delivery and facilitate the establishment of therapeutic trials of treatment to prevent preterm birth. Secondly, the work established that events early in pregnancy had an influence on the later timing of birth. Understanding the regulation of placental CRH expression may therefore provide insights into the determination of gestational length. Recent work in animals has suggested that the nutritional state of the mother at conception can influence the length of gestation (Young et al., 1996; Bloomfield et al., 2003). This is the type of clue such comparative studies can provide; we should not expect the situation in humans to be identical but parallels may exist.

Regulation of placental CRH production

Regulation of CRH production has been explored in human placental tissue (Petraglia et al., 1989). CRH is produced by syncytial cells which can be created in vitro by fusion of purified cytotrophoblast cells. Using cultured placental cells and radioimmuno assays, Robinson et al. (1988) demonstrated a consistent effect of glucocorticoids in stimulation of CRH secretion. Interestingly Mazoub et al. have demonstrated that the exponential increase observed in human pregnancy can be well reproduced using a model which incorporates positive feed-forward between CRH and glucocorticoids (Emanuel et al., 1994). This finding was surprising as glucocorticoids inhibit CRH secretion within the hypothalamus. Using transfections of CRH promoter constructs the stimulatory mechanism has been partially elucidated (Figure 2.4). In placental tissue glucocorticoids stimulate CRH gene expression by interacting with proteins which bind to the cyclic adenosine monophosphate (cAMP) response site (cAMP regulatory element, CRE) of the CRH promoter (Cheng et al., 2000). Evidence indicates that the difference in behavior of the CRH gene in the placenta and hypothalamus is due to the expression of different transcription factors, co-activators and co-repressors in these two tissues (King et al., 2002). In the placenta the transcription factor Jun is found binding to the CRE while in the pituitary cell line AtT10 (in which glucocorticoids stimulate CRH expression) Fos is more prominent in its binding. Estrogens have been shown to inhibit CRH secretion and nitric oxide inhibits CRH secretion but not synthesis (Ni et al., 1997; 2002). cAMP analogues are very potent stimulators of CRH production but it is not clear what external signals may be driving cAMP stimulated CRH production. Presently it appears that conditions at the beginning of pregnancy determine the trajectory of CRH production by the placenta (McGrath et al., 2002). Once established this trajectory of exponential increase is maintained by a positive feed-forward system involving glucocorticoids possibly damped by estrogens. The production of

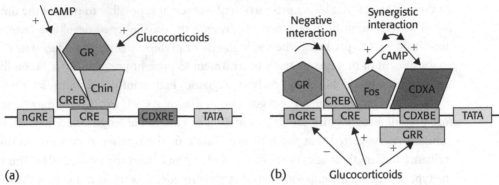

Figure 2.4   Schematic models of CRH gene regulation. Regulatory interactions on the CRH gene promoter are shown for the placenta (a: placental model) and the hypothalamus (b: hypothalamic model). The nGRE is a negative glucocorticoid regulatory element, CRE is the cAMP regulatory element, CDXRE is caudal type homeobox response element, GRR represents the region located between −213 and −99 bps that is stimulated by glucocorticoids in the hypothalamic model, and TATA is the TATA box binding site for basal transcriptional proteins. Stimulatory (+) and inhibitory (−) regulatory effects by cAMP and glucocorticoids through the different elements are shown. The regulatory proteins identified, so far, are represented by different shapes containing their names

estrogens may be regulated by CRH stimulation of dehydroepiandrosterone sulfate (DHEA-S) synthesis by cells of the fetal zone of the adrenal which exhibits CRH receptors (Smith *et al.*, 1998).

Some evidence suggests that the trajectory of CRH production may be increased by an adverse fetal intrauterine environment. Elevated maternal CRH has been observed in pregnancies complicated by pre-eclampsia, reduced umbilical artery flow as reflected in Doppler flow studies and where fetal distress has lead to elective preterm delivery (Giles *et al.*, 1996). Whether these increases are due to increased fetal or maternal cortisol production is unclear. Such increases in maternal CRH may have a protective effect since CRH is a powerful vasodilator in both the maternal and placental vascular trees (Clifton *et al.*, 1995). CRH appears to regulate endothelial function by stimulating mast cell degranulation and increasing release of nitric oxide. The length of gestation may therefore be determined by factors that set the initial rate of production of CRH or by factors later in pregnancy which alter the trajectory of CRH. Not all cases of preterm delivery are associated with elevated concentrations of CRH. It seems likely that the pathway to delivery can be activated independently of CRH. Infection does not appear to be associated with increased CRH production. For these reasons maternal plasma CRH has a relatively high specificity but lower sensitivity (Inder *et al.*, 2001; Ellis *et al.*, 2002). That is if CRH is high it is likely to be associated with preterm delivery but a low CRH does not preclude preterm birth.

Mechanisms proposed to link CRH to the process of parturition

While the association of maternal plasma CRH with preterm birth is robust in published studies it is unclear how CRH may be directly linked to the onset of labor. CRH receptors have been identified on the myometrium, however these are predominantly associated with Gα-s proteins which activate adenylyl cyclase and lead to increased cAMP and pathways which promote relaxation rather than contraction (Grammatopoulos et al., 1998). Work on CRH receptors has suggested that different receptor isoforms may be expressed at the end of pregnancy which are less efficient at stimulating cAMP formation and may therefore move the balance within the myometrial cell towards contraction. Alternatively placental CRH released into the fetal circulation may act on the fetal pituitary to stimulate ACTH production, thereby increasing cortisol synthesis and driving parturition in a manner analogous to that seen in the sheep (possibly by increasing prostaglandin production in the fetal membranes) (Patel et al. 2003). Finally CRH may act on the fetal adrenal, and perhaps the maternal adrenal, to drive DHEA-S production. DHEA-S is an obligate precursor for placental estradiol formation. This mechanism may drive a progressively increasing concentration of estrogen which activates contraction associated genes. However it is also possible that rising concentrations of CRH merely represent a marker of progressive fetoplacental maturation which is itself, through other pathways, associated with the onset of labor. Evidence for the final pathways of human myometrial activation is gradually accumulating through a number of different experimental approaches.

Activation of the human myometrium

In recent years several groups have begun to examine myometrial tissues obtained at caesarian section either prior to, or after, the onset of labor. Using these tissues, and comparing protein and gene expression in the presence and absence of labor, progress in understanding the mechanisms of human labor has occurred. An early report identified a reduction in the expression of the Gas subunit required for pathways leading to myometrial relaxation (Europe-Finner et al., 1993). This suggested a change in the balance of contractile versus relaxatory forces with the onset of labor. A key difficulty in understanding human labor is to determine how labor could occur despite the continued presence of high concentrations of circulating progesterone at the end of pregnancy which would be expected to suppress labor (Figure 2.5). In most mammals labor is associated with a profound fall in circulating progesterone concentrations but this does not occur in humans or other great apes. This conundrum has recently been addressed by Mesiano et al., in Australia and Phil Bennett's group in London, England (Pieber et al., 2001; Mesiano et al.,

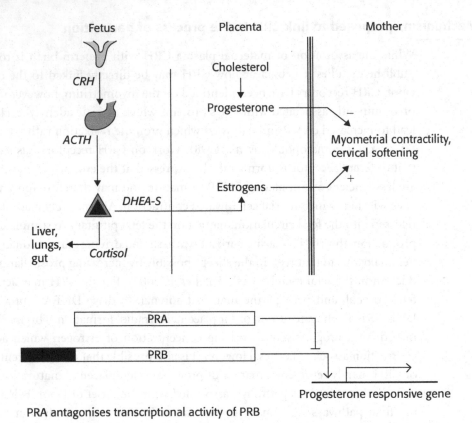

Figure 2.5   Mechanisms leading to production of estrogens and progesterone throughout human pregnancy

2002). There are two isoforms of the progesterone receptor that are splice variants of the single progesterone receptor gene. Progesterone receptor B (PRB) is the usual longer variant which mediates most actions of progesterone, while progesterone receptor A (PRA) is a shortened variant which lacks a key activating domain and acts as a dominant negative or repressor of the PRB activity. Mesiano showed that labor is associated with an increase in myometrial expression of PRA. As the ratio of PRA to PRB increases so more contraction associated genes, such as the estrogen receptor (ER), oxytocin receptor and the prostaglandin synthesizing enzyme COX2 are expressed (Figure 2.6). Thus increased expression of PRA drives the balance towards contraction and reduces the progestational block to contraction. Recent data from Mesiano using a human myometrial cell line suggest that stimulation of PRA expression relative to PRB is via the protein kinase C pathway raising the possibility that prostaglandins or oxytocin may drive this process physiologically.

Using the same myometrial tissue, investigators have also begun to use genomic approaches to identify genes which change with the onset of parturition.

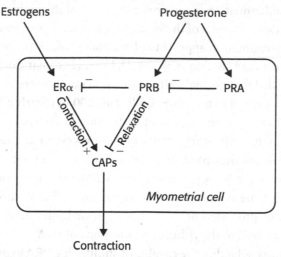

Contraction

Figure 2.6   A model for the interactions between PRA and PRB leading to functional progesterone withdrawal and the onset of parturition in the human myometrium at term

Table 2.1 Genes identified by SSH to be upregulated in labor

Gene	GenBank accession no.
Known genes	
Oxytocin receptor	X64878
MMP9	NM004994
Fibronectin	U60068
IL-8	M28130
Genes not previously linked with labor	
MnSOD	S77127
B23	M23613
IFN 1-8d	X57351
EF1α	J04617
Cyclophilin	Y00052
α-actin	X13839

Four novel genes were also identified with no matching sequences in databases. EF: elongation factor; IFN: interferon; IL: intraleukin MnSOD: manganese superoxide dismutase; SSH: suppression subtractive hybridization.

Chan *et al.* using a subtraction hybridization approach identified a number of genes which were upregulated at the time of labor (Chan *et al.*, 2002). Interestingly many of these genes are known to be involved in inflammatory activation pathways such as intraleukin-8 (IL-8) (see Table 2.1). A school of thought has for many years suggested that inflammation is a major component of the pathway to parturition and that it represents the loss of the immune tolerance shown by the mother for the fetal tissues. Inflammation appears to play a major role in the onset of parturition in the murine model (Bethin *et al.*, 2003). However recent cloning studies in the horse have revealed that normal parturition occurs in this species even when the foal is genetically identical to the mare (Galli *et al.*, 2003). Clearly a breakdown of immune tolerance is not the mechanism of parturition in this species. This does not exclude a role for inflammatory agents in the process of human delivery. Whether inflammation initiates parturition or follows as a consequence of the process remains a hot topic. Progesterone is known to have anti-inflammatory properties and perhaps the pathways may be linked by withdrawal of the anti-inflammatory effects of progesterone as PRA is expressed. Alternatively perhaps inflammatory pathways lead to the rising concentrations of PRA.

Certainly in vitro prostaglandins are capable of stimulating PRA expression and prostaglandins are an element of inflammation. Prostaglandin production is known to play a key role in parturition in many mammals such as the prostaglandin mediated luteolysis which occurs in goats and even in humans prostaglandins are potent stimulators of parturition which are used clinically. Interestingly, administration of progesterone to women at high-risk of preterm delivery, either intramuscularly or intravaginally (Meis *et al.*, 2003; Pomianowski, 2003), appears to increase the response to tocolytics, whether this occurs via an effect on the oxytocin receptor (Zingg *et al.*, 1998) or by the antiinflammatory action of progesterone, or some other mechanism remains unclear. Nevertheless these data may represent an important clue to the nature of human parturition.

Current data support the view that the timing of birth in many women is determined by events at the beginning of pregnancy. Placental CRH production is linked either directly or indirectly to this process and strong statistical relationships exist between maternal plasma concentrations and the timing of birth. At the end of pregnancy labor is associated with a functional progesterone withdrawal leading to the expression of many contraction associated proteins. Many inflammatory genes are activated at the time of labor but it is not yet clear whether the expression of these genes is a consequence of labor or an initiator of the functional progesterone withdrawal. The inevitability of delivery in the human suggests the presence of more than one pathway leading to labor: a failsafe system. Studies to date in humans indicate evidence for inflammatory pathways, oxytocin activated pathways, progesterone withdrawal and a maturational process linked to placental CRH production. Work from Steve Lye's laboratory also suggests that physical factors in the form of stretch may play a role perhaps explaining the earlier onset of labor observed in multigravidas and in the presence of a large fetus (Lye *et al.*, 2001). Although the full picture remains to be assembled the parts are beginning to

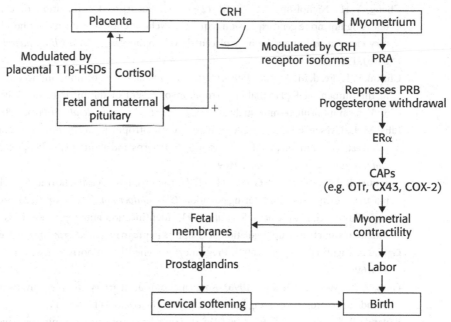

Figure 2.7   Proposed model for control of human parturition. HSD: hydroxysteroid dehydrogenase; CAPs: contraction associated proteins; PRA: progesterone receptor A; PRB: progesterone receptor B; ER: estrogen receptor

take shape (Figure 2.7). Greater understanding of this fundamental aspect of human biology may place our treatment of women in preterm labor on a more rational basis and perhaps reduce the frequency of cerebral palsy and other devastating consequences of preterm birth.

REFERENCES

Bethin, K. E., Nagai, Y. *et al.* (2003). Microarray analysis of uterine gene expression in mouse and human pregnancy. *Mol. Endocrinol.*, **17**(8), 1454–69.

Bloomfield, F. H., Oliver, M. H. *et al.* (2003). A periconceptional nutritional origin for noninfectious preterm birth. *Science*, **300**(5619), 606.

Bowman, M. E., Lopata, A. *et al.* (2001). Corticotropin-releasing hormone-binding protein in primates. *Am. J. Primatol.*, **53**(3), 123–30.

Campbell, E. A., Linton, E. A. *et al.* (1987). Plasma corticotropin-releasing hormone concentrations during pregnancy and parturition. *J. Clin. Endocrinol. Metab.*, **64**(5), 1054–9.

Chan, E. C., Fraser, S. *et al.* (2002). Human myometrial genes are differentially expressed in labor: a suppression subtractive hybridization study. *J. Clin. Endocrinol. Metab.*, **87**(6), 2435–41.

Cheng, Y. H., Nicholson, R. C. *et al.* (2000). Glucocorticoid stimulation of corticotropin-releasing hormone gene expression requires a cyclic adenosine 3′,5′-monophosphate regulatory element in human primary placental cytotrophoblast cells. *J. Clin. Endocrinol. Metab.*, **85**(5), 1937–45.

Clifton, V. L., Read, M. A. *et al.* (1995). Corticotropin-releasing hormone-induced vasodilatation in the human fetal–placental circulation: involvement of the nitric oxide-cyclic guanosine 3′,5′-monophosphate-mediated pathway. *J. Clin. Endocrinol. Metab.*, **80**(10), 2888–93.

Ellis, M. J., Livesey, J. H. *et al.* (2002). Plasma corticotropin-releasing hormone and unconjugated estriol in human pregnancy: gestational patterns and ability to predict preterm delivery. *Am. J. Obstet. Gynecol.*, **186**(1), 94–9.

Emanuel, R. L., Robinson, B. G. *et al.* (1994). Corticotrophin releasing hormone levels in human plasma and amniotic fluid during gestation. *Clin. Endocrinol. (Oxf.)*, **40**(2), 257–62.

Europe-Finner, G. N., Phaneuf, S. *et al.* (1993). Identification and expression of G-proteins in human myometrium: up-regulation of G alpha s in pregnancy. *Endocrinology*, **132**(6), 2484–90.

Galli, C., Lagutina, I. *et al.* (2003). Pregnancy: a cloned horse born to its dam twin. *Nature*, **424**(6949), 635.

Giles, W. B., McLean, M. *et al.* (1996). Abnormal umbilical artery Doppler waveforms and cord blood corticotropin-releasing hormone. *Obstet. Gynecol.*, **87**(1), 107–11.

Goland, R. S., Wardlaw, S. L. *et al.* (1986). High levels of corticotropin-releasing hormone immunoactivity in maternal and fetal plasma during pregnancy. *J. Clin. Endocrinol. Metab.*, **63**(5), 1199–203.

Goland, R. S., Wardlaw, S. L. *et al.* (1992). Plasma corticotropin-releasing factor concentrations in the baboon during pregnancy. *Endocrinology*, **131**(4), 1782–6.

Goldenberg, R. L. (2002). The management of preterm labor. *Obstet. Gynecol.*, **100**(5 Pt 1), 1020–37.

Grammatopoulos, D., Dai, Y. *et al.* (1998). Human corticotropin-releasing hormone receptor: differences in subtype expression between pregnant and nonpregnant myometria. *J. Clin. Endocrinol. Metab.*, **83**(7), 2539–44.

Haig, D. (1993). Genetic conflicts in human pregnancy. *Q. Rev. Biol.*, **68**(4), 495–532.

Inder, W. J., Prickett, T. C. *et al.* (2001). The utility of plasma CRH as a predictor of preterm delivery. *J. Clin. Endocrinol. Metab.*, **86**(12), 5706–10.

King, B. R., Smith, R. *et al.* (2002). Novel glucocorticoid and cAMP interactions on the CRH gene promoter. *Mol. Cell. Endocrinol.*, **194**(1–2), 19–28.

Liggins, G. C. (1973a). Fetal influences on myometrial contractility. *Clin. Obstet. Gynecol.*, **16**(3), 148–65.

Liggins, G. C. (1973b). The physiological role of prostaglandins in parturition. *J. Reprod. Fertil. Suppl.*, **18**, 143–50.

Liggins, G. C. (1994). Mechanisms of the onset of labour: the New Zealand perspective. *Aust. NewZealand J. Obstet. Gynaecol.*, **34**(3), 338–42.

Lye, S. J., Mitchell, J. *et al.* (2001). Role of mechanical signals in the onset of term and preterm labor. *Front. Horm. Res.*, **27**, 165–78.

McGrath, S., McLean, M. *et al.* (2002). Maternal plasma corticotropin-releasing hormone trajectories vary depending on the cause of preterm delivery. *Am. J. Obstet. Gynecol.*, **186**(2), 257–60.

McLean, M., Bisits, A. *et al.* (1995). A placental clock controlling the length of human pregnancy. *Nat. Med.*, **1**(5), 460–3.

Meis, P. J., Klebanoff, M. *et al.* (2003). Prevention of recurrent preterm delivery by 17 alpha-hydroxyprogesterone caproate. *New England J. Med.*, **348**(24), 2379–85.

Mesiano, S., Chan, E. C. *et al.* (2002). Progesterone withdrawal and estrogen activation in human parturition are coordinated by progesterone receptor A expression in the myometrium. *J. Clin. Endocrinol. Metab.*, **87**(6), 2924–30.

Ni, X., Chan, E. C. *et al.* (1997). Nitric oxide inhibits corticotropin-releasing hormone exocytosis but not synthesis by cultured human trophoblasts. *J. Clin. Endocrinol. Metab.*, **82**(12), 4171–5.

Ni, X., Nicholson, R. C. *et al.* (2002). Estrogen represses whereas the estrogen-antagonist ICI 182780 stimulates placental CRH gene expression. *J. Clin. Endocrinol. Metab.*, **87**(8), 3774–8.

Patel, F. A., Funder, J. W. *et al.* (2003). Mechanism of cortisol/progesterone antagonism in the regulation of 15-hydroxyprostaglandin dehydrogenase activity and messenger ribonucleic acid levels in human chorion and placental trophoblast cells at term. *J. Clin. Endocrinol. Metab.*, **88**(6), 2922–33.

Petraglia, F., Sutton, S. *et al.* (1989). Neurotransmitters and peptides modulate the release of immunoreactive corticotropin-releasing factor from cultured human placental cells. *Am. J. Obstet. Gynecol.*, **160**(1), 247–51.

Pieber, D., Allport, V. C. *et al.* (2001). Interactions between progesterone receptor isoforms in myometrial cells in human labour. *Mol. Hum. Reprod.*, **7**(9), 875–9.

Pomianowski, K. (2003). Natural progesterone prevents preterm birth in high-risk pregnancies. *J. Fam. Pract.*, **52**(7), 522–3.

Prickett, T., Ellis, J. *et al.* (2000). *The Utility of Plasma CRH as a Predictor of Premature Labour and Delivery*. Sydney, Australia: ICE.

Robinson, B. G., Emanuel, R. L. *et al.* (1988). Glucocorticoid stimulates expression of corticotropin-releasing hormone gene in human placenta. *Proc. Natl. Acad. Sci. USA*, **85**(14), 5244–8.

Robinson, B. G., D'Angio, Jr., L. A. *et al.* (1989). Preprocorticotropin releasing hormone: cDNA sequence and in vitro processing. *Mol. Cell. Endocrinol.*, **61**(2), 175–80.

Smith, R., Chan, E. C. *et al.* (1993). Corticotropin-releasing hormone in baboon pregnancy. *J. Clin. Endocrinol. Metab.*, **76**(4), 1063–8.

Smith, R., Mesiano, S. *et al.* (1998). Corticotropin-releasing hormone directly and preferentially stimulates dehydroepiandrosterone sulfate secretion by human fetal adrenal cortical cells. *J. Clin. Endocrinol. Metab.*, **83**(8), 2916–20.

Smith, R., Wickings, E. J. *et al.* (1999). Corticotropin-releasing hormone in chimpanzee and gorilla pregnancies. *J. Clin. Endocrinol. Metab.*, **84**(8), 2820–5.

Wolfe, C. D., Patel, S. P. *et al.* (1988). Plasma corticotrophin-releasing factor (CRF) in normal pregnancy. *Br. J. Obstet. Gynaecol.*, **95**(10), 997–1002.

Young, I. R., Loose, J. M. *et al.* (1996). Prostaglandin E2 acts via the hypothalamus to stimulate ACTH secretion in the fetal sheep. *J. Neuroendocrinol.*, **8**(9), 713–20.

Zingg, H. H., Grazzini, E. *et al.* (1998). Genomic and non-genomic mechanisms of oxytocin receptor regulation. *Adv. Exp. Med. Biol.*, **449**, 287–95.

3

Maternal nutrition and metabolic control of pregnancy

Michael L. Power[1] and Suzette D. Tardif[2]

[1] Nutrition Laboratory, Department of Conservation Biology, Smithsonian's National Zoological Park, Washington, DC, USA
[2] Southwest National Primate Research Center, San Antonio, TX, USA

A successful human pregnancy follows a chancy path from fertilization to implantation, through an extended period of placental and fetal growth, to a period of fetal organ maturation that corresponds to a change from uterine quiescence to coordinated uterine contractions, and finally to cervical dilation and parturition. The fate of a fertilized human ovum is far from secure (Figure 3.1). It is estimated that one-third to one-half of human conceptuses either do not implant or are lost shortly after implantation. Among those fertilized ova that successfully implant, as many as one in five succumb before delivery. Even in developed nations, of

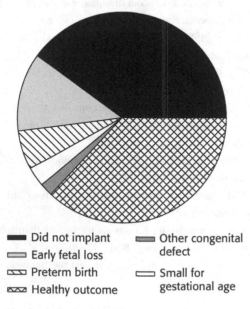

Did not implant
Early fetal loss
Preterm birth
Healthy outcome
Other congenital defect
Small for gestational age

Figure 3.1   The fate of a fertilized human ovum

those fetuses that are delivered, 10% are preterm, 5% are small for their gestational age, and 3% have one or more severe congenital defects (Keen *et al.*, 2003).

A significant proportion of human morbidity and mortality, from neonates to adults, may be attributable to events in utero. Preterm birth and intrauterine growth restriction (IUGR) are significant sources of neonatal morbidity and mortality. In 1947, Eastman (1947) declared, 'Only when the factors underlying prematurity are completely understood can any intelligent attempt at prevention be made.' After considerable research effort since then, our understanding of the causes of preterm labor still is far from complete, and the rate of premature labor and birth has not declined (Goldenberg *et al.*, 2003). Preterm birth and IUGR are associated; preterm delivery is more common in small for gestational age infants. Premature and small for gestational age infants that survive into adulthood have an increased risk of many disabilities and diseases (Ward and Beachy, 2003). Epidemiological studies suggest relations between low birth weight and increased risk for a variety of adult-onset diseases (Barker, 2001). There is convincing evidence that events in utero can have profound effects on fetal development, and on later expression of such traits as blood pressure, insulin/glucose metabolism, and neural function (Seckl, 1998).

All of these adverse outcomes have causes; some are preventable, and some may be an inherent part of the evolved human reproductive strategy that has successfully got us to where we are today. The challenge before us is to understand the biology sufficiently to be able to predict the likely outcome of a pregnancy, and to know whether, and how, to intervene if that predicted outcome is unwanted and can be prevented.

Reproduction is a costly endeavor for mammalian females. Evolution likely has favored mechanisms by which early pregnancy loss will occur if nutritional resources available to the female are inadequate. In most anthropoid primates, the daily energy expenditure for gestation and lactation is not great, especially when compared with other mammals such as rodents. However, this low daily energy expenditure is achieved partly by extending gestation and lactation over considerable lengths of time. Thus, each pregnancy represents a significant proportion of a female's reproductive life span. Early pregnancy loss and preterm birth in humans might represent an adaptive response to circumstances that in our evolutionary past would have led not only to fetal or neonatal demise, but would have adversely affected the mother's future reproduction, for example maternal death.

In this chapter we review the evidence for how inadequate or inappropriate maternal nutrition can affect pregnancy outcome. We consider several possible metabolic signals that might regulate these effects: corticotropin-releasing hormone (CRH), leptin, and the insulin-like growth factor system. The possible role of CRH in normal and adverse pregnancy outcomes is an important focus of this chapter. Humans and other anthropoid primates are the only mammals so far studied known to produce placental CRH (Bowman *et al.*, 2001). In humans, elevated CRH is associated with adverse pregnancy outcomes such as preterm labor and pre-eclampsia (Goland *et al.*, 1995). This suggests that understanding the function and regulation of placental CRH may be a key to understanding human gestation.

Nutrition and pregnancy outcome

The IUGR and early fetal demise are 3–10 times more prevalent in developing countries, with higher incidences of poor maternal nutrition, than they are in developed nations (de Onis *et al.*, 1998). In one study in rural India, 27.4% of neonates had birth weights under 2500 g, although only 6.6% were preterm (Agarwal *et al.*, 2002). In a study of Australian aborigines, low body mass index (BMI $<18.5\,\mathrm{kg/m^2}$) was associated with five times the risk of a low birth weight baby, and 2.5 times the risk of IUGR (Sayers and Powers, 1997). The authors concluded that 28% of low birth weight and 15% of IUGR was attributable to maternal malnutrition. Filipino women with low energy status (as determined by maternal arm fat area) gave birth to male offspring that, 15 years later, had higher total cholesterol and a higher low density lipoprotein (LDL) to high density lipoprotein (HDL) cholesterol ratio than did women in better condition. The findings in the female offspring were less consistent, suggesting a possible sex difference in the relation between fetal nutrition and postnatal lipid metabolism (Kuzawa and Adair, 2003).

Two hypotheses have been proposed to explain the link between low birth weight and later vulnerability to disease: poor fetal nutrition (Barker, 2001) and fetal exposure to excess glucocorticoids (Seckl, 1998). Poor maternal nutrition can contribute towards either mechanism. For example, maternal undernutrition, especially protein-energy malnutrition, appears to down regulate the placental enzyme 11β-hydroxysteroid dehydrogenase type 2, which acts as a barrier to glucocorticoids (Seckl, 1998). This has been shown definitively in the rat (Bertram *et al.*, 2001; Lesage *et al.*, 2001). Thus, maternal malnutrition potentially exposes the fetus to increased maternal glucocorticoids. Seckl and colleagues provide a detailed examination of the evidence for glucocorticoid programming of physiology, and its links to disease in their contribution to this volume.

In contrast to poor women in developing nations, pregnant women in developed nations (and the more 'well-off' segments of the populations in developing nations) are at higher risk of obesity, and its attendant sequelea of metabolic disorders such as gestational diabetes mellitus (GDM). These disorders of 'plenty' also can result in poor fetal outcomes, such as fetal macrosomia, and are associated with a propensity to obesity and type 2 diabetes in later life for the offspring. In a study of pregnant Danish women (Jensen *et al.*, 2003), both overweight and obese women were significantly more at risk for having a large for gestational age infant, in addition to hypertensive disorders during pregnancy, and requiring the induction of labor or Cesarian section. In a study of Australian women, women with non-insulin dependent diabetes during pregnancy were significantly heavier and had greater BMIs than women with uncomplicated pregnancies. In contrast, women in this study with IUGR pregnancies were significantly lighter (McIntyre *et al.*, 2000). Thus, current evidence supports the idea that the risk of an adverse pregnancy outcome is related to BMI by a U-shaped curve.

In addition to maternal energy intake, micronutrient deficiencies (or excess) can adversely affect pregnancy outcome. A prime example is folate deficiency, which is associated with neural tube defects. An early intervention study by Ebbs and colleagues (1941) found that women with a poor diet (defined as low in protein, calcium, and fruits and vegetables) had higher incidences of miscarriages, stillbirths and early neonatal mortality. Inadequate maternal intake of the vitamins B-6, B-12, K, and folate, and the minerals copper, magnesium and zinc, have been associated with abnormal prenatal development, as have excessive maternal intake of vitamins A and D, and of the minerals iodine and iron (Keen *et al.*, 2003). Low maternal intake of vitamin C has been linked with premature rupture of membranes (Siega-Riz *et al.*, 2003).

Micronutrient deficiencies can arise because of poor maternal diet, or secondarily due to genetic factors, nutrient interactions, drug interactions, or alterations of metabolism due to disease. For example, people with Menkes disease suffer from copper deficiency due to genetically based defects in the intracellular transport of copper (Keen *et al.*, 1998). People with phytate-rich diets are susceptible to zinc deficiency due to the mineral-binding capacity of phytate (Hambidge, 2000). Diabetes and hypertension alter the metabolism of zinc, copper and other minerals (Keen *et al.*, 1998).

There are many known risk factors for preterm birth, including previous preterm birth, uterine infection, IUGR and maternal psychosocial stress. Inappropriate maternal nutrition might increase the risk of preterm birth in a number of ways. For example, protein-energy malnutrition and malnutrition in a number of micronutrients (e.g. zinc, vitamins C and E) are known to adversely affect immune status (Goldenberg, 2003). A compromised immune system increases the risk of uterine infection, which in turn is associated with an increased risk of preterm birth. This is a plausible scenario. Infections, parasitic diseases, malnutrition and poor pregnancy outcomes are often associated (Romero *et al.*, 2003; Steketee, 2003). However, evidence is lacking that mineral and vitamin supplementation can improve pregnancy outcomes by reducing infections (Goldenberg, 2003). An overview of randomized controlled trials could not identify any specific nutrient that was asso-ciated with reducing preterm birth (Villar *et al.*, 2003).

Numerous endocrine and exocrine pathways may be involved in the relations among nutritional state and pregnancy outcome. We highlight three potential pathway systems: the CRH-cortisol, leptin and growth hormone insulin-like growth factor (GH-IGF).

CRH-cortisol

Activation of the fetal hypothalamic–pituitary–adrenal (HPA) axis is a common finding at the end of pregnancy in many mammals. It results in increased output of fetal glucocorticoids that contribute to mechanisms that mature fetal organs necessary for life after birth. Steroid production from the fetal adrenal is also important in pathways leading to the ending of uterine quiescence, and the initia-tion of labor and parturition.

The primate has a unique fetal adrenal in function, morphology and maturation (Jaffe *et al.*, 1998). It is characterized by rapid growth, such that it is dispropor-tionately enlarged in late gestation, and high steroidogenic activity. The majority of the primate fetal adrenal consists of a fetal zone that atrophies soon after birth, and has no counterpart postpartum. The primate adrenal fetal zone produces large quantities of dehydroepiandrosterone sulphate (DHEA-S); up to 200 mg/day dur-ing late gestation. DHEA-S is converted to estrogen in the placenta, a vital step in the initiation of the cascade of physiologic events leading to labor. The fetal adre-nal produces cortisol in the transitional zone, which is essential for the mainte-nance of intrauterine homeostasis and induction of enzymes in a variety of organs in preparation for extrauterine existence (Jaffe *et al.*, 1998). The transitional zone production of glucocorticoids increases rapidly at mid-pregnancy and levels remain elevated throughout the remainder of normal pregnancies (Smith *et al.*, 1999; Umezaki *et al.*, 2001). This profile is typical of primates and has been reported for common marmosets (Ziegler and Sousa, 2002), rhesus monkeys (Umezaki *et al.*, 2001), baboons (Pepe *et al.*, 1990), gorillas and chimpanzees (Smith *et al.*, 1999) and humans (Jaffe *et al.*, 1998; Goland *et al.*, 1994).

The CRH is a neuropeptide produced in the brain in hypothalamic regions such as the paraventricular nucleus (PVN), and in extra hypothalamic sites such as the amygdala and the bed nucleus of the stria terminalis. The CRH stimulates adreno-corticotropin-releasing hormone (ACTH) production by the pituitary gland, which in turn stimulates cortisol production in the adrenal glands. Cortisol restrains CRH production by the hypothalamus via a negative feedback mecha-nism. However, cortisol stimulates CRH production in extra hypothalamic sites in

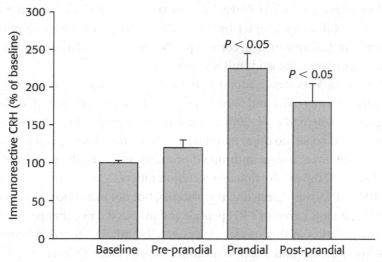

Figure 3.2   CRH response to feeding in central nucleus of the rat amygdala. Mean baseline defined as 100%. Pre-prandial is 30 min prior to feeding; post-prandial is 30 min after feeding. Data obtained using microdialysis. Adapted from Merali et al. (1998) with permission

a feed-forward mechanism that helps sustain central motive states. Detailed information on neural regulation of CRH is reviewed in the chapter by Watts in this volume.

The upregulation of CRH by glucocorticoids in extrahypothalamic regions of the brain is linked to conditions of adversity or stress. It can result in fearful and anxious behaviors (see contribution by Schulkin and colleagues in this volume). However, upregulation of CRH in the amygdala is also seen in appetitive events such as feeding (Merali et al., 1998; Figure 3.2). Some (e.g. Merali et al., 2003) have suggested that the CRH system serves to increase alertness and attention to cues of biological significance. Cues that represent a threat to survival elicit fear; cues that represent aid to survival (e.g. food intake) elicit approach and appetitive behaviors; both types of cue increase CRH in the central nucleus of the amygdala.

Interestingly, sucrose ingestion can down-regulate CRH in the PVN. Sucrose ingestion (and perhaps most feeding?) apparently results in a transient increase in serum cortisol, which then exerts a suppresive effect on hypothalamic CRH. Dallman and colleagues have proposed this as a mechanism to understand 'comfort foods' (Dallman et al., 2003). However, evidence suggests that sucrose ingestion may have direct effects on CRH expression. Adrenalectomized rats given saccharin to drink have higher CRH and lower serum insulin than sham adrenalectomized controls. When adrenalectomized rats are offered sucrose to drink, CRH is lower than in the animals offered saccharin, and indistinguishable from controls, whereas their serum insulin is significantly higher than both groups (Dallman et al., 2003).

Human placental CRH is regulated by cortisol in a similar manner to that of amygdalar CRH (see chapter by Smith and colleagues for a description). Thus, increases in maternal or fetal cortisol production are expected to upregulate CRH messenger ribonucleic acid (mRNA) synthesis.

The available evidence supports the hypothesis that all anthropoid primates produce placental CRH and most produce CRH-binding protein (CRHbp) during pregnancy (Bowman et al., 2001). This sets anthropoid primates apart from other mammals, as, so far, no other mammalian species have been found to produce placental CRH. Even among anthropoid primates, however, the pattern of placental CRH and CRHbp production and secretion differs.

CRH mRNA was detected in the placenta, but not in amnion or chorion, in the rhesus macaque. Levels of CRH peptide and mRNA did not change over the last 18 days of gestation in this species, however, CRH mRNA increased twofold during both spontaneous and androstenedione-induced labor (Wu et al., 1995). In the baboon, there is a peak of maternal serum CRH in early-to-mid-gestation, followed by a gradual decline. Both maternal and fetal CRH remain elevated until term, however (Goland et al., 1992; Smith et al., 1993). In the common marmoset, both CRH and CRHbp are detectable in maternal serum during pregnancy (Bowman et al., 2001), and the pattern of maternal serum CRH is similar to that of the baboon. The common marmoset has a long gestation for its body mass (ca. 350 g; term = 144 days), however, for the first 50–55 days post-fertilization there is little placental or fetal mass accumulation. During this initial quiescent period of gestation CRH is undetectable in maternal serum, but by approximately 55 days gestation maternal serum CRH begins to rapidly rise. This rise in CRH is followed by a rise in maternal cortisol, and shortly thereafter a rise in maternal estradiol. Maternal serum CRH then declines, but remains detectable throughout gestation (Figure 3.3; Tardif et al., unpublished data).

Humans share a pattern of exponentially increasing maternal CRH through pregnancy with our closest relatives, the chimpanzee and gorilla (Smith et al., 1999). Gorillas would appear to be the most similar to humans (Smith et al., 1999; Figure 3.4). Maternal CRH levels in chimpanzees are significantly lower than in humans or gorillas, and chimpanzees do not show a decline in CRHbp at term, in contrast to both humans and gorillas (Smith et al., 1999). The exact function of the early gestational rise in placental CRH production in all anthropoids, and the significance of the differences among monkeys, apes and humans are currently not known.

In humans, placental CRH is secreted into both the maternal and fetal compartments, but cord blood concentrations are significantly lower than maternal concentrations, indicating that it is preferentially secreted into the maternal compartment (Ruth et al., 1993). This also appears to be true in the rhesus macaque, where

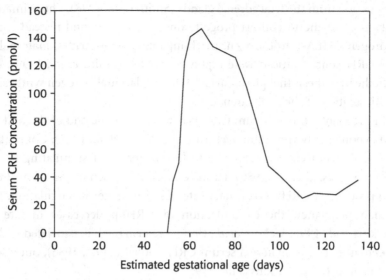

Figure 3.3   Pattern of maternal serum CRH concentration during pregnancy in the common marmoset

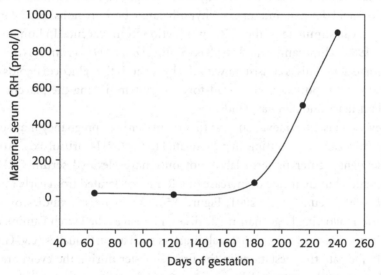

Figure 3.4   The pattern of maternal serum CRH during pregnancy in gorillas. Adapted from Smith
et al. (1999)

fetal CRH concentrations were approximately 1% of maternal concentrations
(Bowman et al., 2001).

Primate placental CRH is as biologically active as CRH produced by the hypothalamus. Placental CRH stimulates ACTH production from the fetal pituitary
gland, which in turn stimulates cortisol and DHEA-S production from fetal adrenal
glands. Placental CRH has been shown to be able to directly stimulate DHEA-S

production from the fetal adrenal glands (Smith *et al.*, 1998). The primate placenta lacks the enzyme to convert progesterone to estrogen, and instead converts the androgen DHEA-S to estrogen. In chimpanzees and gorillas, maternal estradiol and CRH concentrations were highly correlated (Smith *et al.*, 1999), consistent with the hypothesis that placental CRH drives placental estrogen synthesis through its stimulation of the fetal adrenal.

In pregnant women, serum CRH is detectable by the end of the first trimester, and exponentially rises until parturition (McLean *et al.*, 1995). Concentrations of maternal serum CRH quickly rise to levels capable of stimulating the maternal HPA axis (Sasaki *et al.*, 1989). However, through much of gestation the placenta also produces a CRHbp that inactivates CRH in maternal circulation. In normal human pregnancy, the concentration of CRHbp decreases in late gestation (Perkins *et al.*, 1993; McLean *et al.*, 1995). Preterm birth is associated with not only a premature rise in maternal serum CRH (Goland *et al.*, 1986), but also an early decline in CRHbp (Perkins *et al.*, 1993).

The prepartum increase in cortisol production by the fetal adrenal is important for fetal organ maturation, especially of the lungs and kidneys, and also has effects on the fetal HPA axis and on extra hypothalamic brain regions. Fetal cortisol production can stimulate further CRH production from placenta. In humans (Goland *et al.*, 1994), chimpanzees and gorillas (Smith *et al.*, 1999), serum cortisol and CRH are correlated. This is consistent with the hypothesis that glucocorticoids drive placental CRH production via a feed-forward system linking the placenta with the fetal pituitary and adrenal glands.

Several lines of evidence suggest that events early in pregnancy may set the timing of birth and that 'setting' may be related to the CRH-cortisol axis. Women who subsequently enter preterm labor not only have elevated serum CRH at mid-pregnancy, but their rate of increase of CRH is accelerated from early on (McLean *et al.*, 1995; Leung *et al.*, 2001; Figure 3.5). Opportunistic studies of pregnancy duration following large man-made disasters, such as the Dutch Famine in 1944–5 (Stein and Susser, 1975), or natural disasters such as earthquakes (e.g. Glynn *et al.*, 2001) indicate that gestations in the first trimester during the event are the most likely to result in preterm delivery.

Recent, suggestive evidence indicates that an early nutritional insult may also increase the risk of preterm birth in sheep. A study in which 10 ewes were food restricted from 60 days before to 30 days after conception (achieving a 15% reduction in maternal weight), with ad libitum feeding thereafter, resulted in significantly shorter gestation lengths compared with control ewes fed ad libitum throughout (Bloomfield *et al.*, 2004). The evidence (precocial surges in cortisol and ACTH) suggested this early maternal energy restriction resulted in early maturation of the fetal HPA axis. The evidence did not support limited nutrient availability affecting

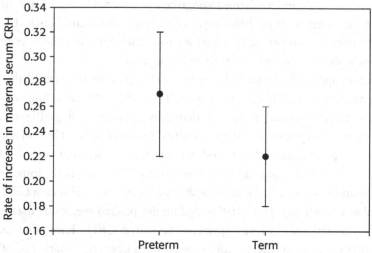

Figure 3.5   The rate of increase in maternal serum CRH concentration is greater in pregnancies destined to deliver preterm. Adapted from Leung *et al.* (2001) with permission

fetal growth, as fetal lambs did not differ in size between the two groups. Thus, an early nutritional insult that did not appear to affect overall fetal growth apparently programmed an accelerated maturation of the fetal HPA axis.

In another study (Whorwood *et al.*, 2001), energy restriction of ewes for the first half of gestation had no effect on length of gestation or birth weight; however, it did have tissue specific effects on the expression of glucocorticoid receptor (GR) and 11β-hydroxy dehydrogenase mRNA in the fetuses. Food restriction during early-to-mid-gestation resulted in increased expression of GR mRNA in fetal organs (adrenal, kidneys, liver, lung, and perirenal adipose tissue), increased 11β-hydroxy dehydrogenase type 1 mRNA in perirenal adipose tissue, and decreased 11β-hydroxy dehydrogenase type 2 mRNA in adrenals and kidney. These differences persisted until birth and were evident in the lambs even though the plane of nutrition was increased to 'normal' for the last half of gestation. In unrestricted ewes, 11β-hydroxy dehydrogenase type 2 was abundant in the placenta at mid-gestation, though absent at term; the placentas of energy restricted ewes had lower 11β-hydroxy dehydrogenase type 2 at mid-gestation.

Feeding, fasting, cortisol, and CRH

Even short-term starvation is known to increase glucocorticoid secretion (Dallman *et al.*, 2003), and energy restriction that results in modest weight loss is known to change the circadian pattern of glucocorticoid secretion (Krieger, 1974). Human pregnancy is associated with a state of hyper secretion of insulin with peripheral insulin resistance and a relative hypoglycemia. Pregnant women are more vulnerable to ketonemia after a brief period of fasting (Felig and Lynch, 1970). This is true of both lean and obese pregnant women (Metzgar *et al.*, 1982). Women appear to have a shorter 'starvation time' when pregnant.

Fasting appears to be an independent risk factor for preterm birth (Hobel and Culhane, 2003). Habitually going more than 13 h without eating was associated with a threefold greater risk of delivering preterm (Siega-Riz *et al.*, 2001). Herrmann and colleagues (2001) examined maternal serum CRH in regard to fasting in 237 pregnancies. They found that women who habitually went 13 h or more without food had significantly higher serum CRH concentrations. In addition, they found an inverse linear relationship between maternal serum CRH and gestational age at delivery. Thus, fasting and an established metabolic marker for pregnancies at risk of delivering preterm (elevated CRH) have now been linked. Whether the elevated CRH is causal of preterm labor, or a marker of other events, perhaps accelerated placental–fetal axis maturation, or merely reflects the activation of the maternal HPA axis, is unknown.

Leptin

Leptin is a molecule intimately linked with nutrition and feeding. Leptin is also an excellent example of the value of animal models in inducing new research pathways. The obese mouse model (ob/ob mouse) was developed over 50 years ago. The evidence quickly supported the hypothesis that the ob/ob mouse lacked a humoral factor that led to unregulated food intake, and thus obesity. However, that humoral factor (leptin) was not identified until recently (Zhang *et al.*, 1994). Adding back leptin to the ob/ob mouse reduced food intake and led to weight loss; but leptin had another effect as well. The obese mouse model was infertile; adding back leptin also reversed the infertility (Chehab *et al.*, 1996). Leptin is now believed to have important functions in many reproductive processes (Castracane and Henson, 2002). This illustrates another biological truism; biologically active molecules often have multiple functions, and are active in many physiological systems.

In addition to its role as a regulator of energy intake and adiposity, leptin appears to have important functions regarding reproduction, though much of the data is open to interpretation. These functions include an association with the onset of puberty, a role in fertility for males and females, a role in ovarian folliculogenesis, and in implantation of the fertilized ovum. Leptin also appears to have important roles in fetal growth and developmental processes. In many instances, such as puberty, the role of leptin may be permissive rather than required. Leptin may serve as a signal to the central nervous system with information on the critical amount of adipose tissue stores that is necessary for gonadotropin-releasing hormone (GnRH) secretion and pubertal activation of the hypothalamic–pituitary–gonadal axis. Leptin also acts at the periphery, directly on the ovary and testis where it may control steroidogenesis (Baldelli *et al.*, 2002).

As leptin is strongly associated with a measure of maternal nutritional status (fat mass), it is a plausible candidate for being an important metabolic signal for the maintenance and duration of pregnancy. Low leptin levels are associated with pregnancy loss in humans. Leptin levels may be abnormally high in pregnancies complicated by conditions such as diabetes mellitus and pre-eclampsia. Leptin is considered to be permissive of pregnancy, but not required. It may serve as a signal that maternal condition is satisfactory for reproduction (Castracane and Henson, 2002; Dumali and Messinis, 2002).

Leptin is produced by the placenta in many species, including humans, baboons, bats, rodents, pigs and sheep. Significant differences in leptin regulation and function during pregnancy exist between rodents and primates. Placental leptin production is greater in primates. In rodents the placenta largely secretes leptin into the fetal compartment, minimally into the maternal compartment. In humans (and baboons) leptin is produced on both sides of the placenta; that is, placental production contributes to both maternal and fetal leptin concentrations (Henson and Castracane, 2002).

In humans, maternal serum leptin concentration is highest at mid-gestation, and then declines. Pregnancy is considered to be a state of hyperleptinaemia with leptin resistance; that is, high maternal leptin does not decrease food intake. Maternal leptin levels drop precipitously at parturition. Serum leptin concentrations are correlated with maternal fat mass, both during pregnancy and postpartum. Figure 3.6 graphically displays regression equations for fasting serum leptin against fat mass during pregnancy and postpartum (Butte *et al.*, 1997). The lines are parallel, implying a consistent effect of fat mass on serum leptin, but the values during pregnancy are shifted upward, suggesting that the excess leptin might be placental in origin.

Placental weight is correlated with placental leptin mRNA (Jakimiuk *et al.*, 2003). Cord serum leptin was correlated with placental leptin mRNA, maternal serum leptin, and with fetal mass (Jakimiuk *et al.*, 2003). Large for gestational age fetuses have higher than normal leptin, small for gestational age fetuses have lower leptin. In twin pregnancies, the larger twin has higher circulating leptin (Sooranna *et al.*, 2001). In humans, cord blood leptin is associated with both length and head circumference of neonates. Evidence supports the hypothesis that most fetal leptin is of placental origin, though some is produced by fetal adipose tissue. Leptin receptors are found in placenta. Human data are lacking, but in rodents, leptin receptors are found in many if not most fetal tissues (e.g. besides

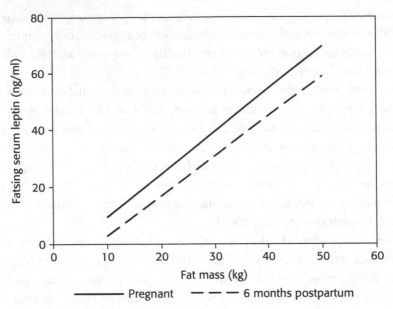

Figure 3.6   Maternal serum leptin concentrations in relation to maternal fat mass during pregnancy and 6 months postpartum. Equations for regression lines from Butte *et al.* (1997)

adopicytes also in hair follicles, cartilage, bone, lung, pancreatic islets cells, kidney, testes, and so forth). Leptin is suspected of having endocrine, autocrine and paracrine effects in placental and fetal tissues. It is hypothesized that leptin has important functions in regulating fetal growth and development. But again, evidence supports the hypothesis that it is permissive but may not be required. Leptin may be a signal/marker of growth and development. Leptin is associated with insulin, insulin-like growth factor, and growth hormone, but appears to be an independent predictor of fetal size in humans.

Interestingly, leptin and CRH appear to have functional interactions. Recent data suggest that CRH serves as a mediator for leptin's anorexigenic effects. In mice the administration of leptin decreased food intake and body weight, however, if a CRH antagonist (alpha-helical CRH 8–41) was also administered this effect was markedly attenuated (Masaki *et al.*, 2003).

Leptin may play a role in the fine-tuning of the timing of parturition in sheep. Intracerebroventricular infusion of leptin into late gestation sheep fetuses inhibits the rise in fetal circulating ACTH and cortisol (Howe *et al.*, 2002). Whether this effect is mediated through CRH is unknown. Energy restriction during pregnancy in sheep and rats results in increased adipose tissue, higher circulating leptin concentrations, and higher food intake in the offspring (Vickers *et al.*, 2000).

GH-IGF

Growth restriction, particularly in energy-restricted pregnancies, is ultimately the result of changes in pathways that control or are responsive to the partitioning of oxygen and fuel molecules between the mother and the fetus. The access of the fetus to oxygen and fuel molecules is determined by the vascular exchange capabilities of the placenta. In a normal pregnancy, overall placental size (amount of exchange surface) increases and the placental vasculature is reorganized, resulting in reduced resistance as gestation progresses (Arduini and Rizzo, 1990). In growth-restricted human and sheep pregnancies, the normal decline in vascular resistance is frequently impaired, reflected in higher pulsatility indices and reduced or absent end diastolic flow in uterine and umbilical arteries (Galan *et al.*, 1998; Harman and Baschat, 2003) and the placenta is frequently smaller (Heinonen *et al.*, 2001).

The IGF system (insulin, GH-, IGFs- and IGF-binding proteins) appears to be a critical link in this process. The principal fetal growth factor in late gestation appears to be IGF-1 produced by fetal liver and other tissues, whereas IGF-2 is the principal embryonic growth factor (Gluckman and Pinal, 2003). In rats, sheep and humans, the size of the fetus/neonate is positively correlated with maternal IGF-1 (Woodall *et al.*, 1999; Verhaeghe *et al.*, 2003). Increasing maternal IGF-1 in food-restricted rat dams does not, however, increase fetal growth (Woodall *et al.*, 1999), suggesting that there is not a direct relation between maternal IGF-1 and placenta function. Fetal IGF-1 is correlated with fetal size and with placental size. Hypoxia induces increases in IGFbp-1 in the fetus, reducing availability of IGF-1, thereby impairing growth – through this mechanism, fetal growth is slowed under conditions that reflect low substrate supply (Nayak and Giudice, 2003; Verhaeghe *et al.*, 2003).

Evidence from studies of human twin pregnancies (e.g. Bajoria *et al.*, 2002) indicate impaired amino acid transport by the placenta and a change in the IGF axis in pregnancies complicated by IUGR. The IUGR twins had lower amino acid concentrations, lower insulin, lower IGF-1, and higher IGFbp-1 than normal for gestational age twins.

There is convincing evidence for placental production of growth hormones (pGH) in sheep and primates (e.g. human and rhesus macaque). The evidence is uncertain for placental production of growth hormones in rodents. In sheep, secretion of growth hormone is into the fetal compartment. The existing evidence suggests that it is unlikely there is any significant secretion into the ovine maternal compartment. In humans, there is evidence of secretion into maternal compartment, but placental growth hormone is not found in fetal blood. It is not known for non-human primates. Humans are the only species for which data on the biologic properties of placental GH exist. Placental GH has high somatogenic and low lactogenic activity, and human pGH has a low affinity for lactogenic receptors (Lacroix *et al.*, 2002).

In humans, from 24 weeks on pituitary GH declines (and becomes effectively non-existent) and pGH takes over its role in maternal physiology; pGH dramatically declines at birth. Placental GH is not regulated by GH-releasing factors, but is suppressed by elevated maternal glucose. The function of pGH is not completely clear, but it likely serves to induce relative maternal insulin resistance, and encourages reliance on lipolysis for maternal energy metabolism (Lacroix *et al.*, 2002).

In sheep, pGH affects placental and fetal physiology, but pGH production is largely restricted to early gestation (until day 50). Fetal pituitary GH expression begins around day 50 of gestation. In humans pGH affects maternal and placental physiology, but does not directly affect fetal physiology. However, IUGR is associated with both reduced placenta size and fewer placental cells expressing pGH, and is associated with lower maternal pGH (Caufriez *et al.*, 1993). In GDM, blood glucose is correlated with pGH in maternal circulation. In a study comparing normal pregnancy with pregnancies complicated by either IUGR or diabetes, maternal serum free pGH at both 28 and 36 weeks gestation was correlated with birth weight (Figure 3.7). Free pGH, IGF-1, and IGF-2 were all significantly lower in IUGR pregnancies at both time periods (McIntyre *et al.*, 2000; Figure 3.8).

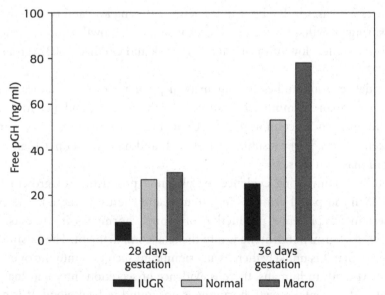

Figure 3.7   Free placental GH in maternal serum at gestational days 28 and 36 by growth category (IUGR <10th percentile; macro >90th percentile)

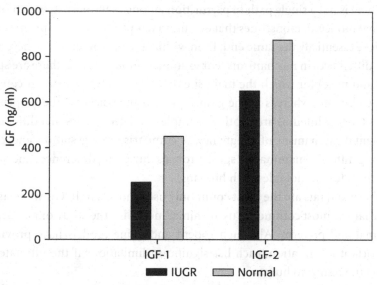

Figure 3.8   IGF-1 and IGF-2 concentrations in maternal serum at 36 days gestation

In a longitudinal study of 89 normal pregnant women, pGH was detectable as early as 5 weeks gestation, and rose to peak values at approximately 37 weeks gestation. Placental GH then decreased until parturition. Interestingly, women who gave birth to the lightest babies had the lowest levels of pGH at term. Also, the gestational age at peak pGH concentration was significantly positively correlated with pregnancy length. In other words, an early peak of pGH was associated with an earlier onset of labor, though all pregnancies were considered full term (Chellakooty *et al.*, 2004).

Animal models: need for diversity

Our understanding of the causes of preterm labor and IUGR remains far from complete. Partly this is due to the difficulties of research in this area. Ethical considerations constrain research on human beings. Experimental manipulations are largely restricted to research on animal models. Numerous animal experiments have documented the detrimental effects of poor maternal nutrition on pregnancy outcome. Animal experiments have also found that maternal overnutrition and/or obesity can adversely affect the offspring (e.g. Daenzer *et al.*, 2002).

However, there are fundamental differences in the regulation of gestation and parturition among mammals that complicate the use of non-human species as models. Potential models for these conditions in humans must be carefully characterized in order to evaluate the insight they can provide.

There is not a single path to parturition among mammals. Research on different animal models demonstrates that evolution has produced multiple mechanisms to achieve essentially the same end. Even within a mammalian order there are important differences in mechanisms. For example, among rodents there are species (e.g. rats and mice) for which the main site of steroidogenesis during pregnancy is the corpus luteum, whereas in the guinea pig it is the placenta. Sheep (placenta) and goats (corpus luteum) are another example of related species that differ in this fundamental mechanism of pregnancy. A comparison of gestation and parturition among different mammalian species reveals intriguing differences and similarities, but finds few homologies with humans.

Sheep and rats are the most commonly used models of IUGR whereas the sheep is by far the most commonly used animal model for the study of parturition, both normal and preterm. Although rodent and ovine models have provided much important information, each has significant limitations if the ultimate goal is to apply the results to humans.

Anthropoid primates would appear to be the non-human species that are the closest analog of human beings, and development of primate models of IUGR and of parturition would be valuable. However, anthropoid primates have disadvantages in terms of costs and potential zoonotic diseases. Their development as models for pathologies of gestation has lagged behind that of non-primate models. For example, in a literature search in August, 2001, Schroder (2003) identified 1406 published animal experiments on fetal growth restriction. Of those experiments, approximately 50.5% were performed on rats, and another 22.3% on mice. Other species used included: sheep (8.7%), pig (8.3%), rabbit (5.7%), guinea pig (2.8%), and horse (1.1%). Only 0.6% (8 out of 1406) of the identified animal experiments were performed on non-human primates.

Recent studies suggest that the common marmoset (*Callithrix jacchus*), a small (circa 350 g) New World monkey (Figure 3.9) may be a useful model in which to examine the effects of nutritional restrictions upon gestation and later health of infants. The common marmoset has many advantages as a non-human primate model. Its small size and low zoonosis factor provide many advantages over other non-human primates in terms of housing and handling, but it retains the advantages of a primate over a similarly sized rodent model. Marmosets offer a particularly valuable opportunity to develop useful primate models of prenatal effects on adult disease risk, given that they have the shortest average and maximum lifespan of any anthropoid primate.

The common marmoset has a higher rate of reproductive output than most anthropoid primates. They are reproductively mature by 2 years of age. Marmosets routinely produce twin fetuses, and often triplets, via multiple ovulations from one or both ovaries. Triplets are more likely to be produced when

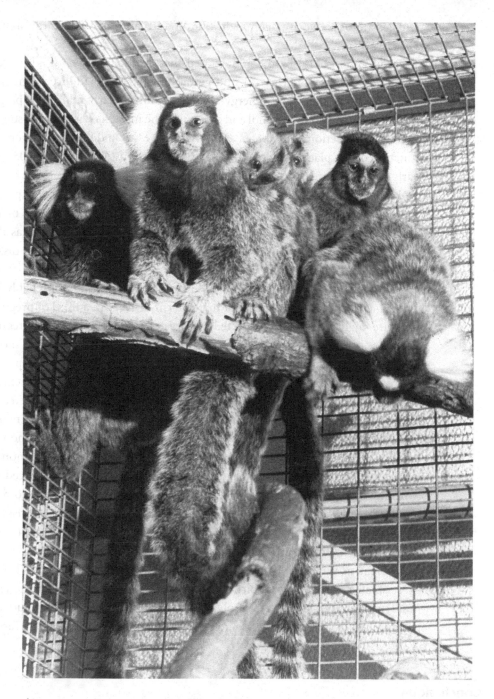

Figure 3.9   The common marmoset (*Callithrix jacchus*)

females are of above average weight (Tardif and Jaquish, 1997; Tardif and Bales, 2004).

Tardif *et al.* (2004) have demonstrated that a modest (75% of ad lib) energy restriction occurring in early-to-mid-gestation will reliably induce pregnancy loss in the common marmoset. Energy restriction during early marmoset pregnancy results in reduced free estradiol and cortisol in the maternal circulation, suggesting that food restriction does not act as a classical stressor and that perhaps endocrine function of the placenta is impaired by the restriction (Tardif *et al.*, 2005). In one early-restricted pregnancy complete aborted material was recovered. The weight and crown-rump length of the collected twin fetuses were less than expected for the estimated gestational age (83 days), based on published measures of fetuses collected at day 80 (Chambers and Hearn, 1985). The placental weight was also less than expected based upon published measures; however, the placental disk areas were similar to the expected area.

The same energy restriction initiated in late pregnancy did not reliably induce pregnancy loss, though it did result in pre-term delivery in a third of pregnancies, a figure higher than that expected in normal, non-manipulated pregnancies (Tardif *et al.*, 2004). These findings contrast with those for rodents and sheep and suggest that the marmoset may be particularly sensitive to early-to-mid-pregnancy energy restrictions. The mechanism behind this sensitivity is not yet elucidated.

In addition, the variation and relationships among maternal parameters, birth condition, infant growth and subsequent adult weight in the common marmoset indicate potential for this species to be a useful model of the links among birth weight, subsequent growth, and latter adult vulnerability to disease. Among marmoset females between 2 and 7 years old, older females generally produced infants with higher birth weights. Low maternal weight was associated with slower early infant growth, but not with low birth weight. This might reflect a greater constraint on females due to the costs of lactation as opposed to the costs of gestation (Tardif *et al.*, 2001). However, long bone growth did appear to be related to maternal weight, as infants of larger mothers had greater knee–heel lengths. Twins that were smaller than average at birth were more likely to be small as adults. This was not true, however, for triplets, implying that the mechanisms that produce a small infant likely differ between twin and triplet pregnancies in this species (Tardif and Bales, 2004).

Conclusions

Maternal nutrient intake and nutritional status can affect pregnancy outcome in a myriad of ways. In the context of this book we have focused on how they might affect the timing of birth and fetal growth and development. There would appear to be a U-shaped distribution relating energy stores in pregnant women and the risk of an adverse pregnancy outcome. Both maternal undernutrition and overnutrition (obesity) can negatively affect later health in offspring.

The metabolic signals and markers of at-risk pregnancy are not well understood. The IGF system plays a major role in fetal growth, and growth hormones produced by the placenta affect maternal and placental physiology in pregnant women. Placental growth hormone is regulated by maternal serum glucose, and maternal serum pGH, IGF-1, and IGF-2 are lower in pregnancies complicated by IUGR. Recent findings indicate that in normal pregnancies the gestational age of peak placental GH concentration in maternal serum is associated with total length of gestation and that women who give birth to lighter children have lower serum pGH concentrations at term (Chellakooty et al., 2004).

Leptin, often primarily considered a hormone of energy homeostasis and a regulator of food intake, appears to have multiple functions in pregnancy, from ovulation through implantation and maintenance of pregnancy. Leptin produced by the placenta is secreted into both maternal and fetal compartments. Low maternal leptin is associated with early pregnancy loss. Leptin may also have important functions in fetal growth and development.

The CRH is perhaps the most intriguing of the hormones discussed in this chapter, at least from an evolutionary perspective. Only anthropoid primates produce placental CRH, and among our anthropoid relatives only our closest relatives, the chimpanzee and gorilla, share the human pattern of exponentially increasing maternal CRH from early-to-mid-pregnancy until parturition (Smith et al., 1999). Preterm birth is associated with both increased maternal serum CRH from early in pregnancy, and an accelerated rate of increase of serum CRH concentration (McLean et al., 1995; Leung et al., 2001). The evidence is consistent with serum CRH concentration functioning as a 'clock', that is set early in pregnancy, and predicts the timing of parturition (McLean et al., 1995).

Placental CRH is secreted into both the maternal and fetal compartments, although fetal concentrations are significantly lower than maternal. Placental CRH may stimulate the maternal pituitary-adrenal axis, and almost certainly stimulates the fetal pituitary-adrenal axis and the fetal adrenal directly (Smith et al., 1998). In vitro studies have shown that human placental CRH can be stimulated by catecholamines (Petraglia et al., 1989). In vivo studies have shown associations between CRH and cortisol and ACTH (Goland et al., 1992; 1994). Thus, it is possible that maternal stress responses can affect and be affected by placental CRH.

The primate fetal adrenal produces cortisol and androgens, primarily DHEA-S, which then feedback to the placenta. Cortisol stimulates placental CRH production, and DHEA-S is converted to estrogen. Thus, a positive feedback loop is established that results in increasing production of estrogen as pregnancy progresses.

Elevated maternal serum CRH appears to signal a metabolic disruption of pregnancy in humans. Whether CRH is merely a marker of an at-risk pregnancy, or an effector molecule that is causal to the pathology is unclear.

Maternal malnutrition could affect placental CRH production in a number of ways. Fetal undernutrition could result in a stress response by the fetal HPA axis, resulting in increased fetal glucocorticoids that would feed back to the placenta and increase CRH production. Maternal malnutrition could down regulate placental 11β-hydroxysteroid dehydrogenase type 2, exposing both the fetus and the placenta to effectively higher concentrations of maternal glucocorticoids. Habitual short-term maternal starvation could increase maternal serum glucocorticoid concentration, stimulating placental CRH production, which then stimulates the fetal adrenals, leading to increased fetal cortisol and DHEA-S production, which in turn stimulates placental CRH production. All of these hypotheses are plausible, if simplistic.

REFERENCES

Agarwal, S., Agarwal, A., Bansal, A. K., Agarwal, D. K. and Agarwal, K. N. (2002). Birth weight patterns in rural undernourished pregnant women. *Indian Pediatr.*, **39**, 244–53.

Arduini, D. and Rizzo, G. (1990). Normal values of pulsatility index from fetal vessels: a cross-sectional study on 1556 health fetuses. *J. Perinat. Med.*, **18**, 165–72.

Bajoria, R., Sooranna, S. R., Ward, S. and Hancock, M. (2002). Placenta as a link between amino acids, insulin-IGF axis, and low birth weight: evidence from twin studies. *J. Clin. Endocrinol. Metab.*, **87**, 308–15.

Baldelli, R., Dieguez, C. and Casanueva, F. F. (2002). The role of leptin in reproduction: experimental and clinical aspects. *Ann. Med.*, **34**(1), 5–18.

Barker, D. J. P. (2001). The malnourished baby and infant. *Br. Med. Bull.*, **60**, 69–88.

Bertram, C., Trowern, A. R., Copin, N., Jackson, A. A. and Whorwood, C. B. (2001). The maternal diet during pregnancy programs altered expression of the glucocorticoid receptor and type 2 11beta-hydroxysteroid dehydrogenase: Potential molecular mechanisms underlying the programming of hypertension in utero. *Endocrinology*, **142**(7), 2841–53.

Bloomfield, F. H., Oliver, M. H., Hawkins, P. *et al.* (2004). Periconceptional undernutrition in sheep accelerates maturation of the fetal hypothalamic-pituitary-adrenal axis in late gestation. *Endocrinology* **145**, 4278–85.

Bowman, M. E., Lopata, A. *et al.* (2001). Corticotropin-releasing hormone-binding protein in primates. *Am. J. Primatol.*, **53**, 123–30.

Butte, N. F., Hopkinson, J. M., Nicolson, M. A. (1997). Leptin in human reproduction: serum leptin levels in pregnant and lactating women. *J. Clin. Endocrinol. Metab.*, **82**, 585–89.

Castracane, V. D. and Henson, M. C. (2002). When did leptin become a reproductive hormone? *Semin. Reprod. Med.*, **20**, 89–92.

Caufriez, A., Frankenne, F., Hennen, G. and Copinschi, G. (1993). Regulation of maternal IGF-I by placental GH in normal and abnormal pregnancy. *Am. J. Physiol.*, **265**, E572–7.

Chambers, P. L. and Hearn, J. P. (1985). Embryonic, foetal and placental development in the common marmoset monkey (*Callithrix jacchus*). *J. Zool. Lond.*, **207**, 545–61.

Chehab, F. F., Lim, M. E. and Lu, R. (1996). Correction of the sterility defect in homozygous obese female mice by treatment with human recombinant leptin. *Nat. Genet.*, **12**, 318–20.

Chellakooty, M., Vansgaard, K., Larsen, T. *et al.* (2004). A longitudinal study of intrauterine growth and the placental growth hormone (GH)-insulin-like growth factor I axis in maternal circulation: association between placental GH and fetal growth. *J. Clin. Endocrinol. Metab.*, **89**, 384–91.

Daenzer, M., Ortmann, S., Klaus, S. and Metges, C. C. (2002). Prenatal high protein exposure decreases energy expenditure and increases adiposity in young rats. *J. Nutr.*, **132**, 142–4.

Dallman, M. F., Pecoraro, N., Akana, S. F. *et al.* (2003). Chronic stress and obesity: a new view of "comfort food". *Proc. Natl. Acad. Sci. USA*, **100**(20), 11696–701.

De Onis, M., Blossner, M. and Villar, J. (1998). Levels and patterns of intrauterine growth restriction in developing countries. *Eur. J. Clin. Nutr.*, **52**(Suppl 1), S5–15.

Domali, E. and Messinis, I. E. (2002). Leptin in pregnancy. *J. Mater. Fetal Neonatal Med.*, **12**(4), 222–30.

Eastman, N. T. (1947). Prematurity from the viewpoint of the obstetrician. *Am. Pract.*, **1**, 343.

Ebbs, J. H., Tisdall, F. F. and Scott, W. A. (1941). The influence of prenatal diet on the mother and child. *J. Nutr.*, **22**, 515–21.

Felig, P. and Lynch, V. (1970). Starvation in human pregnancy: hypoglycemia, hypoinsulinemia, and hyperketonemia. *Science*, **170**, 990–2.

Galan, H. L., Hussey, M. J., Chung, M. *et al.* (1998). Doppler velocimetry of growth-restricted fetuses in an ovine model of placental insufficiency. *Am. J. Obstet. Gynecol.*, **178**, 451–6.

Gluckman, P. D. and Pinal, C. S. (2003). Regulation of fetal growth by the somatotrophic axis. *J. Nutr.*, **133**(Suppl), 1741S–6S.

Glynn, L., Wadhwa, P. D., Dunkel Schetter, C. and Sandman, C. A. (2001). When stress happens matters: the effects of earthquake timing on stress responsivity in pregnancy. *Am. J. Obstet. Gynecol.*, **184**, 637–42.

Goland, R. S., Wardlaw, S. L., Stark, R. I., Brown, L. S. J. and Frantz, A. G. (1986). High levels of corticotropin-releasing hormone immunoreactivity in maternal and fetal plasma during pregnancy. *J. Clin. Endocrinol. Metab.*, **63**, 1199–203.

Goland, R. S., Wardlaw, S. L. and Fortman, J. D. (1992). Plasma corticotropin-releasing factor concentrations in the baboon during pregnancy. *Endocrinology*, **131**, 1782–6.

Goland, R. S., Jozak, S. and Conwell, I. (1994). Placental corticotropin-releasing hormone and the hypercortisolism of pregnancy. *Am. J. Obstet. Gynecol.*, **171**, 1287–91.

Goland, R. S., Tropper, P. J., Warren, W. B., Stark, R. I., Jozak, S. M. and Conwell, I. M. (1995). Concentrations of corticotropin-releasing hormone in the umbilical cord blood of pregnancies complicated by preeclampsia. *Reproduction Fertility and Development*, **7**, 1227–30.

Goldenberg, R. L. (2003). The plausibility of micronutrient deficiency in relationship to perinatal infection. *J. Nutr.*, **133**, 1645S–8S.

Goldenberg, R. L., Iams, J. D., Mercer, B. M. *et al.* (2003). What we have learned about the predictors of preterm birth. *Semin. Perinatol.*, **27**, 185–93.

Harman, C. R. and Baschat, A. A. (2003). Comprehensive assessment of fetal wellbeing: which Doppler tests should be performed? *Curr. Opin. Obstet. Gynecol.*, **15**, 147–57.

Heinonen, S., Taipale, P. and Saarikoski, S. (2001). Weights of placentae from small-for-gestational age infants revisited. *Placenta*, **22**, 399–404.

Henson, M. C. and Castracane, V. D. (2002). Leptin: roles and regulation in primate pregnancy. *Semin. Reprod. Med.*, **20**(2), 113–22.

Herrmann, T. S., Siega-Riz, A. M., Hobel, C. J., Aurora, C. and Dunkel-Schetter, C. (2001). Prolonged periods without food intake during pregnancy increase risk for elevated maternal corticotropin-releasing hormone concentrations. *Am. J. Obstet. Gynecol.*, **185**, 403–12.

Howe, D. C., Gertler, A. and Challis, J. R. (2002). The late gestation increase in circulating ACTH and cortisol in the fetal sheep is suppressed by intracerebroventricular infusion of recombinant ovine leptin. *J. Endocrinol.*, **174**, 259–66.

Jaffe, R. B., Mesiano, S., Smith, R. *et al.* (1998). The regulation and role of fetal adrenal development in human pregnancy. *Endocrin. Res.*, **24**, 919–26.

Jakimiuk, A. J., Skalba, P., Huterski, R., Haczynski, J. and Magoffin, D. A. (2003). Leptin messenger ribonucleic acid (mRNA) content in the human placenta at term: relationship to levels of leptin in cord blood and placental weight. *Gynecol. Endocrinol.*, **17**, 311–16.

Jensen, D. M., Damm, P., Sørenson, B. *et al.* (2003). Pregnancy outcome and prepregnancy body mass index in 2459 glucose-tolerant anish women. *Am. J. Obstet. Gynecol.*, **189**, 239–44.

Keen, C. L., Uriu-Hare, J. Y., Hawk, S. N. *et al.* (1998). Effect of copper deficiency on prenatal development and pregnancy outcome. *Am. J. Clin. Nutr.*, **67**, 1003S–11S.

Keen, C. L., Clegg, M. S., Hanna, L. A. *et al.* (2003). The plausibility of micronutrient deficiencies being a significant contributing factor to the occurrence of pregnancy complications. *J. Nutr.*, **133**, 1592S–6S.

Krieger, D. T. (1974). Food and water restriction shifts corticosterone, temperature, activity and brain amine periodicity. *Endocrinology*, **95**, 1195–1201.

Kuzawa, C. W. and Adair, L. S. (2003). Lipid profiles in adolescent Filipinos: relation to birth weight and maternal energy status during pregnancy. *Am. J. Clin. Nutr.*, **77**, 960–6.

Lacroix, M.-C., Guibourdenche, J., Frendo, J.-L., Pidoux, G. and Evain-Brion, D. (2002). Placental growth hormones. *Endocrine*, **19**, 73–9.

Lesage, J., Blondeau, B., Grino, M., Breant, B. and Dupouy, J. P. (2001). Maternal undernutrition during late gestation induces fetal overexposure to glucocorticoids and intrauterine growth retardation, and disturbs the hypothalamo-pituitary adrenal axis in the newborn rat. *Endocrinology*, **142**, 1692–702.

Leung, T. N., Chung, T. K. H., Madsen, G. *et al.* (2001). Rate of rise in maternal plasma corticotropin-releasing hormone and its relation to gestational length. *Br. J. Obstet. Gynaecol.*, **108**, 527–32.

Masaki, T., Yoshimichi, G., Chiba, S. *et al.* (2003). Corticotropin-releasing hormone-mediated pathway of leptin to regulate feeding, adiposity, and uncoupling protein expression in mice. *Endocrinology*, **144**, 3547–54.

McIntyre, H. D., Serek, R., Crane, D. I. *et al.* (2000). Placental growth hormone (GH), GH-binding protein, and insulin-like growth factor axis in normal, growth-retarded, and diabetic pregnancies: correlations with fetal growth. *J. Clin. Endocrinol. Metab.*, **85**, 1143–50.

McLean, M., Bistis, A., Davies, J. J. *et al.* (1995). A placental clock controlling the length of human pregnancy. *Nat. Med.*, **1**, 460–3.

Merali, Z., McIntosh, J., Kent, P., Michaud, D. and Anisman, H. (1998). Aversive and appetitive events evoke the release of corticotropin-releasing hormone and bombesin-like peptides at the central nucleus of the amygdala. *J. Neurosci.*, **18**, 4758–66.

Merali, Z., Michaud, D., McIntosh, J., Kent, P. and Anisman, H. (2003). Differential involvement of amydaloid CRH system(s) in the salience and valence of the stimuli. *Progress in Neuro-Psychopharmacology & Biological Psychiatry*, **27**, 1201–12.

Metzgar, B. E., Ravnikar, V., Vileisis, R. A. and Freinkel, N. (1982). Accelerated starvation and the skipped breakfast in late normal pregnancy. *Lancet*, **1**, 588–92.

Nayak, N. R. and Giudice, L. C. (2003). Comparative biology of the IGF system in endometrium, deciduas, and placenta and clinical implications for foetal growth and implantation disorders. *Placenta*, **24**, 281–96.

Pepe, G. J., Waddell, B. J. and Albrecht, E. D. (1990). Activation of the baboon fetal hypothalamic–pituitary–adrenocortical axis at midgestation by estrogen-induced changes in placental corticosteroid metabolism. *Endocrinology*, **127**, 3117–23.

Perkins, A. V., Eben, F., Wolfe, C. D., Schulte, H. M. and Linton, E. A. (1993). Plasma measurement of corticotrophin-releasing hormone-binding protein in normal and abnormal human pregnancy. *J. Endocrinol.*, 149–57.

Petraglia, F., Sutton, S. and Vale, W. (1989). Neurotransmitters and peptides modulate the release of immunoreactive corticotropin-releasing factor from cultured human placental cells. *Am. J. Obstet. Gynecol.*, **160**, 247–51.

Romero, R., Chaiworapongsa, T. and Espinoza, J. (2003). Micronutrients and intrauterine infection, preterm birth and the fetal inflammatory response syndrome. *J. Nutr.*, **133**, 1668S–73S.

Ruth, V., Hallman, M. and Laatikainen, T. (1993). Corticotropin-releasing hormone and cortisol in cord plasma in relation to gestational age, labor, and fetal distress. *Am. J. Perinatol.*, **10**, 115–18.

Sasaki, A., Shinkawa, O. and Yoshinaga, K. (1989). Placental coricotropin-releasing hormone may be a stimulator of maternal pituitary adrenocorticotropic hormone secretion in humans. *J Clin. Invest.*, **84**, 1997–2001.

Sayers, S. and Powers, J. (1997). Risk factors for aboriginal low birthweight, intrauterine growth retardation and preterm in the Darwin Health Region. *Aust. New Zeal. J. Public Health*, **21**, 524–30.

Schroder, H. J. (2003). Models of fetal growth restriction. *Eur. J. Obstetr. Gynecol. Reprod. Biol.*, **110**(Suppl 1), S29–39.

Seckl, J. R. (1998). Physiologic programming of the fetus. *Clin. Perinatol.*, **25**, 939–64.

Siega-Riz, A. M., Herrmann, T. S., Savitz, D. A. and Thorp, J. M. (2001). Frequency of eating during pregnancy and its effect on preterm delivery. *Am. J. Epidemiol.*, **153**, 647–52.

Siega-Riz, A. M., Promislow, J. H. E., Savitz, D. A., Thorp, Jr., J. M. and McDonald, T. (2003). Vitamin C intake and the risk of preterm delivery. *Am. J. Obstetr. Gynecol.*, **189**, 519–25.

Smith, R., Chan, E.-C., Bowman, M. E., Harewood, W. J. and Phippard, A. F. (1993). Corticotropin-releasing hormone in baboon pregnancy. *J. Clin. Endocrinol. Metab.*, **76**, 1063–8.

Smith, R., Mesiano, S., Chan, E.-C., Brown, S. and Jaffe, R. B. (1998). Corticotropin-releasing hormone directly stimulates dehydroepiandrosterone sulfate excretion by human fetal adrenal cortical cells. *J. Clin. Endocrinol. Metab.*, **83**, 2916–20.

Smith, R., Wickings, J., Bowman, M. B. *et al.* (1999). Corticotropin-releasing hormone in Chimpanzee and Gorilla pregnancy. *J. Clin. Endocrinol. Metab.*, **84**: 2820–5.

Sooranna, S. R., Ward, S. and Bajoria, R. (2001). Fetal leptin influences birth weight in twins with discordant growth. *Pediatr. Res.*, **49**, 667–72.

Stein, Z. and Susser, M. (1975). The Dutch famine, 1944–1945, and the reproductive process. I. Effects or six indices at birth. *Pediatr. Res.*, **9**, 70–6.

Steketee, R. W. (2003). Pregnancy, nutrition and parasitic diseases. *J. Nutr.*, **133**, 1661S–7S.

Tardif, S. D. and Jaquish, C. E. (1997). Ovulation number in the marmoset monkey (*Callithrix jacchus*): relation to body weight, age and repeatability. *Am. J. Primatol.*, **42**, 323–9.

Tardif, S. D., Power, M., Oftedal, O. T., Power, R. A. and Layne, D. G. (2001). Lactation, maternal behavior and infant growth in common marmoset monkeys (*Callithrix jacchus*): effects of maternal size and litter size. *Behav. Ecol. Sociobiol.*, **51**, 17–25.

Tardif, S. D. and Bales, K. L. (2004). Relations among birth condition, maternal condition, and postnatal growth in captive common marmoset monkeys (*Callithrix jacchus*). *Am. L. Primatol.*, **62**, 83–94.

Tardif, S. D., Power, M., Layne, D., Smucny, D. and Ziegler, T. (2004). Energy restriction initiated at different gestational ages has varying effects on maternal weight gain and pregnancy outcome in common marmoset monkeys (*Callithrix jacchus*). *Br. J. Nutr.*, **92**, 841–9.

Tardif, S. D., Ziegler, T. E., Power, M. and Layne, D. G. (2005). Endocrine changes in full term pregnancies and pregnancy loss due to energy restriction in the common marmoset (*Callithrix jacchus*). *J. Clin. Endocrinol. Metab.*, **90**, 335–9.

Umezaki, H., Hess, D. L., Valenzuela, G. J. and Ducsay, C. A. (2001). Fetectomy alters maternal pituitary-adrenal function in pregnant rhesus macaques. *Biol. Reprod.*, **65**, 1616–21.

Verhaeghe, J., Van Herck, R., Billen, J. *et al.* (2003). Regulation of insulin-like growth factor-1 and insulin-like growth factor binding protein-1 concentrations in preterm fetuses. *Am. J. Obstet. Gynecol.*, **188**, 485–91.

Vickers, M. H., Breier, B. H., Cutfield, W. S., Hofman, P. L. and Gluckman, P. D. (2000). Fetal origins of hyperphagia, obesity, and hypertension and postnatal amplification by hypercaloric nutrition. *Am. J. Physiol. Endocrinol. Metab.*, **279**, E83–7.

Villar, J., Merialdi, M., Gülmezoglu, A. M. *et al.* (2003). Nutritional interventions during pregnancy for the prevention or treatment of maternal morbidity and preterm delivery: an overview of randomized clinical trials. *J. Nutr.*, **133**, 1606S–25S.

Ward, R. M. and Beachy, J. C. (2003). Neonatal complications following preterm birth. *BJOG*, **110**(Suppl 20), 81–6.

Whorwood, C. B., Firth, K. M., Budge, H. and Symonds, M. E. (2001). Maternal undernutrition during early to midgestation programs tissue-specific alterations in the expression of the glucocorticoid receptor, 11 beta-hydroxysteroid dehydrogenase isoforms, and type 1 angiotensin II receptor in neonatal sheep. *Endocrinology*, **142**, 2854–64.

Woodall, S. M., Breier, B. H., Johnston, B. M., Bassett, N. S., Barnard, R. and Gluckman, P. D. (1999). Administration of growth hormone or IGF-1 to pregnant rats on a reduced diet throughout pregnancy does not prevent fetal intrauterine growth retardation and elevated blood pressure in adult offspring. *J. Endocrinol.*, **163**, 69–7.

Wu, W. X., Unno, S., Giussani, D. A. *et al.* (1995). Corticotropin-releasing hormone and its receptor distribution in fetal membranes and placenta of the rhesus monkey in late gestation and labor. *Endocrinology*, **136**, 4621–8.

Zhang, Y., Proenca, R., Maffei, M., Baron, M., Leopold, L. and Friedman, J. M. (1994). Positional cloning of the mouse Obese gene and its human analog. *Nature*, **372**, 425–31.

Ziegler, T. E. and Sousa, M. B. C. (2002). Parent–daughter relationships and social controls on fertility in female common marmosets, *Callithrix jacchus. Horm. Behav.*, **42**, 356–67.

4

Fetal HPA activation, preterm birth and postnatal programming

Deborah M. Sloboda[1], Timothy J. M. Moss[1], John P. Newnham[1] and John R. G. Challis[2]

[1] School of Women's and Infants' Health and the Women and Infants Research Foundation, University of Western Australia, Western Australia
[2] Departments of Physiology, and Obstetrics and Gynaecology, University of Toronto, CIHR Group in Fetal and Neonatal Health and Development, CIHR Institute of Human Development, Child and Youth Health, Canada

Activation of the fetal hypothalamic–pituitary–adrenal (HPA) axis in late gestation is a common characteristic across species resulting in increased output of fetal glucocorticoids, contributing to mechanisms associated with the onset of parturition and maturation of organ systems required for extrauterine survival. The fetus responds to an adverse intrauterine environment with precocious HPA activation, and premature upregulation of critical genes at each level along the axis. Thus in utero the fetus may be exposed inappropriately to sustained elevations of glucocorticoids. In addition, fetal glucocorticoid concentrations may be elevated in circumstances of maternal stress, particularly in association with diminished activity of placental 11β-hydroxysteroid dehydrogenase type 2 (11β-HSD2) activity, or after maternal administration of synthetic glucocorticoids. Animal studies have demonstrated that glucocorticoid administration in late gestation results in intrauterine growth restriction (IUGR) and significant alterations in metabolic and HPA axis function and regulation.

These associations among elevated fetal glucocorticoid concentrations and growth and development may underlie the increased incidence of spontaneous preterm labor in small-for-gestational-age babies. They possibly contribute to mechanisms by which aberrant development in utero predisposes to different pathophysiologies in later life. Over the last 10–15 years epidemiological studies have shown that a suboptimal intrauterine environment is associated with an increased risk of developing cardiovascular disease, hypertension, type 2 diabetes and 'syndrome X' (metabolic syndrome). This chapter will describe animal studies that seek to determine the relationship between fetal HPA axis and metabolic development and function, aberrant postnatal endocrine responsiveness and the risk of developing long-term disease.

The fetal HPA axis

Glucocorticoids are essential for life and have a wide spectrum of effects. In mammals, the primary glucocorticoids are cortisol (primates and sheep) and corticosterone (rodents). Activation of the HPA axis causes the synthesis and release of corticotrophin-releasing hormone (CRH) and/or arginine vasopressin (AVP) from neurosecretory cells of the paraventricular nucleus (PVN) of the hypothalamus into the hypophyseal portal system to target corticotroph cells within the anterior lobe region of the pituitary gland. Here, CRH and AVP stimulate the synthesis of a polypeptide precursor pro-opiomelanocortin (POMC), which is then cleaved by processing enzymes to produce adrenocorticotrophic hormone (ACTH) in addition to smaller molecular weight peptides (Dallman *et al.*, 1987, for detailed review see Matthews and Challis, 1998). ACTH stimulates the synthesis and release of glucocorticoids from the zona fasciculata of the adrenal cortex (Dallman *et al.*, 1987). In turn, glucocorticoids regulate their own release through the action of negative and positive feedback systems. Circulating glucocorticoid levels are maintained through the action of a negative feedback system present within the brain (hippocampus and hypothalamus) and pituitary via corticosteroid receptors (Keller-Wood and Dallman, 1984).

The hippocampus exerts an inhibitory influence on basal, circadian and stress-induced HPA activity (Jacobson and Sapolsky, 1991). Central corticosteroid receptors in the hippocampus are thought to play a critical role in the regulation of HPA activity (De Kloet *et al.*, 1990; 1998; Meijer and De Kloet, 1998). Two corticosteroid receptors are present in the hippocampus: type 1, mineralocorticoid receptor (MR), identical to the kidney MR; and type 2, the classic glucocorticoid receptor (GR). MR-bind cortisol/corticosterone with an affinity that is, 10-fold greater ($Kd \sim 0.5\,nM$) than that of GR ($Kd \sim 5.0\,nM$) (Bamberger *et al.*, 1996; De Kloet *et al.*, 1998). In most species, the hippocampus exhibits the highest levels of corticosteroid receptors of any brain region (Jacobson and Sapolsky, 1991; De Kloet *et al.*, 1998) and is one of the few regions to express both MR and GR (Reul and De Kloet, 1985). Under most circumstances MR are thought to regulate basal or circadian trough levels of ACTH and cortisol. GR mediate the effects of circadian peak or stress-induced increases in HPA activity (Reul and De Kloet, 1985; Jacobson and Sapolsky, 1991). Alterations in MR and GR expression therefore influence basal and stress-induced increases in HPA activity.

The hypothalamus is divided into several nuclei including the paraventricular and supraoptic nuclei (PVN and SON, respectively). The PVN is a highly differentiated nucleus containing discrete regions of neurons that can be classified into three groups; those that project to the posterior pituitary, those associated with the autonomic nervous system, and those that project to the median eminence and affect anterior pituitary function. It is within this nucleus that CRH and AVP neurons are primarily localized in discrete areas. In fetal sheep CRH and AVP are considered to be primary factors driving ACTH release from the anterior pituitary corticotroph in vivo (Norman and Challis, 1987) and in vitro (Durand *et al.*, 1986; Matthews and Challis, 1997). Hypothalamic PVN lesions in fetal sheep have been shown to prevent the normal gestational rise in circulating ACTH and cortisol levels and decrease the ACTH and cortisol response to hypotensive stress (McDonald *et al.*, 1988; 1991). Immunoreactive (ir)-CRH and CRH bioactivity have been detected in hypothalamic extracts from human fetuses by 12–13 weeks of gestation (Ackland *et al.*, 1986) and CRH synthesis and secretion in the fetal hypothalamus increases with advancing gestation.

Anatomical maturation of corticotrophs within the anterior pituitary during development parallels a change in corticotroph function. Ir-ACTH levels increase with advancing gestation in both fetal plasma and in the anterior pituitary of fetal sheep (Norman *et al.*, 1985; Perry *et al.*, 1985; McMillen *et al.*, 1995). Corticotroph maturation appears to be regulated by the fetal hypothalamus and adrenal (McDonald *et al.*, 1992). Hypothalamic PVN lesions in fetal sheep delay fetal corticotroph maturation (McDonald *et al.*, 1992) and fetal adrenalectomy at 120 days of gestation resulted in a delay in the maturation of corticotrophs. This effect was reversed with cortisol infusion (Antolovich *et al.*, 1989).

In the human, rapid growth of the adrenal begins at ∼10 weeks of gestation and continues to term. The primate adrenal, unlike that of the fetal sheep, primarily secretes androgens, specifically dehydroepiandrostendione (DHEA) due to the low expression of 3β-HSD in the fetal zone of the adrenal. In primates, the placenta lacks the enzyme $P450_{C17}$ (17-hydroxylase, 17,20 desmolase) and therefore is dependant upon the production of DHEA from the fetal adrenal as the substrate for the synthesis of estrogens (Mesiano and Jaffe, 1997). The fetal sheep adrenal is somewhat different. In the fetal sheep, the adrenal gland is present by 28 days of gestation (Wintour *et al.*, 1975) and two distinct zones within the cortex are observed by day 60 (term is approximately 150 days) (Webb, 1980). Maturation of these zones begins later in gestation and although the outer zone resembles a mature zona glomerulosa and the inner zone resembles the zona fasciculata, the zona reticularis does not develop until postnatal life (Robinson *et al.*, 1979; Webb, 1980). Fetal adrenal responsiveness to ACTH changes over the course of gestation. Glickman and Challis (1980) demonstrated that basal cortisol output by cultured fetal sheep adrenal cells was significantly greater on day 50 of gestation than at day 100 or 130, but not different from term (150 days) adrenal tissue. In addition, adrenal responsiveness to ACTH stimulation followed a similar profile, in that adrenal cells responded to exogenous ACTH with elevated cortisol output early in gestation (50–60 days) followed by a loss in responsiveness at midgestation (90–125 days)

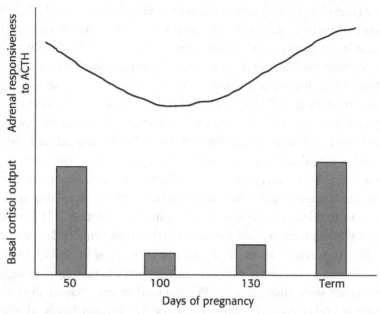

Figure 4.1   Schematic representation of basal cortisol output and adrenal responsiveness to ACTH in cultured fetal sheep adrenal cells with advancing gestation. Adapted from Glickman and Challis (1980)

and a re-emergence of responsiveness towards term (Wintour *et al.*, 1975; Glickman and Challis, 1980; Figure 4.1). Altered adrenal responsiveness has been attributed to an increase in ACTH receptor number (Durand *et al.*, 1980), enhanced sensitivity to ACTH via increased adenylyl cyclase activity, increased cyclic adenosine monophosphate (cAMP) levels (Durand *et al.*, 1981), or enhanced steroidogenic enzyme expression and activity (Durand *et al.*, 1982; Challis *et al.*, 1986).

In several species, normal fetal HPA axis function is essential for growth, development and for the onset of labor (Liggins, 1994). Glucocorticoids generally promote tissue and organ maturation at the expense of cellular proliferation, and are therefore responsible for the maturational changes of a variety of organ systems preparing the fetus for extrauterine life (Liggins, 1994; Fowden *et al.*, 1998). Most of these changes can be induced prematurely by exogenous glucocorticoid administration (Fowden, 1993; Liggins, 1994). In most species so far studied glucocorticoid concentrations in the fetus increase with advancing gestation (Fowden *et al.*, 1998) and negative feedback capability is apparent in the last third of gestation (Norman and Challis, 1985; Wintour *et al.*, 1985). In sheep, over the last 15 days of gestation the negative feedback effects of glucocorticoids on HPA function are attenuated, permitting concomitant increases in fetal plasma ACTH and cortisol levels (Challis and Brooks, 1989). Even in species that give birth to very immature young (including marsupials), the neonates have well developed adrenals and synthesize cortisol by 22 days of the 26 days gestation (Shaw and Renfee, 2001). It is this increase in circulating fetal cortisol concentrations that provides the stimulus for organ maturation and the trigger for parturition (Liggins, 1994; Challis *et al.*, 2000).

Placental-derived prostaglandin (PG) E_2 (PGE_2) has been shown to play a role in the activation of fetal HPA function. Fetal plasma PGE_2 concentrations rise progressively in late gestation with a time course that is similar to that seen in fetal plasma cortisol (Challis *et al.*, 1978). Infusion of PGE_2 into catheterized fetal sheep resulted in a significant elevation in circulating ACTH and cortisol concentrations (Louis *et al.*, 1976; Young *et al.*, 1996). PGE_2 infusion into hypophysectomized fetal sheep was not associated with changes in either ACTH or cortisol concentrations suggesting that PGs act via the hypothalamus to stimulate ACTH secretion (Young *et al.*, 1996). At term cortisol can act directly on placental PGH_2 synthase type 2 (PGHS2) to further increase PGE_2 output (Whittle *et al.*, 2000). Placental PGE_2 may represent a positive feed-forward mechanism whereby an increase in fetal glucocorticoids stimulates placental PG production and PGs further stimulate an increase in fetal HPA activity (Brooks *et al.*, 1996). Glucocorticoids can also act on PG metabolizing enzymes (15-OH PG dehydrogenase, PGDH) to alter local levels of PGs.

The developmental programming of adult disease

Subtle changes in the intrauterine environment are important in determining the health and development of the fetus and can result in effects that are seen much later in adulthood. The fetal programming hypothesis outlines the possibility of an intrauterine factor mediating cellular growth and development at a vulnerable time in gestation, subsequently resulting in permanent alterations in tissue and organ function that are apparent later in life (Barker, 1994; Seckl, 1997). IUGR is associated with an increased incidence of developing an array of diseases in adulthood including coronary artery disease, hypertension, insulin resistance and type 2 diabetes.

Glucocorticoids late in gestation provide maturational signals to many fetal organ systems and are imperative for the onset of parturition in most species. Alterations in the level of glucocorticoid exposure could potentially disrupt the balance of HPA development and function. It is therefore critical for the fetus to strictly control the levels and timing of the pre-partum increase in glucocorticoids. There are several features of fetal exposure to elevated levels of glucocorticoids that support its role in the programming of adult disease (Seckl, 1997). Human studies have shown that fetal levels of ACTH and cortisol are increased in association with IUGR (Goland *et al.*, 1993). Glucocorticoids increase blood pressure in adults (Tonolo *et al.*, 1988) and cortisol infusion into the fetal sheep results in elevated fetal blood pressure (Dodic and Wintour, 1994). Prenatal stress or glucocorticoid administration has

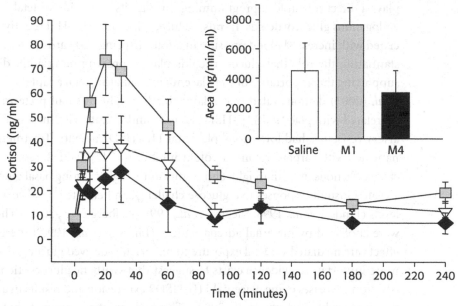

Figure 4.2   One single dose of betamethasone administered to ewes at 104 days of gestation
resulted in significant increases in cortisol responsiveness to a CRH with AVP challenge
in their lambs at 1 year of postnatal age. M1 (shaded squares) represents animals that
received one single dose of betamethasone at 104 days of gestation followed by 3 weekly
injections of saline. M4 (black diamonds) represents animals that received 4 weekly doses
of maternal betamethasone beginning at 104 days of gestation. MS (open triangles)
represents animals that received four doses of saline at weekly intervals starting at 104
days of gestation. Histograms represent the area under the cortisol response curves.
All values are expressed at mean ± SEM. Adapted from Sloboda et al. (2002a)

been shown by numerous studies to alter growth and HPA activity as well as glucose tolerance (Uno et al., 1990; Weinstock et al., 1992; Lindsay et al., 1996; Welberg
and Seckl, 2001; Figure 4.2). Low birth weight in humans correlates with increased
adult cortisol levels as well as insulin resistance and elevated blood pressure
(Phillips et al., 1998; Levitt et al., 2000; Reynolds et al., 2001).

Prenatal glucocorticoid exposure and fetal programming

The placenta and prenatal stress

The placental enzyme 11β-HSD2 acts as a dehydrogenase enzyme, rapidly converting
active glucocorticoids to inactive metabolites (Edwards et al., 1993; Krozowski, 1999)
and represents a barrier reducing fetal exposure to elevated levels of maternally-
derived glucocorticoids (Brown et al., 1993). As a result placental 11β-HSD2

plays a direct role in fetal programming through its regulation of fetal exposure to endogenous glucocorticoids. In rats, reduced placental 11β-HSD2 activity is associated with increased blood pressure in adult offspring (Edwards *et al.*, 1993), substantiating the role that glucocorticoids play in programming adult disease and supporting the importance of the placenta in regulating fetal adaptations. Kajantie *et al.* (2003) demonstrated that relative birth weight in small preterm infants is correlated with placental 11β-HSD2 activity and infants with increased umbilical artery resistance had lower total placental 11β-HSD2 activity. Treatment of pregnant rats with carbenoxolone, a potent inhibitor of 11β-HSD2, results in significant reductions in birth weight, and significantly higher fasting basal glucose levels, elevated insulin responses to a glucose challenge and elevated basal corticosterone levels (Lindsay *et al.*, 1996; Saegusa *et al.*, 1999; Welberg *et al.*, 2000). These results were abolished by maternal adrenalectomy (Lindsay *et al.*, 1996); therefore these effects are mediated via fetal exposure to maternally-derived glucocorticoids. Even more importantly, evidence exists to suggest that synthetic glucocorticoid administration decreases ovine placental 11β-HSD2 expression and results in a reduction in fetal weight (Kerzner *et al.*, 2002). These observations suggest that following synthetic glucocorticoid administration the fetus is not only exposed to exogenous glucocorticoids, but also may be exposed to increased levels of maternally-derived endogenous glucocorticoids.

Prenatal maternal stress increases maternal endogenous glucocorticoid levels potentially resulting in fetal exposure to elevated levels of glucocorticoid during development. Prenatal stress has been shown to permanently program the pattern of HPA and metabolic responses, even though these relationships are complex, and subtle differences in stimuli exert different effects (Seckl, 1997). Most human data come from retrospective studies on children whose mothers experienced psychological stress during pregnancy (Weinstock, 1996; Austin and Leader, 2000; Niederhofer and Reiter, 2000). Some of these children have delayed motor development and abnormal behavioral characteristics (Weinstock, 1996). Experimental evidence suggests that stress increases both maternal and fetal glucocorticoid levels and that maternally-derived glucocorticoids may program postnatal HPA activity (Barbazanges *et al.*, 1996; Takahashi, 1998). Stress during pregnancy in the rat has resulted in offspring with elevated basal plasma ACTH and corticosterone levels (Takahashi and Kalin, 1991), increased corticosterone and ACTH responses to a stressor (Takahashi and Kalin, 1991; Weinstock *et al.*, 1992; Barbazanges *et al.*, 1996) and altered anxiety behavior (Weinstock *et al.*, 1992). It has been shown that postnatal responses of prenatally stressed offspring can be suppressed by maternal adrenalectomy, further supporting the observation that maternally-derived glucocorticoids program postnatal alterations in HPA function (Barbazanges *et al.*, 1996).

A substantial body of evidence exists describing HPA function after postnatal manipulations in the neonatal rat (Meaney *et al.*, 1985; 1989; Liu *et al.*, 1997; Avishai-Eliner *et al.*, 2001). The rodent gives birth to immature offspring and the period of rapid brain growth associated with HPA development occurs in the first 2 weeks of postnatal life (Rosenfeld *et al.*, 1992). Therefore, the rat HPA axis is susceptible to programming in the early postnatal period. Early postnatal events such as maternal separation or neonatal handling, result in significant elevations in hippocampal GR-binding capacity and number (Meaney *et al.*, 1985; 1989), reduced plasma ACTH and corticosterone responses to stress and enhanced glucocorticoid feedback sensitivity (Liu *et al.*, 1997). These occur at a time in which the HPA axis is relatively quiescent in the developing neonate (Rosenfeld *et al.*, 1992). Therefore, neonatal handling during a critical developmental window (1–3 weeks postnatally) in the rat results in permanent alterations in HPA function as a result of alterations in hippocampal corticosteroid receptors. Several studies have shown that the prenatal effects of stress are reversible by early postnatal manipulations. Prenatally stressed rats exposed to postnatal handling exhibited significantly lower corticosterone responses to stress as adults (Vallee *et al.*, 1996). Postnatal adoption that encourages maternal interaction with pups also reverses the effects of prenatal stress, decreasing stress-induced corticosterone peak levels in adult offspring (Maccari *et al.*, 1995). These observations highlight the importance of different developmental windows, during which exposure to elevated glucocorticoid levels may produce permanent effects. It has been suggested that in the rat prenatal stress may have to occur several days beyond birth in order to cause permanent effects (Takahashi, 1998). This concept is somewhat different in mammals that exhibit HPA axis development and brain growth in the prenatal or perinatal period such as in the primate or sheep.

Antenatal administration of glucocorticoids

Over 30 years ago, Liggins (1969) demonstrated that lambs delivered prematurely (118–123 days of gestation) after fetal infusions of ACTH, cortisol or dexamethasone exhibited advanced alveolar stability in their lungs and suggested that the maturational properties of glucocorticoids caused premature pulmonary development and maturation. Subsequently, Liggins and Howie (1972) were the first to demonstrate that the administration of maternal glucocorticoids to women at risk of preterm delivery significantly enhanced fetal lung maturation and reduced neonatal morbidity and mortality. In this study, women in premature labor at 24–34 weeks of gestation were admitted into the first controlled trial of antepartum glucocorticoid treatment for the prevention of respiratory distress syndrome (RDS) in premature infants (Liggins and Howie, 1972). The administration protocol consisted of an intramuscular injection of a mixture of 6 mg of betamethasone phosphate and 6 mg of betamethasone acetate or a control injection, followed by a second injection 24 hours later. The incidence of RDS in preterm infants was reduced by 50% and neonatal death in the first 7 days of life was significantly less frequent, although the maximum effects were seen if delivery occurred more than 24 hours and less than 7 days after treatment (Liggins and Howie, 1972). Synthetic glucocorticoids such as betamethasone and dexamethasone are 25–30 times more potent glucocorticoids than cortisol with insignificant mineralocorticoid action (Speight, 1987). Furthermore, synthetic glucocorticoids do not bind to circulating binding proteins (corticosteroid binding protein/corticosteroid binding globulin, CBG) (Pugeat *et al.*, 1981) and are poor substrates for metabolism by placental 11β-HSD2 (Siebe *et al.*, 1993) making synthetic glucocorticoids prime candidates for clinical management of women at risk of preterm delivery.

Since the first report by Liggins and Howie (1972), multiple trials have demonstrated a decrease in the number of cases of RDS and mortality among treated infants (Kari *et al.*, 1994; Ballard and Ballard, 1996; Anyaegbunam *et al.*, 1997; Ee *et al.*, 1998). In 1995, The National Institutes of Health (NIH) Consensus Developmental Conference on the Effects of Corticosteroid for Fetal Maturation concluded that antenatal corticosteroid therapy for fetal lung maturation reduced mortality, RDS and intraventricular hemorrhage in preterm infants (NIH Consensus, 1995). According to the panel, corticosteroids should be administered to women at risk of preterm birth between 24 and 34 weeks of gestation and in a treatment window of 24 hours to 7 days prior to delivery. Since 1972, the administration of synthetic glucocorticoids to women threatened with preterm delivery has become routine practice. Until recently many medical practitioners assumed that more may be better. By the late 1990s surveys demonstrated that a high percentage of obstetricians prescribed repeat doses in cases of pregnant women who had a persisting risk of preterm delivery (Quinlivan *et al.*, 1998; Brocklehurst *et al.*, 1999). However, the mechanisms regulating the onset of preterm labor are poorly understood and as a result preterm labor is difficult to diagnose accurately. Given the increasing evidence suggesting that excessive fetal glucocorticoid exposure has long term consequences, it is worrying that women who are not in preterm labor may be receiving unnecessary corticosteroid administration.

There is substantial evidence from animal studies demonstrating that fetal exposure to elevated levels of glucocorticoids alters fetal growth and has long-term effects on cardiovascular, HPA and metabolic function. Early studies with rhesus monkeys demonstrated that maternal intramuscular betamethasone administration at 120–133 days of gestation (term = 167 days) resulted in significant reductions in fetal body weight of ~23% at 133 and 167 days of gestation. In addition, brain, cerebellar, pancreatic, adrenal and pituitary weights were all significantly reduced with treatment (Johnson *et al.*, 1981). Significant growth restriction has also been shown in most animal models studied (Bakker *et al.*, 1995; Levitt *et al.*, 1996; Nyirenda *et al.*, 1998; Newnham *et al.*, 1999; Thakur *et al.*, 2000; Sloboda *et al.*, 2000).

Some time ago, our research group developed a model to investigate the effects of maternal synthetic glucocorticoid administration on the developing fetal lung (Jobe *et al.*, 1993; Ikegami *et al.*, 1997). In this model intramuscular injections of betamethasone (0.5 mg/kg) are administered to the pregnant sheep, beginning at 104 days of gestation (term = 150 days), with repeated injections given again at 111, 118 and 125 days. This dose has been shown to be the minimal dose required for maximal fetal lung maturation in this model. In our model of maternal administration of synthetic glucocorticoids, fetal weight is significantly reduced in a dose dependant manner (Ikegami *et al.*, 1997, Newnham *et al.*, 1999; Figure 4.3), persisting until 3 months of postnatal age (Moss *et al.*, 2001). These alterations in body weight have been associated with significant reductions in whole brain and cerebellum weights, as well as reductions in the myelination of axons located in the optic nerve and the corpus callosum (Dunlop *et al.*, 1997; Huang *et al.*, 1999). Prenatal glucocorticoid exposure has long-term effects on brain growth, reducing brain weight in adult animals aged 3.5 years (Moss *et al.*, 2005). Such observations have important implications for the 'hard-wiring' of the brain and suggest that long-term brain function may be quite vulnerable to glucocorticoid administration. French *et al.* (1999) demonstrated a dose dependant reduction in neonatal head circumference with increasing doses of maternal corticosteroids in a geographical based cohort of preterm infants. Further, re-evaluation of these infants at 3 and 6 years of age demonstrated that children who had received 3 or more

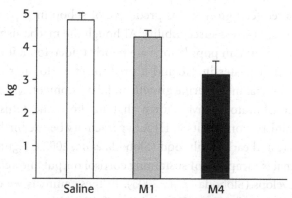

Figure 4.3   Betamethasone administration in ewes significantly reduces lamb birth weight in a dose-dependent manner. M1 represents animals that received one single dose of betamethasone at 104 days of gestation followed by three weekly injections of saline. M4 represents animals that received 4 weekly doses of maternal betamethasone beginning at 104 days of gestation. Adapted from Newnham *et al.* (1999)

courses of antenatal corticosteroids had significantly higher relative risks of demonstrating externalizing behavioral disorders (French *et al.*, 2003). This effect was specific to behavior with no differences in intelligence testing.

Adult disease and programming HPA axis function: human and animal evidence

Growth restricted babies have elevated levels of cord plasma CRH, ACTH and cortisol (Economides *et al.*, 1991; Goland *et al.*, 1993). In addition, increases in urinary glucocorticoid metabolites in children of 9 years of age were associated with reduced birth weight (Clark *et al.*, 1996). Recent epidemiological studies have begun to establish a strong correlation between circulating cortisol levels and the incidence of hypertension and diabetes. Phillips *et al.* (1998) have shown that fasting plasma cortisol levels in men aged 64 years were inversely related to birth weight, independent of body mass index (BMI), and that elevated cortisol levels were significantly associated with higher blood pressure, plasma glucose levels, fasting triglyceride levels and insulin resistance. More recently, low birth weight has been associated with elevated fasting and stimulated cortisol concentrations in adult human beings (Levitt *et al.*, 2000; Phillips *et al.*, 2000; Reynolds *et al.*, 2001). In each case, cortisol levels were positively associated with high-blood pressure and in some populations, associated with glucose intolerance (Levitt *et al.*, 2000; Reynolds *et al.*, 2001). These observations support a role for the programming of HPA axis function in the predisposition to adult disease. Nilsson *et al.* (2001) found that men with lower birth weight and a small head circumference at birth scored poorly on psychological assessment surveys compared to their heavier counterparts. It was suggested that impaired fetal growth was predictive of suboptimal psychological functioning and increased stress susceptibility. Although the mechanisms regulating these associations in human populations are poorly understood, it is apparent that elevated HPA activity later in life and a predisposition to later disease are linked to alterations in fetal intrauterine growth and development.

Studies from our laboratory have shown that in the ovine fetus maternal betamethasone administration results in HPA hyperactivity before birth (Sloboda *et al.*, 2000; Table 4.1) and early adulthood (Sloboda *et al.*, 2002a; Figure 4.2), but later in life the adrenal is incapable of sustaining cortisol output and relative adrenal insufficiency develops (Sloboda *et al.*, 2003). In these animals we observed a dose dependant increase in basal ACTH levels in adulthood, associated with significant reductions in basal cortisol levels. Although alterations in HPA function exist in offspring exposed in utero to either single or multiple doses of maternal betamethasone, the changes were most pronounced in offspring that were exposed to multiple doses. Our observations suggest that prenatal betamethasone exposure

Table 4.1 Betamethasone administration in ewes at 3 weekly doses beginning at 104 days of gestation significantly alters cortisol-binding capacity (CBC) at 125 days of gestation and increases fetal HPA activity at 146 days of gestation

Variables	125 days of gestation		146 days of gestation	
	Control ($n = 5$)	Betamethasone ($n = 6$)	Control ($n = 7$)	Betamethasone ($n = 8$)
ACTH (pg/ml)	29.5 ± 3.0	36.0 ± 10.1	54.6 ± 5.2	$82.1 \pm 6.7^*$
Cortisol (ng/ml)	3.2 ± 0.6	1.9 ± 0.3	12.5 ± 2.2	35.7 ± 17.8
CBC (ng/ml)	17.3 ± 3.2	$47.9 \pm 10.7^*$	57.3 ± 17.7	54.3 ± 14.4

All values are mean $\pm$ SEM, $^*P < 0.05$.
Source: Adapted from Sloboda *et al.* (2000).

in the sheep results in a dynamic sequence of altered adrenal function after birth beginning with hyper- and ending with hypo-responsiveness by adulthood. A single cross-sectional study after birth therefore, may provide a misleading impression of life-long consequences. The exact mechanisms regulating this evolution in HPA responsiveness are unknown; however it seems likely that adrenal receptor and/or steroidogenic enzyme expression or activity are likely to be altered in these animals.

The potential impact of fetal glucocorticoid exposure on the developing HPA axis may occur via the GR, which is expressed at every level of the axis. Synthetic glucocorticoids can potentially impact at the level of the brain, hypothalamus, pituitary and/or the adrenal. Remarkably little is known regarding the mechanisms that regulate alterations in HPA function following maternal glucocorticoid administration and their relationship to postnatal disease. In most models, programming of the HPA axis has been associated with alterations in hippocampal corticosteroid receptor populations (Uno *et al.*, 1994; Levitt *et al.*, 1996; Dean and Matthews, 1999). Negative feedback at the level of the hippocampus results in an inhibition of HPA activity, therefore reduced glucocorticoid feedback through alterations in receptor number would elevate HPA activity (Jacobson and Sapolsky, 1991). HPA hyperactivity has been demonstrated following prenatal undernutrition in the guinea pig (Lingas *et al.*, 1999), prenatal stress in the rat (Takahashi and Kalin, 1991; Weinstock *et al.*, 1992) as well as maternal glucocorticoid administration in the rat (Levitt *et al.*, 1996), rhesus monkey (Uno *et al.*, 1994) and sheep (Sloboda *et al.*, 2000).

Maternal administration of dexamethasone in the rhesus monkey at 132 and 133 days of gestation (term = 165 days) results in significant alterations in the cytoarchitechtural development of hippocampal neurons at 135 days of gestation

(Uno *et al.*, 1990). Degeneration of neurons and a significant reduction in the size of the whole hippocampal formation were observed in dexamethasone-treated fetuses at 135 and 162 days of gestation. Those fetuses that received multiple injections showed more severe damage, suggesting that these effects were dose dependant (Uno *et al.*, 1990). Furthermore, at 10 months of postnatal age, dexamethasone-treated offspring demonstrated higher basal cortisol levels and higher plasma cortisol levels following stress (Uno *et al.*, 1994). In other experiments maternal dexamethasone treatment in the guinea pig on 50–51 days of gestation (term = 70 days) resulted in significant increases in basal cortisol levels in female fetuses but not male fetuses. Furthermore, dexamethasone exposure resulted in significant increases in MR and GR messenger ribonucleic acid (mRNA) in the hippocampus of female fetuses but not in males (Dean and Matthews, 1999).

Prenatal glucocorticoid exposure and postnatal metabolic function: type 2 diabetes

Many studies have proposed that the increased incidence of glucose intolerance and insulin resistance associated with type 2 diabetes later in life may be programmed in utero (Ravelli *et al.*, 1998). In human beings, low birth weight has been associated with a higher incidence of syndrome X; a cluster of risk factors including insulin resistance, glucose intolerance, hyper-insulinemia, hyper-triglyceridemia, decreased high-density lipoprotein cholesterol, and hypertension (syndrome X; Reaven, 1988). This syndrome is accompanied by alterations in the HPA axis and cortisol metabolism. Early studies found the risk of developing glucose intolerance and diabetes later in life was double in men who had low birth weights (Ravelli *et al.*, 1998). Low birth weight in the rat has also been correlated with a reduction in pancreatic function and impaired β-cell growth and function (Berney *et al.*, 1997).

Recent studies suggest that the effects of prenatal growth restriction in combination with accelerated postnatal growth may have important metabolic implications. Girls born within the lowest birth weight tertile that end up with a BMI in the highest tertile have a 30% increased risk of developing syndrome X (Yarbrough *et al.*, 1998). The presence of prenatal growth restriction in combination with increased postnatal weight gain or velocity has serious effects on carbohydrate metabolism even in young children. Bavdekar *et al.* (1999) demonstrated that the highest incidence of insulin resistance, high plasma total and low-density lipid (LDL) cholesterol and fasting insulin levels, were observed in children who had been of low birth weight and at 8 years of age were of high fat mass and height. Others suggest that insulin resistance and pancreatic β-cell activity/dysfunction may be regulated by growth velocity between birth and 7 years of age (Crowther *et al.*, 2000). Small for gestational age neonates also exhibit insulin resistance, especially those children with catch-up growth and increases in BMI (Veening *et al.*, 2002).

The relationship between low birth weight and type 2 diabetes in adult life has been described by the *thrifty phenotype hypothesis* (Hales *et al.*, 1992). This hypothesis proposes that the metabolic development of the fetus is programmed in utero in a way that influences postnatal metabolic responses. The developmental mechanisms that underpin the *thrifty phenotype hypothesis* are multifactorial. Although much of the hypothesis was formulated around prenatal undernutrition, current evidence points to prenatal exposure to elevated levels of glucocorticoids as a major contributor in fetal programming. In the rat, maternal treatment with carbenoxolone, a placental 11β-HSD2 inhibitor, allows increased passage of maternal glucocorticoids to the fetus and resulted in reduced birth weight and glucose intolerance in offspring (Lindsay *et al.*, 1996). We have shown previously that as little as one dose of maternally administered betamethasone in the sheep results in insulin responses to a glucose challenge that are similar to those seen in type 2 diabetes (Moss *et al.*, 2001; Figure 4.4).

Although the mechanisms are unclear, prenatal glucocorticoid overexposure can potentially program a number of organ systems regulating glucose homeostasis. Glucocorticoids regulate skeletal muscle glucose transporter expression (Coderre *et al.*, 1996), reduce basal and insulin stimulated glucose uptake and impair glucose transporter recruitment (Weinstien *et al.*, 1995; 1998). Glucocorticoids have been shown to regulate insulin secretion (Lambillote *et al.*, 1997) and the expression of factors regulating pancreatic growth and remodelling, such as pancreatic duodenal homeobox-1 (Pdx-1) and insulin-like growth factor 2 (IGF2) (Sander *et al.*, 1997; Hill, 1999). Fetal rat corticosteroid concentrations are negatively correlated with pancreatic insulin content, and β-cell mass increased when fetal steroid production was impaired (Blondeau *et al.*, 2001). It is unknown if fetal glucocorticoid exposure permanently alters fetal β-cell development in a way that alters life-long adult pancreatic morphology and function. It seems likely however, that altered pancreatic function would impair postnatal metabolic function. Expression of hepatic gluconeogenic enzymes (phosphophenolpyruvate carboxykinase, PEPCK) in offspring of dexamethasone-treated pregnant rats is increased, an effect that persists up to 8 months of postnatal age. These rats demonstrated a significant reduction in birth weight as well as fasting hyperglycemia and elevated glucose and insulin responses to glucose loading (Nyirenda *et al.*, 1998). Such observations may have important relevance in terms of hepatic insulin resistance, since transgenic mice over-expressing PEPCK exhibit increases in hepatic glucose output, increases in glucose-6 phosphatase levels, decreased insulin receptor substrate 2 (IRS-2) levels and decreased phosphatidyl inositol 3 (PI_3) kinase activity. Recent data suggest that programming of GR expression in rats prenatally

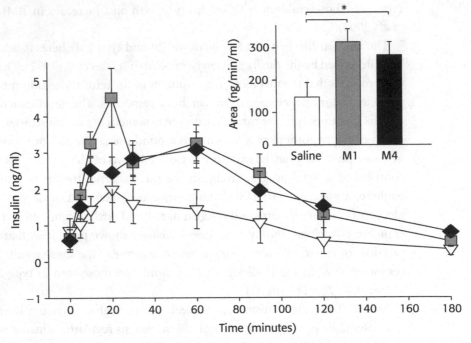

Figure 4.4   Maternal betamethasone administered at 104 days of gestation (M1) or on 4 occasions at weekly intervals (M4) resulted in significant increases in insulin responsiveness to a glucose challenge at 6 months of postnatal age, compared with saline administration (MS). M1 (shaded squares) represents animals that received one single dose of betamethasone at 104 days of gestation followed by 3 weekly injections of saline. M4 (black diamonds) represents animals that received 4 weekly doses of maternal betamethasone beginning at 104 days of gestation. MS (open triangles) represents animals that received 4 doses of saline at weekly intervals starting at 104 days of gestation. Histograms represent the area under the insulin response curves. Values are expressed as mean ± SEM. *P < 0.05. Adapted from Moss *et al.* (2001)

overexposed to glucocorticoids may be a primary mechanism of insulin resistance (Cleasby *et al.*, 2003). We have previously shown that repeated exposure of the fetal sheep to glucocorticoids results in significant increases in hepatic 11β-HSD1 and CBG levels (Sloboda *et al.*, 2002a) (Figures 4.5 and 4.6). These data suggest that glucocorticoids may not only directly program metabolic enzymes, but also program intra-hepatic levels of glucocorticoids, thus providing a feed-forward loop of glucocorticoid effects. The gluconeogenic responses of 11β-HSD1 knockout mice were attenuated after stress and these animals resist hyperglycemia induced by chronic high-fat feeding. These observations support 11β-HSD1 as an important amplifier of intra-hepatic glucocorticoid action in vivo (Kotelevtsev *et al.*, 1997).

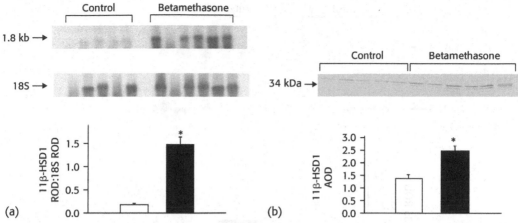

Figure 4.5   Repeated doses of maternally administered betamethasone significantly increased fetal
sheep hepatic 11β-HSD1 mRNA and protein levels at 125 days of gestation. Fetal sheep
hepatic 11β-HSD1 mRNA (a) and protein (b) levels following either saline (open bar) or
maternal betamethasone (shaded bars) administration are represented in histograms.
The relative optical density (ROD) of 11β-HSD1 mRNA was expressed as a ratio 11β-HSD1
ROD:18S ROD. 11β-HSD1 protein levels are expressed as arbitrary optical density
(AOD) units. Values presented as mean ± SEM. *$P < 0.05$. Adapted from Sloboda
et al. (2002a)

Glucocorticoids may program postnatal metabolism through an increase in
postnatal accumulation of visceral fat. The risk factors for diabetes rise as body fat
content increases and visceral fat depots are strongly linked to insulin resistance
and syndrome X (Kahn *et al.*, 2000). In cases of glucocorticoid excess, such as
Cushing's syndrome, visceral adiposity is increased (Wolf, 2002) and tissue specific
changes in peripheral cortisol metabolism have been suggested to play a central
role. 11β-HSD1 is localized specifically to omental adipose cells, regulating the
conversion of inactive cortisone to active cortisol (Bujalska *et al.*, 1999). 11β-
HSD1 expression and activity are associated with an increased incidence of central
obesity and glucose intolerance (Rask *et al.*, 2002). The expression of 11β-HSD1 in
cultured omental adipose cells is elevated with cortisol treatment (Bujalska *et al.*,
1997). Although there are no data regarding the effects of prenatal glucocorticoids
on postnatal cortisol metabolism in adipocytes, it is possible that prenatal glucocorticoids may program intra-adipocyte cortisol levels via effects on 11β-HSD.

Recently, it has been shown that cortisol is necessary for promoting fetal ovine
adipose tissue maturation (Mostyn *et al.*, 2003), but the mechanisms remain unclear.
GRs have been localized to pre-adipocytes in both visceral and subcutaneous fat and
glucocorticoids have been shown to enhance pre-adipocyte differentiation (Joyner
et al., 2000). Excess cortisol in adipose tissue counteracts the insulin inhibition of

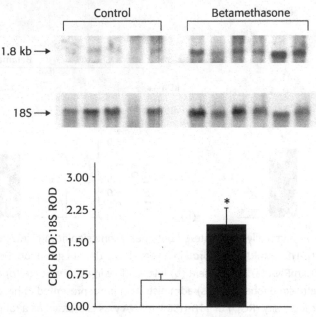

Figure 4.6   Repeated doses of maternally administered betamethasone significantly increased fetal sheep hepatic CBG mRNA levels at 125 days of gestation. Fetal sheep hepatic CBG mRNA levels at 125 days of gestation following either saline (open bar) or maternal betamethasone (shaded bars) administration. The ROD of CBG mRNA was expressed as a ratio CBG ROD:18S ROD. Values presented as mean ± SEM. $^{*}P < 0.05$. Adapted from Sloboda *et al.* (2002a)

lipolysis and has been shown to cause insulin resistance (Brindley, 1995). These observations are important since we have shown previously that prenatal gluco-corticoid administration in the sheep significantly affects long-term postnatal HPA function (Sloboda *et al.*, 2002a; 2003) and results in patterns of insulin resistance at 1 year of age (Moss *et al.*, 2001). Although it is unknown whether prenatal glucocorticoid treatment alters postnatal adiposity, our observations suggest prenatal programming of postnatal HPA function is closely linked with postnatal metabolism. It is possible that this association may be through prenatal programming of postnatal adiposity.

Research into the role of leptin in obesity has verified a link between adipose tissue, the brain and the endocrine system. Leptin, a polypeptide encoded by the Ob gene, is secreted by adipose tissue and is believed to regulate energy balance, feeding behavior and adiposity. The adipoinsular axis is a complex feedback system between the brain, adipocytes and pancreatic β cells. Leptin sensitive neurons in the arcuate nucleus of the hypothalamus that express neuropeptide Y (NPY), among other neuropeptides, are central in the regulation of food intake and satiety

(Ahima and Flier, 2000). NPY stimulates food intake, inhibits sympathetic nervous activity, lowers energy expenditure and increases HPA activity. This integrated response promotes fat accumulation and storage (Schwartz et al., 1997). Leptin inhibits NPY release and reduces appetite and food intake, therefore in cases of leptin deficiency or dysfunction, NPY release is increased, increasing food intake. Leptin sensitive neurons project to the PVN and may regulate HPA axis activity. The exact pathways by which leptin regulates HPA activity are controversial. There is evidence that leptin can stimulate and inhibit CRH release from the PVN, thereby altering downstream glucocorticoid release from the adrenal (Schwartz et al., 1997). Furthermore, leptin acts on a number of tissues (skeletal muscle, liver, etc.) regulating glucose production and uptake, lipid metabolism and insulin secretion (Fruhbeck and Salvador, 2000), complicating the pathway even further.

Obesity is characterized by high circulating leptin levels and increased adipose expression of leptin. Hyperleptinemia is considered to be an indication of leptin resistance (Ahima and Flier, 2000; Speigelman and Flier, 2001). Although the concept of leptin resistance is poorly understood, it appears that defects in leptin synthesis, receptors and/or defects in downstream mediators of leptin action result in a dysregulation of energy balance, food intake and body weight (Speigelman and Flier, 2001; Bowen et al., 2003). Central leptin resistance (hypothalamus) may contribute to alterations in satiety accompanied by changes in food intake and peripheral leptin resistance may contribute to hyperinsulinemia and adiposity (Ahima and Flier, 2000; Breier et al., 2001). Therefore leptin resistance may be one important factor in the development of obesity and type 2 diabetes. Recent reports suggest that leptin resistance may be programmed in utero (Breier et al., 2001). Vickers et al. (2000; 2001) were the first to describe the possibility of programming leptin resistance. In these rat studies, offspring from undernourished mothers were smaller at birth and exhibited elevated plasma insulin and leptin levels. Offspring exhibited a significant elevation in food intake and obesity. Recently Cleasby et al. (2003) have demonstrated that prenatal exposure to glucocorticoids results in changes in GR expression levels in muscle and fat in rats at 6 months of postnatal age. These offspring also exhibited alterations in factors that regulate free fatty acid uptake. Although the mechanisms are poorly understood, these observations suggest that intrauterine events can permanently alter the regulation of the adipoinsular axis.

Concluding remarks

In this chapter we have highlighted the importance of normal development and maturation of the fetal HPA axis for extrauterine survival. Increased levels of cortisol are necessary for normal growth and development and also provide a component of the

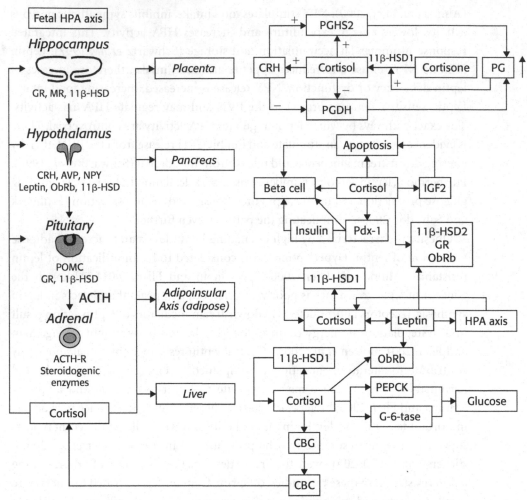

Figure 4.7   Schematic representation laying out glucocorticoid sensitive placental-fetal pathways hypothesized to be involved in programming HPA function and metabolic regulation. Adapted from data based on Ahima and Flier (2000), Challis *et al.* (2002), Sloboda *et al.* (2000; 2002a)

stimulus to the onset of parturition. Fetal exposure to elevated levels of glucocorticoids (either endogenous or exogenous) at inappropriate times of development however, has serious consequences on organ development and life-long health. The potential effects of elevated circulating glucocorticoids can be seen in most endocrine axes. Those organ systems are vulnerable that possess high levels of the GR and 11β-HSD, since both circulating concentrations of cortisol and intra-tissue concentrations of cortisol can have long-term effects on glucocorticoid sensitive genes (see Figure 4.7). Furthermore, the association between an adverse intrauterine environment and fetal hypercortisolemia may underlie the increased incidence of spontaneous preterm labor in small-for-gestational-age babies (see Figure 4.7). This may contribute to mechanisms by which aberrant development in utero predisposes to different pathophysiologies in later life. Clinically, preterm birth represents a human model whereby fetuses are often exposed to high levels of synthetic glucocorticoids prior to birth. The diagnosis of preterm birth is often difficult and in recent times women may have received repeated courses of antenatal glucocorticoids when administration may have been unnecessary. Basic science research has already made significant progress in changing clinical practice in an effort to minimize fetal exposure to synthetic glucocorticoids. Recently, an NIH Consensus Statement (2001) recommended that repeated courses of maternal synthetic glucocorticoid should not be administered to women threatened with preterm delivery, except for those enrolled in randomized controlled trials currently underway in North America, the United Kingdom and Australia. Health care providers and basic science research share a partnership in the management of preterm delivery to improve clinical care and investigate the mechanisms regulating preterm delivery and the management of preterm and term infants as newborns and adults.

REFERENCES

Ackland, J. F., Ratter, S., Bourne, G. L. and Rees L. H. (1986). Corticotrophin-releasing factor – like immunoreactivity and bioactivity of human fetal and adult hypothalami. *J. Endocrinol.*, **108**, 171–80.

Antolovich, G. C., Perry, R. A., Trahair, J. F., Silver, M. and Robinson, P. M. (1989). The development of corticotrophs in the fetal sheep pars distalis; the effect of adrenalectomy or cortisol infusion. *Endocrinology*, **124**, 1333–9.

Ahima, R. S. and Flier, J. S. (2000). *Leptin. Annu. Rev. Physiol.*, **62**, 413–37.

Anyaegbunam, W. I. and Adetona, A. B. (1997). Use of antenatal corticosteroids for fetal maturation in preterm infants. *Am. Fam. Physician*, **56**, 1093–6.

Austin, M. P. and Leader, L. R. (2000). Maternal stress and obstetric and infant outcomes: epidemiological findings and neuroendocrine mechanisms. *Aust. NZ. Obstet Gyn.*, **40**, 331–7.

Avishai-Eliner, S., Eghbal-Ahmadi, M., Tabachnik, E., Brunson, K. L. and Baram, T. Z. (2001). Down-regulation of hypothalamic corticotropin-releasing hormone messenger ribonucleic acid (mRNA) precedes early life experience – induced changes in hippocampal glucocorticoid receptor mRNA. *Endocrinology*, **142**, 89–97.

Bakker, J. M., Schmidt, E. D., Kroes, H. *et al.* (1995). Effects of short-term dexamethasone treatment during pregnancy on the development of the immune system and the hypothalamo–pituitary adrenal axis in the rat. *J. Neuroimmunol.*, **63**, 183–191.

Ballard, R. A. and Ballard, P. L. (1996). Antenatal hormone therapy for improving the outcome of the preterm infant. *J. Perinatol.*, **16**, 390–6.

Bamberger, C. M., Schulte, H. M. and Chrousos, G. P. (1996). Molecular determinants of gluco-corticoid receptor function and tissue sensitivity to glucocorticoids. *Endocr. Rev.*, **17**, 245–60.

Barbazanges, A., Piazza, P. V., Le Moal, M. and Maccari, S. (1996). Maternal glucocorticoid secretion mediates long-term effects of prenatal stress. *J. Neurosci.*, **16**, 3943–9.

Barker, D. J. P. (1994). The fetal origins of adult disease. *Fetal Matern. Med. Rev.*, **6**, 71–80.

Bavdekar, A., Yajnik, C. S., Fall, C. H. *et al.* (1999). Insulin resistance syndrome in 8-year-old Indian children: small at birth, big at 8 years, or both? *Diabetes*, **48**, 2422–9.

Berney, D. M., Desai, M., Greenwald, S. *et al.* (1997). The effects of maternal protein deprivation on the fetal rat pancreas: major structural changes and their recuperation. *J. Pathol.*, **183**, 109–15.

Blondeau, B., Lesage, J., Czernichow, P., Dupouy, J. P. and Breant, B. (2001). Glucocorticoids impair fetal beta-cell development in rats. *Am. J. Physiol. Endocrinol. Metab.*, **281**, E592–9.

Bowen, H., Mitchell, T. D. and Harris, R. B. (2003). Method of leptin dosing, strain, and group housing influence leptin sensitivity in high-fat-fed weanling mice. *Am. J. Physiol. Regul. Integr. Comp. Physiol.*, **284**(1), R87–100.

Breier, B. H., Vickers, M. H., Ikenasio, B. A., Chan, K. Y. and Wong, W. P. (2001). Fetal programming of appetite and obesity. *Mol. Cell. Endocrinol.*, **185**, 73–9.

Brindley, D. N. (1995). Role of glucocorticoids and fatty acids in the impairment of lipid metabolism observed in the metabolic syndrome. *Int. J. Obes. Relat. Metab. Disord.*, **19**(Suppl 1), S69–75.

Brocklehurst, P., Gates, S., McKenzie-McHarg, K., Alfirevic, Z. and Chamberlain, G. (1999). Are we prescribing multiple courses of antenatal corticosteroids? A survey of practice in the UK. *Br. J. Obstet. Gyn.*, **106**, 977–9.

Brooks, A. N., Hagan, D. M. and Howe, D. C. (1996). Neuroendocrine regulation of pituitary–adrenal function during fetal life. *Eur. J. Endocrinol.*, **135**, 153–65.

Brown, R. W., Chapman, K. E., Edwards, C. R. W. and Seckl, J. R. (1993). Human placental 11β hydroxysteroid dehydrogenase: evidence for and partial purification of a distinct NAD-dependant isoform. *Endocrinology*, **132**, 2614–21.

Bujalska, I. J., Kumar, S., Stewart, P. M. (1997). Does central obesity reflect 'Cushing's disease of the omentum'? *Lancet*, **349**, 1210–13.

Bujalska, I. J., Kumar, S., Hewison, M. and Stewart, P. M. (1999). Differentiation of adipose stromal cells: the roles of glucocorticoids and 11beta-hydroxysteroid dehydrogenase. *Endocrinology*, **140**, 3188–96.

Challis, J. R. G., Carson, G. D. and Naftolin, F. (1978). Effect of prostaglandin E_2 on the concentration of Cortisol in the plasma of newborn lambs. *J. Endocr.*, **76**, 177–8.

Challis, J. R. G., Lye, S. J. and Welsh, J. (1986). Ovine fetal adrenal maturation at term and during fetal ACTH administration: evidence that the modulating effect of cortisol may involve cAMP. *Can. J. Physiol. Pharm.*, **64**, 1085–90.

Challis, J. R. G. and Brooks, A. N. (1989). Maturation and activation of hypothalamic–pituitary–adrenal function in fetal sheep. *Endocr. Rev.*, **10**, 182–204.

Challis, J. R. G., Sloboda, D. M., Matthews, S. G. *et al.* (2000). Fetal hypothalamic–pituitary adrenal (HPA) development and activation as a determinant of the timing of birth, and of postnatal disease. *Endocr. Res.*, **26**, 489–504.

Clark, P. M. S., Hindmarsh, P. C., Shiell, A. W. *et al.* (1996). Size at birth and adrenocortical function in childhood. *Clin. Endocrinol.*, **45**, 721–6.

Cleasby, M. E., Livingstone, D. E., Nyirenda, M. J., Seckl, J. R. and Walker, B. R. (2003). Is programming of glucocorticoid receptor expression by prenatal dexamethasone in the rat secondary to metabolic derangement in adulthood? *Eur. J. Endocrinol.*, **148**, 129–38.

Coderre, L., Vallega, G. A., Pilch, P. F. and Chipkin, S. R. (1996). In vivo effects of dexamethasone and sucrose on glucose transport (GLUT-4) protein tissue distribution. *Am. J. Physiol.*, **271**, E643–8.

Crowther, N. J., Trusler, J., Cameron, N., Toman, M. and Gray, I. P. (2000). Relation between weight gain and beta-cell secretory activity and non-esterified fatty acid production in 7-year-old African children: results from the Birth to Ten study. *Diabetologia*, **43**, 978–85.

Dallman, M. F., Akana, S. F., Jacobson, L. *et al.* (1987). Characterization of corticosterone feedback regulation of ACTH secretion. *Ann. N. Y. Acad. Sci.*, **512**, 402–14.

Dean, F. and Matthews, S. G. (1999). Maternal dexamethasone treatment in late gestation alters glucocorticoid and mineralocorticoid receptor mRNA in the fetal guinea pig brain. *Brain Res.*, **846**, 253–9.

De Kloet, E. R., Reul, J. M. H. M. and Sutanto, W. (1990). Corticosteroids and the brain. *J. Steroid Biochem. Mol. Biol.*, **37**, 387–94.

De Kloet, E. R., Vreugdenhil, E., Oitzl, M. S. and Joels, M. (1998). Brain corticosteroids receptor balance in health and disease. *Endocr. Rev.*, **19**, 269–301.

Dodic, M. and Wintour, E. M. (1994). Effects of prolonged (48 h) infusion of cortisol on blood pressure, renal function and fetal fluids in the immature ovine foetus. *Clin. Exp. Pharmacol. Physiol.*, **21**, 971–80.

Dunlop, S. A., Archer, M. A., Quinlivan, J. A., Beazley, L. D. and Newnham, J. P. (1997). Repeated prenatal corticosteriods delay myelination in the ovine central nervous system. *J. Matern.–Fetal Med.*, **6**, 309–13.

Durand, P., Bosc, M. J. and Locatelli, A. (1980). Adrenal maturation of the sheep fetus during late pregnancy. *Reprod. Nutr. Develop.*, **20**, 339–47.

Durand, P., Locatelli, A., Cathiard, A. M., Dazord, A. and Saez, J. M. (1981). ACTH induction of the maturation of ACTH-sensitive adenylate cyclase system in the ovine fetal adrenal. *J. Steroid Biochem.*, **15**, 445–8.

Durand, P., Cathiard, A. M., Locatelli, A. and Saez, J. M. (1982). Modifications of the steroidogenic pathway during spontaneous and adrenocorticotropin-induced maturation of ovine fetal adrenal. *Endocrinology*, **110**, 500–5.

Durand, P., Cathiard, A. M., Dacheux, F., Naaman, E. and Saez, J. M. (1986). *In vitro* stimulation and inhibition of adrenocorticotropin release by pituitary cells from ovine fetuses and lambs. *Endocrinology*, **118**, 1387–94.

Economides, D. L., Nicolaides, K. H. and Campbell, S. (1991). Metabolic and endocrine findings in appropriate and small for gestational age fetuses. *J. Perinat. Med.*, **19**, 97–105.

Edwards, C. R. W., Benediktsson, R., Lindsay, R. M. and Seckl, J. R. (1993). Dysfunction of placental glucocorticoid barrier: link between fetal environment and adult hypertension? *FEBS J.*, **341**, 355–7.

Ee, L., Hagan, R., Evans, S. and French, N. P. (1998). Antenatal steroid, condition at birth and respiratory morbidity and mortality in very preterm infants. *J. Pediat. Child Health*, **34**, 377–83.

Fowden, A. L., Mijovic, J. and Silver, M. (1993). The effects of cortisol on hepatic and renal gluconeogenic enzyme activities in the sheep fetus during late gestation. *J. Endocrinol.*, **137**, 213–22.

Fowden, A. L., Li, J., Forhead, A. J. (1998). Glucocorticoids and the preparation for life after birth: are there long-term consequences of the life insurance? *Proc. Nutr. Soc.*, **57**, 113–22.

French, N. P., Evans, S. F., Godfrey, K. M. and Newnham, J. P. (1999). Repeated antenatal corticosteroids: size at birth and subsequent development. *Am. J. Obstet. Gynecol.*, **180**, 114–21.

French, N. P., Evans, S. F., Godfrey, K. M. and Newnham, J. P. (2004). Repeated antenatal corticosteroids: size at birth and subsequent development. *Am. J. Obstet. Gynecol.*, **190**, 588–95.

Fruhbeck, G. and Salvador, J. (2000). Relation between leptin and the regulation of glucose metabolism. *Diabetologia*, **43**, 3–12.

Glickman, J. A. and Challis, J. R. G. (1980). The changing response pattern of sheep fetal adrenal cells throughout the course of gestation. *Endocrinology*, **106**, 1371–6.

Goland, R. S., Jozak, S., Warren, W. B., Conwell, I. M. *et al.* (1993). Elevated levels of umbilical cord plasma corticotropin-releasing hormone in growth retarded fetuses. *J. Clin. Endocrinol. Metab.*, **77**, 1174–9.

Hales, C. N. and Barker, D. J. P. (1992). Type 2 (non-insulin-dependent) diabetes mellitus: the thrifty phenotype hypothesis. *Diabetologia*, **35**, 595–601.

Hill, D. J. (1999). Fetal programming of the pancreatic β cells and the implications for postnatal diabetes. *Semin. Neonatol.*, **4**, 99–113.

Huang, W. L., Beazley, L. D., Quinlivan, J. A. *et al.* (1999). Effect of corticosteroids on brain growth in fetal sheep. *Obstet. Gynecol.*, **94**, 213–18.

Ikegami, M., Jobe, A. H., Newnham, J. *et al.* (1997). Repetitive prenatal glucocorticoids improve lung function and decrease growth in preterm lambs. *Am. J. Resp. Crit. Care*, **156**, 178–84.

Jacobson, L. and Sapolsky, R. M. (1991). The role of the hippocampus in feedback regulation of the hypothalamic–pituitary–adrenocortical axis. *Endocr. Rev.*, **12**, 118–34.

Jobe, A. H., Polk, D., Ikegami, M. *et al.* (1993). Lung responses to ultrasound-guided fetal treatments with corticosteroids in preterm lambs. *Appl. Physiol.*, **75**(5), 2099–105.

Johnson, J. W. C., Mitzner, W., Beck, J. C. *et al.* (1981). Long-term effects of betamethasone on fetal development. *Am. J. Obstet. Gynecol.*, **141**, 1053–64.

Joyner, J. M., Hutley, L. J. and Cameron, D. P. (2000). Glucocorticoid receptors in human preadipocytes: regional and gender differences. *J. Endocrinol.*, **166**, 145–52.

Kahn, B. B. and Flier, J. S. (2000). Obesity and insulin resistance. *J. Clin. Invest.*, **106**, 473–81.

Kajantie, E., Dunkel, L., Turpeinen, U. *et al.* (2003). Placental 11{beta}-hydroxysteroid dehydrogenase-2 and fetal cortisol/cortisone shuttle in small preterm infants. *J. Clin. Endocrinol. Metab.*, **88**, 493–500.

Kari, M. A., Hallman, M., Eronen, M. *et al.* (1994). Prenatal dexamethasone treatment in conjunction with rescue therapy of human surfactant: a randomized placebo-controlled multicenter study. *Pediatrics*, **93**, 730–6.

Keller-Wood, M. E. and Dallman, M. F. (1984). Corticosteroid inhibition of ACTH secretion. *Endocr. Rev.*, **5**, 1–24.

Kerzner, L. S., Stonestreet, B. S., Wu, K. Y., Sadowska, G. and Malee, M. P. (2002). Antenatal dexamethasone: effect on ovine placental 11beta-hydroxysteroid dehydrogenase type 2 expression and fetal growth. *Pediatr. Res.*, **52**, 706–12.

Kotelevtsev, Y. V., Holmes, M. C., Burchell, A. *et al.* (1997). 11β hydroxysteroid dehydrogenase type 1 knockout mice show attenuated glucocorticoid inducible responses and resist hyperglycemia on obesity or stress. *Proc. Natl. Acad. Sci. USA*, **94**, 14924–9.

Krozowski, Z. (1999). The 11beta hydroxysteroid dehydrogenases: functions and physiological effects. *Mol. Cell. Endocrinol.*, **25**, 121–7.

Lambillotte, C., Gilon, P. and Henquin, J. C. (1997). Direct glucocorticoid inhibition of insulin secretion. *J. Clin. Invest.*, **99**, 414–23.

Levitt, N. S., Lindsay, R. S., Holmes, M. C. and Seckl, J. R. (1996). Dexamethasone in the last week of pregnancy attenuates hippocampal glucocorticoid receptor gene expression and elevates blood pressure in the adult offspring in the rat. *Neuroendocrinology*, **64**, 412–19.

Levitt, N. S., Lambert, E. V., Woods, D. *et al.* (2000). Impaired glucose tolerance and elevated blood pressure in low birth weight, nonobese, young South African adults: early programming of cortisol axis. *J. Clin. Endocr. Metab.*, **85**, 4611–18.

Liggins, G. C. (1969). Premature delivery of fetal lambs infused with glucocorticoids. *J. Endocrinol.*, **45**, 515–23.

Liggins, G. C. and Howie, R. N. (1972). A controlled trial of antepartum glucocorticoid treatment for prevention of the respiratory distress syndrome in premature infants. *Pediatrics*, **50**, 515–25.

Liggins, G. C. (1994). The role of cortisol in preparing the fetus for birth. *Reprod. Fert. Develop.*, **6**, 141–50.

Lindsay, R. S., Lindsay, R. M., Waddell, B. J. and Seckl, J. R. (1996). Prenatal glucocorticoid exposure lead to offspring hyperglycemia in the rat: studies with the 11β hydroxysteroid dehydrogenase inhibitor carbenoxolone. *Diabetologia*, **39**, 1299–305.

Lingas, R., Dean, F. and Matthews, S. G. (1999). Maternal nutrient restriction (48H) modifies brain corticosteroid receptor expression and endocrine function in the fetal guinea pig. *Brain Res.*, **846**, 236–42.

Liu, D., Diorio, J., Tannembaum, B. *et al.* (1997). Maternal care, hippocampal glucocorticoid receptors and hypothalamic pituitary adrenal responses to stress. *Science*, **277**, 1659–62.

Louis, T. M., Challis, J. R. G., Robinson, J. S. and Thorburn, G. D. (1976). Rapid increase of fetal corticosteroids after prostaglandin E$_2$. *Nature*, **264**, 797–9.

Maccari, S., Piazza, P. V., Kabbaj, M. *et al.* (1995). Adoption reverses the long-term impairment in glucocorticoid feedback induced by prenatal stress. *J. Neurosci.*, **15**, 110–16.

Matthews, S. G. and Challis, J. R. G. (1997). CRH and AVP-induced changes in synthesis and release of ACTH from the ovine fetal pituitary in vitro: negative influences of cortisol. *Endocrine*, **6**, 293–300.

McDonald, T. J., Rose, J. C., Figueroa, J. P., Gluckman, P. D. and Nathaneilsz, P. W. (1988). The effect of hypothalamic paraventricular nuclear lesions placed at 108–110 days gestational age on plasma ACTH concentrations in the fetal sheep. *J. Develop. Physiol.*, **10**, 191–200.

McDonald, T. J. and Nathaneilsz, P. W. (1991). Bilateral destruction of the fetal paraventricular nuclei prolongs gestation in sheep. *Am. J. Obstet. Gynecol.*, **165**, 764–70.

McDonald, T. J., Hoffman, G. E. and Nathaneilsz, P. W. (1992). Hypothalamic paraventricular nuclear lesions delay corticotroph maturation in the fetal sheep anterior pituitary. *Endocrinology*, **131**, 1101–6.

McMillen, I. C., Merei, J. J., White, A. and Schwartz, J. (1995). Increasing gestational age and cortisol alter the ratio of ACTH precursors: ACTH secreted from the anterior pituitary of the fetal sheep. *J. Endocrinol.*, **144**, 569–76.

Meaney, M. J., Sapolsky, R. M. and McEwen, B. S. (1985). The development of the glucocorticoid receptor system in the rat limbic brain. I. Ontogeny and autoregulation. *Develop. Brain Res.*, **18**, 159–64.

Meaney, M. J., Aitken, D. H., Viau, V., Sharma, S. and Sarrieau, A. (1989). Neonatal handling alters adrenocortical negative feedback sensitivity and hippocampal type II glucocorticoid receptor binding in the rat. *Neuroendocrinology*, **50**, 597–604.

Meijer, O. and De Kloet, E. R. (1998). Corticosterone and serotonergic neurotransmission in the hippocampus: functional implications of central corticosteroid receptor diversity. *Crit. Rev. Neurobiol.*, **12**, 1–20.

Mesiano, S., Jaffe, R. B. (1997). Developmental and functional biology of the primate fetal adrenal cortex. *Endocr. Rev.*, **18**, 378–403.

Moss, T. J. M., Sloboda, D. M., Gurrin, L. C. *et al.* (2001). Programming effects in sheep of prenatal growth restriction and glucocorticoid exposure. *Am. J. Physiol.*, **281**, R960–70.

Moss, T. J. M., Doherty, D. A., Nitsos, I. *et al.* (2005). Effects into adulthood of single or repeated antenatal corticosteroids in sheep. *Am. J. Obstet. Gynecol.*, **192**, 146–52.

Mostyn, A., Pearce, S., Budge, H. *et al.* (2003). Influence of cortisol on adipose tissue development in the fetal sheep during late gestation. *J. Endocrinol.*, **176**, 23–30.

Newnham, J. P., Evans, S. F., Godfrey, M. *et al.* (1999). Maternal, but not fetal, administration of corticosteroids restricts fetal growth. *J. Matern. Fetal. Med.*, **8**, 81–7.

Niederhofer, H. and Reiter, A. (2000). Maternal stress during pregnancy, its objectivation by ultrasound observation of fetal intrauterine movements and child's temperament at 6 months and 6 years of age: pilot study. *Psychol. Rep.*, **86**, 526–8.

Nilsson, P. M., Nyberg, P. and Ostergren, P. (2001). Increase susceptibility to stress at a psychological assessment of stress tolerance is associated with impaired fetal growth. *Intern. J. Epidemiol.*, **30**, 75–80.

Norman, L. J., Lye, S. J., Wlodek, M. E. and Challis, J. R. G. (1985). Changes in pituitary responses to synthetic ovine corticotrophin releasing factor in fetal sheep. *Can. J. Physiol. Pharmacol.*, **63**, 1398–403.

Norman, L. J. and Challis, J. R. G. (1987). Synergism between systemic corticotropin-releasing factor and arginine vasopressin on adrenocorticotropin release *in vivo* varies as a function of gestational age in the ovine fetus. *Endocrinology*, **120**, 1052–8.

Nyirenda, M. J., Lindsay, R. M., Kenyon, C. J., Burchell, A. and Seckl, J. R. (1998). Glucocorticoid exposure in late gestation permanently programs rat hepatic phosphoenolpyruvate carboxykinase and glucocoritcoid receptor expression and causes glucose intolerance in adult offspring. *J. Clin. Invest.*, **101**, 2174–81.

Perry, R. A., Mulvogue, H. M., McMillen, I. C. and Robinson, P. M. (1985). Immunohistochemical localization of ACTH in the adult and fetal sheep pituitary. *J. Develop. Physiol.*, **7**(6), 397–404.

Phillips, D. I. W., Barker, D. J. P., Fall, C. H. D. *et al.* (1998). Elevated plasma cortisol concentrations: a link between low birth weight and the insulin resistance syndrome. *J. Clin. Endocrinol. Metab.*, **83**, 757–60.

Phillips, D. I. W., Walker, B. R., Reynolds, R. M. *et al.* (2000). Low birth weight predicts elevated plasma cortisol concentrations in adults from 3 populations. *Hypertension*, **36**, 1301–6.

Pugeat, M. M., Dunn, J. F. and Nisula, B. C. (1981). Transport of steroid hormones: interaction of 70 drugs with testosterone binding globulin and corticosteroid binding globulin in human plasma. *J. Clin. Endocrinol. Metab.*, **53**, 69–75.

Quinlivan, J. A., Evan, S. F., Dunlop, S. A., Beazley, L. D. and Newnham, J. (1998). Use of corticosteroid by Australian obstetricians–a survey of clinical practice. *Aust. NZ. Obstet. Gynecol.*, **38**, 1–7.

Rask, E., Walker, B. R., Soderberg, S. *et al.* (2002). Tissue-specific changes in peripheral cortisol metabolism in obese women: increased adipose 11{beta}-hydroxysteroid dehydrogenase type 1 activity. *J. Clin. Endocrinol. Metab.*, **87**, 3330–6.

Ravelli, A. C. J., van der Meulen, J. H. P., Michels, R. P. J. *et al.* (1998). Glucose tolerance in adults after prenatal exposure to famine. *Lancet*, **351**, 173–7.

Reaven, G. M. (1988). Role of insulin resistance in human disease. *Diabetes*, **37**, 1595–607.

Reul, J. M. H. M., De Kloet, E. R. (1985). Two receptor systems for corticosterone in rat brain: microdistribution and differential occupation. *Endocrinology*, **117**, 2505–11.

Reynolds, R. M., Walker, B. R., Syddall, H. E. *et al.* (2001). Altered control of cortisol secretion in adult men with low birth weight and cardiovascular risk factors. *J. Clin. Endocrinol. Metab.*, **86**, 245–50.

Robinson, P. M., Rowe, E. J. and Wintour, E. M. (1979). The histogenesis of the adrenal cortex in the fetal sheep. *Acta Endocrinol.*, **91**, 134–49.

Rosenfeld, P., Suchecki, D. and Levine, S. (1992). Multifactoral regulation of the hypothalamic–pituitary–adrenal axis during development. *Neurosci. Biobehav. Rev.*, **16**, 553–68.

Saegusa, H., Nakagawa, Y., Liu, Y. J. and Ohzeki, T. (1999). Influence of placental 11β-hydroxysteroid dehydrogenase (11β HSD) inhibition on glucose metabolism and 11β HSD regulation in adult offspring of rats. *Metabolism*, **48**, 1584–8.

Sander, M. and German, M. S. (1997). The β cell transcription factors and development of the pancreas. *J. Mol. Med.*, **75**, 327–40.

Schwartz, M. W., Strack, A. M. and Dallman, M. F. (1997). Evidence that elevated plasma corticosterone levels are the cause of reduced hypothalamic corticotorphin-releasing hormone gene expression in diabetes. *Regul. Peptides*, **72**, 105–12.

Seckl, J. R. (1997). Glucocorticoids, feto–placental 11β-hydroxysteroid dehydrogenase type 2, and the early life origins of adult disease. *Steroids*, **62**, 89–94.

Shaw, G. and Renfee, M. B. (2001). Fetal control of parturition in marsupials. *Reprod. Fert. Develop.*, **13**, 653–9.

Siebe, H., Baude, G., Lichtenstein, I. *et al.* (1993). Metabolism of dexamethasone: sites and activity in mammalian tissues. *Renal Physiol. Biochem.*, **16**, 79–88.

Sloboda, D. M., Newnham, J. and Challis, J. R. G. (2000). Effects of repeated maternal betamethasone administration on growth and hypothalamic–pituitary–adrenal function of the ovine fetus at term. *J. Endocrinol.*, **165**, 79–91.

Sloboda, D. M., Moss, T. J., Gurrin, L. C., Newnham, J. and Challis, J. R. G. (2002a). The effect of prenatal betamethasone administration on postnatal ovine hypothalamic–pituitary–adrenal function. *J. Endocrinol.*, **172**, 71–81.

Sloboda, D. M., Newnham, J. P. and Challis, J. R. G. (2002b). Effects of repeated maternal betamethasone administration the development of the fetal liver. *J. Endocrinol.*, **175**, 535–43.

Sloboda, D. M., Moss, T., Doherty, D., Challis, J. R. G. and Newnham, J. P. (2003). Antenatal glucocorticoid treatment in sheep results in adrenal suppression in adulthood. *J. Soc. Gynecol. Invest.*, **10**(2).

Speight, T. M. (1987). Endocrine diseases. Avery's drug treatment. Speight T. M. eds., *Principles and Practice of Clinical Pharmacology and Therapeutics*. ADIS Press Ltd., Auckland, p. 564.

Spiegelman, B. M. and Flier, J. S. (2001). Obesity and the regulation of energy balance. *Cell.* **104**(4), 531–43.

Takahashi, L. K. and Kalin, N. H. (1991). Early developmental and temporal characteristics of stress-induced secretion of pituitary adrenal hormones in prenatally stressed rat pups. *Brain Res.*, **558**, 75–8.

Takahashi, L. K. (1998). Prenatal stress: consequences of glucocorticoids on hippocampal development and function. *Intern. J. Neurosci.*, **16**, 199–207.

Thakur, A., Sase, M., Lee, J. J., Thakur, V. and Buchmiller, T. L. (2000). Effect of dexamethasone on insulin-like growth factor-1 expression in a rabbit model of growth retardation. *J. Pediat. Surg.*, **35**, 898–905.

Tonolo, G., Fraser, G., Connell, J. M. and Kenyon, C. J. (1988). Chronic low dose infusions of dexamethasone in rats: effects on blood pressure, body weight and plasma atrial natriuretic peptide. *J. Hypertens.*, **6**, 25–31.

Uno, H., Lohmiller, L., Thieme, C. *et al.* (1990). Brain damage induced by prenatal exposure to dexamethasone in fetal rhesus macaques. I. Hippocampus. *Develop. Brain Res.*, **53**, 157–67.

Uno, H., Eisele, S., Sakai, A. *et al.* (1994). Neurotoxicity of glucocorticoids in the primate brain. *Horm. Behav.*, **28**, 336–48.

Vallee, M., Mayo, W., Maccari, S., Le Moal, M. and Simon, H. (1996). Long-term effects of prenatal stress and handling on metabolic parameters: relationship to corticosterone secretion response. *Brain Res.*, **712**, 287–92.

Veening, M. A., van Weissenbruch, M. M. and Delemarre-van de Waal, H. A. (2002). Glucose tolerance, insulin sensitivity, and insulin secretion in children born small for gestational age. *J. Clin. Endocrinol. Metab.*, **87**, 4657–61.

Webb, P. D. (1980). Development of the adrenal cortex in the fetal sheep: an ultrastructural study. *J. Dev. Physiol.*, **2**(3), 161–81.

Weinstein, S. P., Paquin, T., Pritsker, A. and Haber, R. S. (1995). Glucocorticoid-induced insulin resistance: dexamethasone inhibits the activation of glucose transport in rat skeletal muscle by both insulin- and non-insulin-related stimuli. *Diabetes*, **44**, 441–5.

Weinstein, S. P., Wilson, C. M., Pritsker, A. and Cushman, S. W. (1998). Dexamethasone inhibits insulin-stimulated recruitment of GLUT4 to the cell surface in rat skeletal muscle. *Metabolism*, **47**, 3–6.

Weinstock, M., Matlina, E., Maor, G. I., Rosen, H. and McEwen, B. S. (1992). Prenatal stress selectively alters the reactivity of the hypothalamic-pituitary adrenal system in the female rat. *Brain Res.*, **595**, 195–200.

Weinstock, M. (1996). Does prenatal stress impair coping and regulation of hypothalamic–pituitary–adrenal axis. *Neurosci. Biobehav. Rev.*, **21**, 1–10.

Welberg, L. A. M., Seckl, J. R. and Holmes, M. C. (2000). Inhibition of 11β-hydroxysteroid dehydrogenase, the fetal-placental barrier to maternal glucocorticoids, permanently programs amygdala GRmRNA expression and anxiety-like behaviour in the offspring. *Eur. J. Neurosci.*, **12**, 1047–54.

Welberg, L. A. M. and Seckl, J. R. (2001). Prenatal stress, glucocorticoids and the programming of the brain. *J. Neuroendocrinol.*, **13**, 113–28.

Whittle, W. L., Holloway, A. C., Lye, S. J., Gibb, W. and Challis, J. R. G. (2000). Prostaglandin production at the onset of ovine parturition is regulated by both estrogen-independent and estrogen-dependent pathways. *Endocrinology*, **141**, 3783–91.

Wintour, E. M., Brown, E. H., Denton, D. A., Hardy, K. J., McDougall, J. G., Oddie, C. J. and Whipp, G. T. (1975). The ontogeny and regulation of corticosteroid secretion by the ovine foetal adrenal. *Acta. Endocrinol. (Copenh).*, **79**(2), 301–16.

Wintour, E. M., Smith, M. B., Bell, R. J., McDougall, J. G. and Cauchi, M. N. (1985). The role of fetal adrenal hormones in the switch from fetal to adult globin synthesis in the sheep. *J. Endocrinol.*, **104**(1), 165–70.

Wolf, G. (2002). Glucocorticoids in adipocytes stimulate visceral obesity. *Nutr. Rev.*, **60**, 148–51.

Yarbrough, D. E., Barrett-Connor, E., Kritz-Silverstein, D. and Wingard, D. L. (1998). Birth weight, adult weight, and girth as predictors of the metabolic syndrome in postmenopausal women: the Rancho Bernardo Study. *Diabetes Care*, **21**, 1652–8.

Young, I. R., Loose, J. M., Kleftogiannis, F. and Canny, B. J. (1996). Prostaglandin E_2 acts via hypothalamus to stimulate ACTH secretion in the fetal sheep. *J. Neuroendocrinol.*, **8**, 713–20.

5

Prenatal glucocorticoids and the programming of adult disease

Jonathan R. Seckl, Amanda J. Drake and Megan C. Holmes

Endocrinology Unit, University of Edinburgh, Western General Hospital, Edinburgh, UK

'*The Child is Father of the Man*', wrote British poet William Wordsworth (1807), reflecting upon the consistency of an individual's emotional responses through the long human lifespan. Soon afterwards, Mendelian and Darwinian genetics and the still controversial concept of *early life programming* indicated plausible biological bases for Wordsworth's artistic muse. Now, nearly two centuries later, many readily accept that part of our individual emotional compass is constrained by events affecting the development of the brain before birth, effects that persist for life, defining parameters upon which nurture and the adult environment exert their modifying effects. For genetics, the effects of classically inherited genes and chromosomal variation confirm the fundamental nature of inheritance of traits. Here we address the role of a specific aspect of the early life environment upon the lifelong characteristics of an individual, a much more recent addition to understanding of 'ease or disease' through our span.

Epidemiology and the concept of 'programming'

To begin, in appropriate recent historical sequence, with human epidemiology. Numerous studies, initially in the UK and then encompassing much of the world, have demonstrated an association between lower birth weight and the subsequent development of the common cardiovascular and metabolic disorders of adult life, namely hypertension, insulin resistance, type 2 diabetes and cardiovascular disease deaths (Barker, 1991; Barker *et al.*, 1993a, b; Fall *et al.*, 1995; Yajnik *et al.*, 1995; Curhan *et al.*, 1996a, b; Leon *et al.*, 1996; Lithell *et al.*, 1996; Moore *et al.*, 1996; Forsen *et al.*, 1997; RichEdwards *et al.*, 1997). The association between birth weight and later cardio-metabolic disease appears to be largely independent of classical lifestyle risk factors such as smoking, adult weight, social class, alcohol and lack of exercise, which are additive to the effect of birth weight (Barker *et al.*, 1993a). The studies suggest that these relationships are generally continuous and represent birth weights within the normal range, rather than severe intrauterine growth retardation, multiple births or very premature babies (Barker, 1991; Barker *et al.*, 1993a; Curhan *et al.*, 1996a, b). However, premature babies also have increased cardiovascular risk in adult life (Irving *et al.*, 2000). Additionally, postnatal catch-up growth also appears to be predictive of the risk of adult cardiovascular disease (Barker, 1991; Osmond *et al.*, 1993; Levine *et al.*, 1994; Leon *et al.*, 1996; Forsen *et al.*, 1997; Bavdekar *et al.*, 1999; Law *et al.*, 2002), suggesting that it is the restriction of intrauterine growth rather than smallness itself which is important. Whilst such effects might reflect classical genetic actions, some work has suggested that the smaller of twins at birth has higher blood pressure in later life (Levine *et al.*, 1994), although this has not been a consistent finding (Baird *et al.*, 2001).

These early life effects are important predictors of adult morbidity (Barker *et al.*, 1990; Curhan *et al.*, 1996a, b). In the Preston study, a small baby with a large placenta had three times the relative risk of adult hypertension compared with a large baby with a normal placenta (Barker *et al.*, 1990). In a study of 22,000 American men, those born lighter than 5.5 lb had increased relative risks of adult hypertension (1.26) and type 2 diabetes (1.75) compared with average birth-weight adults (Curhan *et al.*, 1996b). Similarly, lighter but otherwise normal babies of 71,000 US nurses had a relative risk of 1.43 of developing adult hypertension (Curhan *et al.*, 1996a). Whilst there is still debate as to the importance of birth weight in determining later disease (Huxley *et al.*, 2002) as well as the magnitude of any such effect (it has been suggested that some studies linking lower birth weight with higher adult blood pressure fail to take into account the impact of random error and may involve inappropriate adjustment for confounding factors (Huxley *et al.*, 2002)), the mass of human epidemiological data and the production of animal models show that early life environmental manipulations produce persisting adult effects in both inbred and outbred species under controlled conditions, which suggest that discrete prenatal events may have permanent effects on adult biology.

It is also important to consider that birth weight is an unsophisticated and blunt measure of a disadvantageous intrauterine environment. It is therefore not surprising that birth weight associates poorly with adult pathophysiology in some studies. Indeed the remarkable thing is that any link has been established at all, given the crude measure of fetal challenge employed, its typically inaccurate assessment in practice and the extensive time span between the early life insult and the adult pathology examined. So how can we mechanistically explain such an unanticipated association between events at either end of the lifespan?

Programming

To explain the apparent association of fetal growth and later disease, the idea of early life physiological 'programming' or 'imprinting' has been advanced (Barker *et al.*, 1993a; Edwards *et al.*, 1993; Seckl, 1998). Programming reflects the action of a factor during sensitive periods or 'windows' of development to exercise organizational effects upon developing tissues that persist throughout life. Of course, different cells and tissues are sensitive at different times, so the effects of environmental challenges will have distinct effects depending not only the challenge involved but also upon its timing.

Two major environmental hypotheses have been proposed to explain the mechanism by which low birth weight is associated with adult disease: fetal undernutrition and overexposure of the fetus to glucocorticoids (Barker *et al.*, 1993a; Edwards *et al.*, 1993; Seckl, 1998). A third perhaps complementary hypothesis suggests that genetic factors may lead to both low birth weight and subsequent risk of cardiovascular disease (Figure 5.1). Indeed, loci have been described which may link smallness at birth with adult disease (Dunger *et al.*, 1998; Hattersley *et al.*, 1998; Vaessen *et al.*, 2001). Whilst the putative loci implicated relate to biologically plausible candidate genes such as insulin, insulin-like growth factors (IGF) and their signalling pathways, as well as other key metabolic regulators such as β3-adrenoceptors, peroxisome proliferator-activated receptor (PPARγ) and tumour necrosis factor alpha (TNFα) (Jaquet *et al.*, 2002), there remains debate as to reproducibility of findings (Frayling *et al.*, 2002), perhaps because studies have been underpowered (Frayling and Hattersley, 2001). So the relative importance of genetic and environmental factors in the 'low-birth-weight baby syndrome' remains unknown. However, the occurrence of associations between early life environmental manipulations and later physiology–disease risk in isogenic rodent models and, less certainly, the birth-weight–adult-disease associations in human twins implicate environmental factors, at least in part, in aetiology. Here the specific issue of hormonal programming by glucocorticoids is considered.

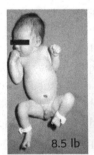 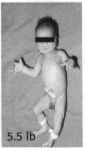

8.5 lb   5.5 lb

Two full-term babies born to healthy, non-smoking, unmedicated mothers on the same day in the same hospital. The smaller, thinner baby on the right has a substantially increased risk of cardio-metabolic disease in adulthood

Possible mechanisms (non-exclusive)

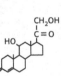

- Genetics
- Uterine size
- Maternal malnutrition
- Growth factors (IGFs, insulin)
- Glucocorticoids
  - Reduce birth weight in mammals
  - Alter organ maturation
  - Directly cause: hypertension, diabetes, osteoporosis, etc.
  - Sex steroids 'programme'

CH_2OH
$C=O$
HO

Figure 5.1   Birth weight and adult disease: possible mechanisms

Glucocorticoid programming

Steroids and organizational effects

Steroid hormones have long been associated with organizational actions. It is well documented that neonatal exposure to androgens programme expression of hepatic steroid metabolizing enzymes, the development of sexually dimorphic structures in the anterior hypothalamus and sexual behaviour in many vertebrate species including mammals (Arai and Gorski, 1968; Gustafsson et al., 1983). Estrogens also exert organizational effects on the developing central nervous system (CNS) (Simerly, 2002). Critically, these effects can only be exerted during specific perinatal periods, but then persist throughout life, largely irrespective of any subsequent sex steroid manipulations. The mechanisms reflect sex steroid actions on the growth, maturation and remodelling of organs during critical perinatal periods. In the rat, the sexually dimorphic nucleus of the preoptic hypothalamic area is larger in males. Testosterone inhibits apoptosis specifically between postnatal days 6 and 10 and selectively in this locus, thus producing the male adult phenotype (Davis et al., 1996).

Why glucocorticoids?

Glucocorticoids and birth weight

In addressing the link between birth weight, which surely is merely a marker of an adverse intrauterine environment, and adult cardio-metabolic disorders, glucocorticoids are attractive candidate aetiological factors (Seckl, 1994; 1998) (Figure 5.1). For decades it has been observed that glucocorticoid therapy during pregnancy reduces birth weight in animal models, including non-human primates (Reinisch et al., 1978; Ikegami et al., 1997; Nyirenda et al., 1998; French et al., 1999; Newnham et al., 1999; Newnham and Moss, 2001). Such effects are the most powerful in the latter stages of pregnancy (Nyirenda et al., 1998), presumably reflecting the catabolic actions of these steroids, which is most manifest during the phases of maximum fetal somatic growth.

In human pregnancy, glucocorticoids are now only widely used in the management of women at risk of preterm delivery and in the antenatal management of fetuses at risk of congenital adrenal hyperplasia. In some such populations antenatal glucocorticoids are associated with a reduction in birth weight (French et al., 1999; Bloom et al., 2001), although normal birth weight has been reported in infants at risk of congenital adrenal hyperplasia whose mothers received low-dose dexamethasone in utero from the first trimester (Forest et al., 1993b; Mercado et al., 1995b). A recent study of pregnant women with asthma did not find changes in birth weight with use of inhaled and/or episodic oral glucocorticoids. Indeed, a lack of glucocorticoid treatment was associated with a reduction in offspring birth weight (Murphy *et al.*, 2002). However, the effects on placental function of inflammatory mediators in poorly controlled asthma, the predominant topical route of steroid administration and the use of prednisolone which is rapidly inactivated by placental 11β-hydroxysteroid dehydrogenase type 2 (HSD-2) and poorly accesses the fetal compartment (see below) might explain these findings.

For endogenous glucocorticoids, human *fetal* plasma cortisol levels are increased in intrauterine growth retardation or in pre-eclampsia, implicating endogenous cortisol in retarded fetal growth (Goland *et al.*, 1993; 1995). Cortisol also affects placental size, at least in animals, the effect dependent of the dose and timing of exposure (Gunberg, 1957).

Glucocorticoids and tissue maturation

Glucocorticoids have potent effects upon tissue development. Indeed it is the accelerated maturation of organs notably the lung (Ward, 1994) which underpins their widespread use in obstetric and neonatal practice in threatened or actual preterm delivery.

Underpinning such actions, glucocorticoid receptors (GR), which are members of the nuclear hormone receptor superfamily of ligand-activated transcription factors, are expressed in most fetal tissues from early embryonal stages (Cole, 1995). Expression of the closely related, higher-affinity mineralocorticoid receptor (MR) has a more limited tissue distribution in development and is only present at later gestational stages, at least in rodents (Brown *et al.*, 1996a). Additionally, GR are highly expressed in the placenta (Sun *et al.*, 1997) where they mediate metabolic and anti-inflammatory actions. Clearly systems to transduce glucocorticoid actions upon the genome exist from early developmental stages, with complex cell-specific patterns of expression and presumably sensitivity to the steroid ligands.

Glucocorticoids and the low-birth-weight baby syndrome

The major systems affected in the 'low-birth-weight baby syndrome' are glucocorticoid-sensitive targets. Notably the syndrome is broadly familiar to endocrinologists since it resembles the Cushing's syndrome/metabolic syndrome continuum of inter-associated cardiovascular risk factors (type 2 diabetes/insulin resistance, dyslipidemia, hypertension) linked by circulating or tissue glucocorticoid excess (Seckl and Walker, 2001). Even the less well-recognized components of the small baby syndrome such as osteoporosis (Gale *et al.*, 2001) are also key features of Cushing's syndromes. Moreover, at least a proportion of these physiological systems are also glucocorticoid sensitive in early life since cortisol also elevates fetal blood pressure when infused directly in utero in sheep (Tangalakis *et al.*, 1992) and at birth in sheep (Berry *et al.*, 1997) and humans (Kari *et al.*, 1994).

Physiology: placental 11β-HSD-2

All the points above relate to pharmacological glucocorticoid exposures or tissue sensitivity. However, study of the latter led to an understanding of a possible physiological basis of glucocorticoid overexposure in utero.

Whilst lipophilic compounds such as steroids are thought to cross the placenta rapidly, fetal glucocorticoid levels are much lower than maternal levels (Beitens et al., 1973; Klemcke, 1995). This is thought to be due to 11β-HSD-2 (Figure 5.2) which is highly expressed in the placenta. 11β-HSD-2 is an NAD-dependent 11β-dehydrogenase which catalyses the rapid metabolism of the active physiological glucocorticoids cortisol and corticosterone to their inert 11-keto forms, cortisone and 11-dehydrocorticosterone (White et al., 1997). It is 11β-HSD-2 that excludes glucocorticoids from intrinsically non-selective MR in the distal nephron where the enzyme forms a complete barrier to glucocorticoid access (White et al., 1997; Kotelevtsev et al., 1999). In the placenta, however, the enzyme is not a complete barrier to maternal steroids (Benediktsson et al., 1997) and in rodents the peak of the circadian rhythm of plasma corticosterone is able to penetrate the 11β-HSD-2 barrier to some extent (Venihaki et al., 2000), presumably adding to the provision of glucocorticoids to the fetus for normal key developmental processes such as maturation of the lung. However, dexamethasone readily passes the placenta as it is a poor 11β-HSD-2 substrate (Albiston et al., 1994; Brown et al., 1996b). Betamethasone is presumed a similarly poor substrate, but 11β-HSD-2 rapidly inactivates prednisolone to inert prednisone.

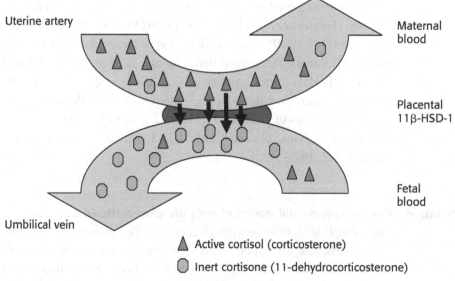

▲ Active cortisol (corticosterone)

⬭ Inert cortisone (11-dehydrocorticosterone)

Figure 5.2   Physiology: placental 11β-HSD-2 converts glucocorticoids to inert forms thus excluding *active* maternal steroids from the fetal compartment

Placental 11β-HSD-2 and birth weight

Observational studies have suggested that placental 11β-HSD-2 relates to birth weight. The activity of placental 11β-HSD-2 near term shows considerable inter-individual variation in humans and rats (Benediktsson *et al.*, 1993; Stewart *et al.*, 1995). A relative deficiency of 11β-HSD-2, with consequent reduced placental inactivation of maternal steroids, may lead to overexposure of the fetus to gluco-corticoids, retard fetal growth and programme responses leading to later disease (Edwards *et al.*, 1993). Studies in rats have demonstrated that lower placental 11β-HSD-2 activity is seen in the smallest fetuses with the largest placentas (Benediktsson *et al.*, 1993). Similar associations have been reported in humans (Stewart *et al.*, 1995; Shams *et al.*, 1998; McTernan *et al.*, 2001; Murphy *et al.*, 2002), although not all studies have reproduced this finding (Rogerson *et al.*, 1996; 1997). Additionally, markers of fetal exposure to glucocorticoids such as cord blood levels of osteocalcin (a glucocorticoid-sensitive osteoblast product that does not cross the placenta), also correlate with placental 11β-HSD-2 activity (Benediktsson *et al.*, 1995).

Rare human cases of 11β-HSD-2 deficiency are described, with homozygotes (or compound heterozygotes) substantially deficient in 11β-HSD-2 activity due to mutations in the encoding gene. Whilst children and adults exhibit 'apparent miner-alocorticoid excess' due to illicit activation of renal MR by cortisol (Stewart *et al.*, 1988), and an identical adult phenotype is seen in 11β-HSD-2 knockout mice (Kotelevtsev *et al.*, 1999), affected individuals have very low birth weight (Dave-Sharma *et al.*, 1998), averaging 1.2 kg less than their heterozygote siblings. Though an initial report suggested that 11β-HSD-2 null mice have normal fetal weight in late gestation (Kotelevtsev *et al.*, 1999), this appears to have reflected the 'genetic noise' of the crossed (129 $\times$ MF1) strain background of the original 11β-HSD-2 null mouse. Indeed preliminary data suggest that in congenic mice on the C57Bl/6 strain back-ground 11β-HSD-2 nullizygosity lowers birth weight (Holmes *et al.*, 2002). Additionally, there may also be species differences. Thus, the mouse shows dramatic late gestational loss of placental 11β-HSD-2 gene expression (Brown *et al.*, 1996a), whereas in humans, placental 11β-HSD-2 activity increases through gestation (Stewart *et al.*, 1995).

An introduction to experimental studies of early life glucocorticoid exposure

Given the plausible links between glucocorticoid excess and the epidemiological find-ings, a causal role was hypothesized soon after the initial human observations were reported (Edwards *et al.*, 1993). This notion has been addressed in a variety of experi-mental models. Importantly, the animal data have also been used to re-examine mechanisms and the phenotype of human low-birth-weight populations to 'complete

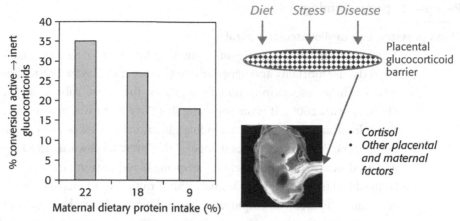

Figure 5.3   Placental 11β-HSD-2 is downregulated by maternal dietary protein restriction. This may be one common mechanism linking the maternal and fetal environments. Adapted from Langley-Evans *et al.* (1996b)

the circle'. Broadly, two approaches have been employed. Most workers have used synthetic glucocorticoids such as dexamethasone and betamethasone that relatively freely cross the placenta as they are poor substrates for 11β-HSD-2. Such agents are also used clinically in obstetric practice. In addition, some studies have exploited drugs such as carbenoxolone that inhibit 11β-HSD-2 thus increasing feto-placental exposure to endogenous steroids. The data from both approaches are in general complementary and here the key findings are reviewed.

It is noteworthy that a common mechanism may underlie fetal programming through maternal undernutrition and glucocorticoid exposure (Figure 5.3). Dietary protein restriction during rat pregnancy selectively attenuates 11β-HSD-2, but apparently not other placental enzymes (Langley-Evans *et al.*, 1996b; Bertram *et al.*, 2001; Lesage *et al.*, 2001). Indeed in the maternal protein restriction model, offspring hypertension can be prevented by treating the pregnant dam with glucocorticoid synthesis inhibitors, and can be recreated by concurrent administration of corticosterone, at least in female offspring (Langley-Evans, 1997).

As the maternal glucocorticoid levels are much higher than those of the fetus, subtle changes in placental 11β-HSD-2 activity may have profound effects on fetal glucocorticoid exposure (Lopez-Bernal *et al.*, 1980; Lopez Bernal and Craft, 1981). A relative deficiency of placental 11β-HSD-2 therefore has far greater potential consequences in terms of the fetal glucocorticoid load than any alteration in fetal adrenal steroid production, once the capacity of the fetal hypothalamic–pituitary–adrenal (HPA) axis to suppress fetal adrenal output has been overwhelmed.

Peripheral programming

Blood pressure and cardiovascular control

The human epidemiology began by showing low birth weight associates with adult heart disease mortality and hypertension (Barker *et al.*, 1989a, b; RichEdwards *et al.*, 1997). These associations remain arguably the most robust in the literature (Huxley *et al.*, 2000). It is unsurprising therefore that investigators have addressed the role of antenatal insults, including glucocorticoid excess, upon cardiovascular parameters. From these studies it appears that prenatal glucocorticoid exposure usually produces permanently elevated offspring blood pressure in later life, as assessed by the direct (semi-restrained animals with chronically catheterized vessels) and indirect (tail cuff) methods employed. It should be noted that these techniques involve an inherent component of stress in their measurement and true basal pressures (using 'gold standard' telemetric approaches) remain as yet unreported.

In utero, cortisol infusion into the fetus elevates blood pressure in sheep (Tangalakis *et al.*, 1992). Betamethasone given to pregnant baboons has similar hypertensive effects on the fetuses (Koenen *et al.*, 2002). Excess cortisol also directly elevates blood pressure at birth in humans (Kari *et al.*, 1994) and sheep (Berry *et al.*, 1997). Such effects appear to persist.

Thus, treatment of pregnant rats with dexamethasone, a synthetic glucocorticoid used in obstetric practice which readily crosses the placenta, reduces birth weight, a deficit reversed by weaning. Both male and female adult offspring of dexamethasone-treated pregnancies have elevated blood pressures (Benediktsson *et al.*, 1993). Similarly, adult hypertension is produced in sheep exposed to excess glucocorticoid in utero, either as maternally administered dexamethasone or as a maternal cortisol infusion (Dodic *et al.*, 1998; 1999; 2002a, b; Jensen *et al.*, 2002). The timing of glucocorticoid exposure appears to be important; exposure to glucocorticoids during the final week of pregnancy in the rat is sufficient to produce permanent adult hypertension (Levitt *et al.*, 1996; Sugden *et al.*, 2001), whereas the sensitive window for such effects in sheep are earlier in gestation (Gatford *et al.*, 2000). Such differences may be primarily due to the complex species-specific patterns of expression of GR, MR and the isoenzymes of 11β-HSD, which are crucial in both the regulation of maternal glucocorticoid transfer to the fetus, and in modulating glucocorticoid action at the tissue level. So, excess exposure to exogenous glucocorticoid can programme cardiovascular physiology, but outside obstetric pharmacotherapy does this matter to the majority of low-birth-weight babies?

Inhibition of 11β-HSD by treatment of pregnant rats with carbenoxolone has effects similar to dexamethasone, leading to offspring of modestly reduced birth weight. This associates with increased passage of maternal corticosterone to the fetal plasma. Although the weight deficit is typically regained by weaning, as with dexamethasone, prenatal carbenoxolone-exposed rats develop adult hypertension (Lindsay *et al.*, 1996a). These effects of carbenoxolone are independent of changes in maternal blood pressure or electrolytes, but require the presence of maternal glucocorticoids; the offspring of adrenalectomized pregnant rats are protected from carbenoxolone actions upon birth weight or adult physiology. It must be noted that carbenoxolone is non-selective and inhibits the other 11β-HSD isozyme (type 1) (HSD-1) and related dehydrogenases. However, congenic 11β-HSD-2 null mice also have low birth weight and preliminary data suggest that they show programming of CNS development and adult functions such as anxiety-related behaviours (see below).

Mechanisms of cardiovascular programming by prenatal glucocorticoids

Exploring such rodent models, the mechanisms of glucocorticoid-programmed adult hypertension have been studied. These are thought to involve a variety of processes that are also likely to have distinctive windows of sensitivity. Thus, prenatal glucocorticoids lead to reductions in nephron number (Ortiz *et al.*, 2001) which are largely irreversibly determined around birth. In addition, antenatal glucocorticoid exposure affects fetal and adult vascular responses to vasoconstrictors, enhancing endothelin-induced vasoconstriction in association with abnormal endothelium-dependent relaxation at least in sheep (Molnar *et al.*, 2002; 2003), indicating microvascular dysfunction. Analogous findings occur in rats (Hadoke *et al.*, unpublished data). The vascular changes may reflect the programming of receptors and post-receptor mechanisms in the vascular wall and other cardiovascular structures. These effects appear to be vascular bed specific (Docherty *et al.*, 2001), underlining the exquisite complexity of the systems involved. Also, renin–angiotensin system (RAS) parameters including receptor density and tissue RAS component synthesis are affected by antenatal steroid exposure (Dodic *et al.*, 2001), notably within the fetal kidney (Moritz *et al.*, 2002) where angiotensinogen, the AT1 and AT2 receptors are increased after dexamethasone, accompanied by a reduced glomerular filtration rate response to angiotensin II. Finally, key brain stem barocontrol centres are altered by prenatal glucocorticoid exposure (Dodic *et al.*, 1999). These actions may combine to form an adult with multiple processes contributing to hypertension. Which processes are key remains to be discerned and may, of course, differ between species and the timing of the exposure. Thus, the same apparent adult phenotype may clearly be underpinned by distinct 'programmed' processes, a notion we return to below when addressing neuroendocrine programming.

Programming the heart?

A key component of the human early life origins phenomenon is an increased risk of cardiovascular death in adults who were of low birth weight (Barker *et al.*, 1989b;

RichEdwards *et al.*, 1997). This may merely reflect the sum of increased cardiovascular risk factors such as hypertension and metabolic disorders, but primary cardiac programming may also be involved. In support of the latter possibility, prenatal glucocorticoid exposure alters the trajectory of development of cardiac noradrenergic innervation and sympathetic activity (Bian *et al.*, 1993), increases cardiac adenylate cyclase reactivity to a range of stimuli (Bian *et al.*, 1992) and alters key cardiac metabolic regulators such as the glucose transporter 1, *akt*/protein kinase B, specific uncoupling proteins (UCP) and the nuclear receptor for fatty acids PPARγ (Langdown *et al.*, 2001a, b). Perhaps crucially, given the documented association between overexpression of cardiac calreticulin and cardiac dysfunction and death, antenatal glucocorticoid exposure increases calreticulin levels markedly in the adult heart (Langdown *et al.*, 2003). Thus, these experimental models teach that increased coronary heart disease in low-birth-weight populations may reflect both an increased prevalence of major cardiovascular risk factors as well as primary cardiac dysfunction.

Programming of glucose–insulin homoeostasis and metabolic functions

Prenatal glucocorticoid overexposure also 'programmes' permanent hyperglycaemia and, particularly, hyperinsulinaemia in the adult offspring in the rat (Nyirenda *et al.*, 1998; Sugden *et al.*, 2001), effects delimited to the last third of gestation. Gestational 11β-HSD inhibition has similar adult hyperglycaemic effects (Lindsay *et al.*, 1996b). Earlier gestational dexamethasone exposures or post-partum steroids do not programme hypergylcaemia/hyperinsulinaemia in the rat, defining a tight window for this effect (Nyirenda *et al.*, 1998; 2001). Maternal glucocorticoid administration has an effect on cord glucose and insulin levels in the ovine fetus (Sloboda *et al.*, 2002b). Adult glucose–insulin dyshomoeostasis also occurs in sheep exposed to dexamethasone in utero (Dodic *et al.*, 1998; Gatford *et al.*, 2000), though the sensitive 'windows' again appear to be earlier than in the rat and can be dissociated from those producing with hypertension. Importantly, in the ovine model, antenatal glucocorticoid exposure alters adult glucose metabolism whether or not there is prior fetal growth restriction (Moss *et al.*, 2001). Specifically, maternal but not fetal injections of betamethasone restrict fetal growth (Newnham *et al.*, 1999); however, offspring of both the groups have altered adult glucose dynamics (Moss *et al.*, 2001). Thus, it appears that the programming effects on glucose–insulin homoeostasis in this model relate to fetal exposure to excess glucocorticoids in utero, rather than any primary effect of intrauterine growth retardation per se.

Mechanisms of glucocorticoid-programmed hyperglycaemia/insulin resistance

Several important hepatic metabolic systems are regulated by glucocorticoids, including key enzymes of carbohydrate metabolism such as phosphoenolpyruvate carboxykinase (PEPCK), a rate-limiting enzyme in gluconeogenesis. In rats, exposure

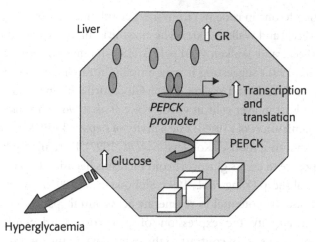

Figure 5.4   Liver programming by glucocorticoids. Prenatal dexamethasone permanently increases PEPCK gene expression. This appears to be driven by increased GR and thus increased sensitivity to glucocorticoid-mediated hyperglycaemia

to excess glucocorticoid in utero leads to offspring with permanent elevations in PEPCK mRNA and enzyme activity from a few days postnatally to midlife. This occurs selectively in the gluconeogenic periportal region of the hepatic acinus (Nyirenda *et al.*, 1998). This finding, which appears specific to PEPCK since other hepatic enzymes examined were unaltered, may be of pathogenic importance (Figure 5.4). Thus, overexpression of PEPCK in a rat hepatoma cell line impairs suppression of gluconeogenesis by insulin (Rosella *et al.*, 1993) and transgenic mice with overexpression of hepatic PEPCK have impaired glucose tolerance (Valera *et al.*, 1994). In terms of molecular mechanisms, PEPCK is regulated by a host of transcription factors (Duong *et al.*, 2002), but intriguingly, it is increased expression of GR itself that occurs in the livers of prenatal dexamethasone-programmed rats (Nyirenda *et al.*, 1998; Cleasby *et al.*, 2003b) in a pattern congruent with the periportal rise in PEPCK gene expression (Nyirenda *et al.*, 1998). This increase in GR may be crucial, since animals exposed to dexamethasone in utero have greater plasma glucose responses to exogenous corticosterone suggesting a specific increase in tissue sensitivity to the glycemic effects of the steroid (Nyirenda *et al.*, 1998). Thus, the observed glucose intolerance in rats exposed to excessive glucocorticoids in utero may be explained in part by programmed hepatic PEPCK overexpression leading to increased gluconeogenesis. Similar increases in hepatic GR are seen in the offspring of undernourished ewes (Whorwood *et al.*, 2001) suggesting the process is conserved.

Programming of hepatic 11β-HSD-1?

The 11β-HSD-1 is an NADPH-associated 11-keto reductase in intact cells and organs such as liver (Jamieson *et al.*, 1995; 2000). This functions to catalyse the reactivation of cortisol (corticosterone in rodents) from inert circulating cortisone (11-dehydro-corticosterone) (Seckl and Walker, 2001). The enzyme is highly expressed in liver and adipose tissue (Seckl and Walker, 2001). 11β-HSD-1 often co-localizes with GR (Whorwood et al., 1991) suggesting it may amplify intracellular ligands and their access to the receptor (Seckl and Walker, 2001). Glucocorticoids in turn regulate 11β-HSD-1 activity at least in liver cells in vitro (Voice et al., 1996), although this is less certain in vivo (Jamieson et al., 1999). The activity of hepatic PEPCK is decreased in the 11β-HSD-1 knockout mouse (Kotelevtsev et al., 1997). Intriguingly, both mater-nal and fetal exposure to excess glucocorticoid increases hepatic 11β-HSD-1 mRNA and protein in fetal sheep (Yang et al., 1995; Sloboda et al., 2002b). Such changes in 11β-HSD-1 increase the potential to regenerate active intrahepatic glucocorticoids, and may further amplify the expression of glucocorticoid-dependent hepatic enzymes of gluconeogenesis. In contrast to the ovine data, in the rat antenatal dexa-methasone has no effect on adult liver 11β-HSD-1 (Nyirenda et al., 1998) and ante-natal carbenoxolone actually reduces adult liver 11β-HSD-1 levels (Saegusa et al., 1999). So the jury remains out on this issue.

Programming the pancreas

In utero undernutrition impairs rat β-cell development (Garofano et al., 1997; 1998), resulting in reduced β-cell mass and subsequent glucose intolerance. Recent evidence suggests that glucocorticoids may play an important part in this (Blondeau et al., 2001). In rats with normal nutrition, fetal pancreatic-insulin content is nega-tively correlated with fetal corticosterone levels, and β-cell mass increases when fetal steroid production is impaired (Blondeau et al., 2001). Maternal malnutrition in the rat is associated with elevated maternal and fetal corticosterone levels in addition to decreased fetal pancreatic-insulin content and β-cell mass. Preventing the cortico-sterone increase in food-restricted dams by adrenalectomy with corticosterone replacement restores β-cell mass (Blondeau et al., 2001). The mechanisms by which glucocorticoids modulate pancreatic development are not fully discerned, but dexa-methasone downregulates β-cell Pdx-1 and induces C/EBPβ, key factors in the induction and repression (respectively) of insulin gene expression (Shen et al., 2003). Further, glucocorticoids influence the expression of IGF-2, a key peptide growth factor in pancreatic development, in addition to the IGF receptor and several IGF-binding proteins (Hill and Duvillie, 2000).

Adipose tissue and programming: an emerging area?
Muscle and fat

Exposure to antenatal dexamethasone in rats is also associated with programming of fat and muscle metabolism (Cleasby et al., 2003a). In skeletal muscle the pheno-type is subtle; prenatal glucocorticoid exposure decreases GR selectively in the type

2 fibre-enriched soleus muscle, but not in muscles rich in type 1 or glycolytic fibres. In contrast, prenatal glucocorticoid exposure causes a striking increase of GR expression in visceral but not peripheral adipose tissue in adult rats (Cleasby et al., 2003a) and sheep (Whorwood et al., 2001). Elevated GR expression in visceral adipose tissue in the presence of circulating hypercorticosteronaemia suggests increased glucocorticoid action in visceral fat. This may contribute to both adipose and hepatic-insulin resistance. These changes in GR expression do not appear to be the result of metabolic derangement in the adult animal, correction of the hypercorticosteronaemia and insulin sensitization are not sufficient to normalize the programmed changes in GR (Cleasby et al., 2003b). However, intriguingly, metformin selectively normalized the elevated GR in dexamethasone-programmed liver, an effect apparently distinct from insulin sensitization since a thiazolidinedione (PPARγ agonist) did not exert the selective effect.

Leptin

Leptin, an adipose gene product that signals both centrally and peripherally, where it plays a role in insulin sensitivity, is present in the circulation of human and porcine fetuses from midgestation (Jaquet et al., 1998; Chen et al., 2000), and in adipose tissue of human fetuses by 20 weeks gestation (Lepercq et al., 2001). Additionally, mRNA for leptin and leptin receptors, have been detected in the fetal tissues of many other species (Yuen et al., 1999; Hoggard et al., 2000; Lepercq et al., 2001; Mostyn et al., 2001; Thomas et al., 2001). In the human fetus, circulating leptin levels increase towards term, associated with a significant increase in body fat after 34 weeks of gestation (Jaquet et al., 1998; Geary et al., 1999; Cetin et al., 2000) and in fetal sheep, leptin mRNA increases in adipose tissue with increasing gestational age (Yuen et al., 1999). Intriguingly, leptin concentrations in human fetal cord blood correlate directly with body weight and adiposity at birth (Koistinen et al., 1997; Schubring et al., 1997; Jaquet et al., 1998; Ong et al., 1999; Lepercq et al., 2001) indicating a potential role for leptin in linking fetal growth and metabolic programming.

In rats, antenatal treatment of the pregnant mother with dexamethasone reduces fetal plasma and placental levels of leptin, while maternal plasma leptin levels remain unchanged or increase (Sugden et al., 2001; Smith and Waddell, 2002). Dexamethasone also reduces placental expression of the leptin receptor isoform Ob-Rb, which mediates leptin action (Smith and Waddell, 2002), while levels of the isoform ObR-S (the proposed transport form of the receptor) are modestly increased (Sugden et al., 2001). In the adult offspring, antenatal glucocorticoids lead to increased leptin levels (Sugden et al., 2001), which may contribute to the cardiometabolic phenotype produced. Of course, the glucocorticoid-sensitive leptin transcript (Slieker et al., 1996) may in part be driven by the higher expression of adipose tissue GR in adult prenatal glucocorticoid-programmed rats, though leptin is mainly produced in peripheral depots whereas GR expression was mainly elevated in visceral fat (Cleasby et al., 2003a). Most intriguingly, concomitant treatment of malnourished pregnant and lactating rats with leptin appears to reverse, in part, the adult metabolic effects of antenatal challenge, at least for maternal malnutrition (Stocker et al., 2003).

However, the same may not pertain in the sheep, in which exogenous cortisol or dexamethasone administration directly to the fetus increases rather than reduces plasma leptin concentrations, albeit transiently (Forhead et al., 2002; Mostyn et al., 2003). The differences between these studies may reflect the route of glucocorticoid administration, species, fetal body fat levels and/or maternal nutrient intake.

Adiponectin

Adiponectin (acrp30, adipoQ) is an abundant, adipose-specific protein which is secreted into the blood. Adiponectin is negatively associated with fat mass (Hu et al., 1996) and positively associated with insulin sensitivity (Weyer et al., 2001) and may mediate obesity-related resistance to insulin. Lower plasma adiponectin levels appear to predict the later occurrence of type 2 diabetes (Lindsay et al., 2002). Adiponectin is strikingly regulated by hormones and other factors during postnatal development (Combs et al., 2003). Given the emerging biology of the adipocyte and its important role in some programming phenomena (Cleasby et al., 2003a), it is likely to be of interest. However, a recent study in humans found no association between birth weight and adiponectin levels (Lindsay et al., 2003).

Glucocorticoid programming of the brain

'We all are born mad. Some remain so', Samuel Beckett, Waiting for Godot (1955). The CNS has long been subject to scrutiny for organizational influences in early life upon adult function and the pathogenesis of neuropsychiatric disorders. Many studies have exploited maternal and/or fetal stressors to alter developmental trajectories of specific CNS structures or gene products and reported persistent effects (Weinstock, 2001). While the effects of stress are in part mediated by glucocorticoid secretion, steroids are by no means the only efferent effector pathway of the stress response and other hormones (catecholamines are obvious candidates), neurotransmitters, vascular and metabolic systems are altered as well in a stressor and strain-specific manner. Nonetheless, studies of antenatal stress in animals have clearly documented long-term effects upon a host of CNS functions (reviewed in Weinstock, 2001; Welberg and Seckl, 2001) and have laid the foundations for studies of more specific programming agents including glucocorticoids.

Glucocorticoids are important for normal brain maturation, exerting a range of effects in most regions of the developing CNS (Meaney et al., 1996; Korte, 2001;

Weinstock, 2001; Welberg and Seckl, 2001) including the initiation of post-mitotic terminal maturation, axo-dendritic remodelling and the modulation of neonatal brain cell death (Meyer, 1983). Prenatal glucocorticoid administration retards brain weight at birth in sheep, with a suggestion of dose dependency (Huang *et al.*, 1999). This is associated with delays in the cellular maturation of neurones, glia and cerebral vasculature (Huang *et al.*, 2001a) and retarded CNS myelination (Huang *et al.*, 2001b). Given such widespread effects of glucocorticoids it is unsurprising that GR and MR are highly expressed in the developing brain with complex locus-specific ontogenies to allow selectivity of effects (Fuxe *et al.*, 1985; Diaz *et al.*, 1996; Kitraki *et al.*, 1997).

However, whether these receptors are occupied by endogenous glucocorticoids until late gestation is not clear, because there is also plentiful 11β-HSD-2 in the CNS at midgestation (Brown *et al.*, 1996a; Diaz *et al.*, 1996; Robson *et al.*, 1998). This presumably functions to 'protect' vulnerable developing cells from premature glucocorticoid actions. Strikingly, 11β-HSD-2 expression is dramatically switched-off in a CNS locus-specific manner, mainly at the end of midgestation in the rat and mouse brain. Possibly this widespread gene silencing in the CNS coincides with the terminal stage of brain nucleus development (Brown *et al.*, 1996a; Diaz *et al.*, 1998). At birth in the rat the main areas of residual 11β-HSD-2 expression are in the thalamus and cerebellum, areas exhibiting substantial postnatal development. At least in the cerebellum this is highly sensitive to glucocorticoids (Bohn and Lauder, 1978; 1980). By weaning at postnatal day 21, CNS 11β-HSD-2 expression is confined to those few areas seen in the adult (Robson *et al.*, 1998). Similarly, in human fetal brain 11β-HSD-2 appears to be silenced between gestational weeks 19 and 26 (Stewart *et al.*, 1994; Brown *et al.*, 1996b). So, there appears to be an exquisitely timed system of protection and then exposure of developing brain regions to circulating glucocorticoids.

The HPA axis and its limbic system connections (hippocampus, amygdala) are also particularly sensitive to endogenous and exogenous glucocorticoids during perinatal development (Bohn, 1980; Gould *et al.*, 1991a, b) and indeed to perinatal glucocorticoids or stress programme-specific effects in these regions of the brain (Welberg and Seckl, 2001). Programming of neuroendocrine and limbic systems appears conserved and is observed across a range of experimental species and, less certainly, in humans.

Programming the HPA axis

Studies in animal models indicate that the HPA axis is an important target for glucocorticoid programming. The HPA axis is controlled by a negative feedback system. Glucocorticoids from the adrenal cortex activate GR in the pituitary and paraventricular nucleus (PVN) of the hypothalamus as well as to extrahypothalamic CNS feedback sites. The latter include the hippocampus (Jacobson and Sapolsky, 1991) which highly expresses both GR and the higher-affinity MR in rodents (Reul and de Kloet, 1985) and probably humans (Seckl *et al.*, 1991). Overactivity at any point along the pathway results in negative feedback to decrease the amount of corticotrophin-releasing hormone (CRH) released from the PVN, and thus decrease adrenocorticotrophic hormone (ACTH) release from the pituitary and hence the synthesis and secretion of glucocorticoids.

Prenatal dexamethasone exposure or 11β-HSD-2 inhibition permanently increases basal plasma corticosterone levels in adult rats (Levitt *et al.*, 1996; Welberg *et al.*, 2001). Whilst the mechanism of hypercorticosteronaemia is not fully understood, the density of GR and MR in the hippocampus are reduced in this model. This would be anticipated to attenuate feedback sensitivity which may well explain basal hypercorticosteronaemia. Moreover, the glucocorticoid excess may drive, at least in part, the hypertension and hyperglycaemia observed in this and other prenatal environmental programming models (Langley-Evans, 1997). Of course, this will be amplified by the documented increase in hepatic (and presumably visceral adipose tissue) glucocorticoid sensitivity (Nyirenda *et al.*, 1998; Cleasby *et al.*, 2003a). Similarly, in sheep, exposure to betamethasone in utero alters HPA responsiveness in the offspring at up to 1 year of age, though earlier exposure to dexamethasone has no persisting HPA effects in this species (Dodic *et al.*, 2002c). Intriguingly, the outcomes vary according to the time of gestational exposure to steroid (Figure 5.5), and whether it was administered to the mother or directly to the fetus (Sloboda *et al.*, 2002a). Thus, maternal administration of betamethasone elevates basal and stimulated cortisol levels in the offspring, whereas betamethasone directly to the fetus attenuates offspring

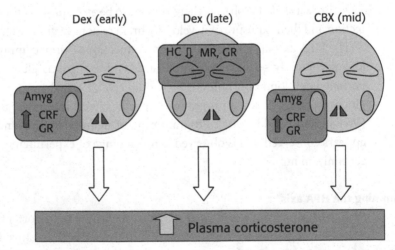

Figure 5.5   Timing of glucocorticoid exposure upon programming of the HPA axis. The same adult phenotype can arise by distinct central mechanisms. HC: hippocampus; Amyg: amygdala; CRF: corticotrophin-releasing factor; Dex: dexamethasone; CBX: carbenoxolone

ACTH responses to CRH with arginine vasopressin (AVP) (Sloboda *et al.*, 2002a); whether this discrepancy reflects relative dose, duration or perhaps indirect effects of maternally administered steroids remains to be determined. Maternal undernutrition in rats (Langley-Evans *et al.*, 1996a) and sheep (Hawkins *et al.*, 2000) also affects adult HPA axis function, suggesting that HPA programming may be a common outcome of prenatal environmental challenge, perhaps acting in part via alterations in placental 11β-HSD-2 activity which is selectively downregulated by maternal dietary constraint (Langley-Evans *et al.*, 1996b; Bertram *et al.*, 2001).

Further evidence for the importance of the details of exposure in determining the long-term effects of glucocorticoid programming comes from recent studies in guinea pigs. These animals are relatively glucocorticoid resistant because of a mutant GR gene (Keightley and Fuller, 1994). Perhaps in consequence, prenatal glucocorticoid exposure has smaller effects on the HPA axis in guinea pig offspring (Dean *et al.*, 2001; Liu *et al.*, 2001). The duration of exposure and the sex of the offspring also have an impact in this species as in others. In males, short-term exposure to dexamethasone (2 days) leads to significantly elevated basal plasma cortisol levels; whereas repeated doses reduce basal and stimulated plasma cortisol levels in adults. In contrast, juvenile females exposed for 2 days have reduced HPA responses to stress, whereas adult females exposed to repeated antenatal doses of dexamethasone have higher plasma cortisol levels in the follicular and early luteal phases. Similar sex-specific programming of the HPA axis have been reported for prenatal stress in rats (Weinstock *et al.*, 1992; McCormick *et al.*, 1995).

A study of the effects of glucocorticoid programming in primates showed that the offspring of mothers treated with dexamethasone during late pregnancy had elevated basal and stress-stimulated cortisol levels and a 30% reduction in hippocampal size (Uno *et al.*, 1994). These studies in rodents, guinea pigs, sheep and primates indicate that exposure to excess glucocorticoids in utero can programme HPA axis function. The data addressing HPA programming in humans are discussed at the end of this review.

Programming behaviour

Overexposure to glucocorticoids in utero, as a result of either prenatal dexamethasone administration or 11β-HSD inhibition leads to alterations in adult behaviour. Administration of dexamethasone to rats for all 3 weeks of gestation or only in the last week reduces ambulation and rearing in the open field in adult animals (Figure 5.6; Welberg *et al.*, 2001), although another study did not find this (Holson *et al.*, 1995). These studies employed subtly different timings of exposure, again suggesting that very specific time windows exist for the effects of prenatal treatments (Figure 5.5). Additionally, late gestation administration of dexamethasone alters exploration on an elevated plus maze and reduces immobility both in the acquisition and the

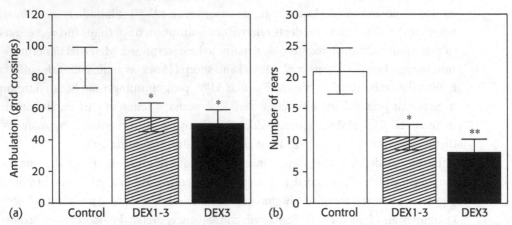

Figure 5.6   Administering dexamethasone to pregnant rats reduced ambulation and rearing of their offspring in the open field. Adapted from Welberg *et al.* (2001)

retrieval phase of a forced-swim test, implying impaired coping and a reduced capacity for acquisition, consolidation and/or retrieval of information under stressful circumstances (Welberg *et al.*, 2001). This suggests that fetal glucocorticoid exposure, especially during the last week of gestation, may programme 'behavioural inhibition' and reduced coping in aversive situations later in life. Intriguingly, inhibition of 11β-HSD, which is most highly expressed in midgestation, produces a phenotype intermediate between continuous and final week dexamethasone exposure (Welberg *et al.*, 2000). Prenatal glucocorticoid exposure also affects the developing dopaminergic system (Diaz *et al.*, 1995; 1997) with clear implications for proposed developmental contributions to schizo-affective, attention-deficit hyperactivity and extrapyramidal disorders. Indeed, stressful events in the second trimester of human pregnancy associate with an increased incidence of schizophrenia in the offspring (Koenig *et al.*, 2002).

Structural effects of antenatal glucocorticoids on the CNS

Exposure to glucocorticoids in utero has widespread acute effects upon neuronal structure and synapse formation (Antonow-Schlorke *et al.*, 2003), and may permanently alter brain structure (Matthews, 2000). Studies in young and aged animals and humans have demonstrated that stress and increased glucocorticoid concentrations can lead to changes in hippocampal structure (Bremner *et al.*, 1995; Sheline *et al.*, 1996; Stein *et al.*, 1997; Sapolsky, 1999). In rhesus monkeys, treatment with antenatal dexamethasone caused a dose-dependent neuronal degeneration of hippocampal neurones and reduced hippocampal volume in the fetuses, which persisted at 20 months of age (Uno *et al.*, 1990). Fetuses receiving multiple lower-dose injections showed more severe damage than those receiving a single-large injection. Human and animal studies have demonstrated that altered hippocampal structure may be associated with a number of consequences for memory and behaviour (Bremner *et al.*, 1995; Sheline *et al.*, 1996; Stein *et al.*, 1997).

In mice, prenatal treatment with prednisolone appears to lead to delayed motor development, offspring have delayed eye opening and delayed development of lifting, walking and gripping skills (Gandelman and Rosenthal, 1981). In rhesus monkeys, prenatal dexamethasone was not associated with delayed motor development (Uno *et al.*, 1994). In sheep, betamethasone exposure in utero is associated with delayed myelination in areas of the brain undergoing active myelination at the time of exposure, such as the optic nerve (Dunlop *et al.*, 1997), with unknown consequences.

Intriguing recent data suggest that deleterious developmental effects of excess glucocorticoids upon the CNS are even more widespread. Prenatal exposure to dexamethasone increases the susceptibility of the cochlea to acoustic noise trauma in adulthood. Interestingly, the mechanism involves increased susceptibility to oxidative stress, and can be treated effectively with antioxidants (Canlon *et al.*, 2003).

CNS programming mechanisms

The brain is clearly important as a target for glucocorticoid programming. Its mechanisms have been examined at a variety of levels, from structural to gene expression, for instance recently exploiting emerging microarray technology (Kinnunen *et al.*, 2003). However, a caution is required since the mechanisms of programming appear to differ somewhat depending on the timing of the exposure and the species involved. Nevertheless, some headway has been made.

Indications of the molecular mechanisms by which early life environmental factors may programme offspring physiology come from the studies of the processes underpinning postnatal environmental programming of the HPA axis in the 'neonatal handling' paradigm (Levine, 1957; 1962; Meaney *et al.*, 1988; 1996). In this model, 15 min of daily handling of rat pups during the first 2 weeks of life (Meaney *et al.*, 1988) permanently increases GR density in the hippocampus and prefrontal cortex, but not in other brain regions. This increase in receptor density potentiates the HPA axis sensitivity to glucocorticoid negative feedback and results in lower plasma glucocorticoid levels throughout life, a state compatible with a good adjustment to environmental stress (Meaney *et al.*, 1989; 1992). Neonatal glucocorticoid exposure may have similar effects (Catalani *et al.*, 1993). The neonatal handling model appears to be of physiological relevance, since handling enhances maternal care-related behaviours and natural variation in such maternal behaviour correlates similarly with the offspring HPA physiology and hippocampal GR expression (Liu *et al.*, 1997). The long-term manifestations of some prenatal programming can be substantially modified by the immediate postnatal environment (Maccari *et al.*,

1995), suggesting that distinct 'windows' occur and showing that apparently similar early life events may produce different responses depending upon their degree, duration, developmental timing or sequence. Again, the implications for human epidemiology are that distinct offspring pathophysiologies may be determined merely by the timing and severity of the stimulus/stress involved.

For prenatal glucocorticoid exposure, in the rat, while both long- and short-term exposure to prenatal dexamethasone result in adults with elevated basal corticosterone levels, the underlying mechanisms differ depending on the timing of exposure. Exposure to dexamethasone during the last third of pregnancy reduces MR and GR levels in the hippocampus and increases CRH mRNA in the hypothalamic PVN (Welberg *et al.*, 2001). In contrast, dexamethasone throughout gestation does not alter hippocampal GR or MR, but increases receptor expression in the amygdala, a structure which stimulates the HPA axis (Welberg *et al.*, 2001). Thus in the rat, late gestational dexamethasone exposure may permanently alter the 'set point' of the HPA axis at the level of the hippocampus, reducing feedback sensitivity, whereas continuous exposure may increase forward drive of the HPA axis through the amygdala. By implication, distinct neural mechanisms underlie the common outcome of altered HPA axis activity following prenatal glucocorticoid exposure. This rather fundamental idea may underlie the subtle but important differences in outcome phenotypes seen in various perinatal programming models and may involve more than the HPA axis. GR and MR programming by antenatal glucocorticoid exposure also occurs in sheep though the effects appear less robust (Matthews, 2002).

CRH programming in the amygdala?

The behavioural changes observed in prenatal glucocorticoid-exposed offspring may be associated with altered functioning of the amygdala, a structure involved in the expression of fear and anxiety. Intra-amygdala administration of CRH is anxiogenic (Dunn and Berridge, 1990). Prenatal dexamethasone or 11β-HSD inhibition increases CRH mRNA levels specifically in the central nucleus of the amygdala (Figure 5.7), a key locus for the effects of the neuropeptide on the expression of fear and anxiety (Welberg *et al.*, 2000; 2001). Prenatal stress similarly programmes increased anxiety-related behaviours along with elevated CRH expression and release in the amygdala (Cratty *et al.*, 1995). Indeed, corticosteroids facilitate CRH mRNA expression in this nucleus (Makino *et al.*, 1994; Hsu *et al.*, 1998) and increase GR and/or MR in the amygdala (Welberg *et al.*, 2000; 2001). The amygdala stimulates the HPA axis via a CRH signal (Feldman and Weidenfeld, 1998), thus an elevated corticosteroid signal in the amygdala consequent on the hypercorticosteronaemia in the adult offspring of dexamethasone-treated dams, may produce the increased CRH levels in adulthood. CRH, arising from the forebrain, is also important in the

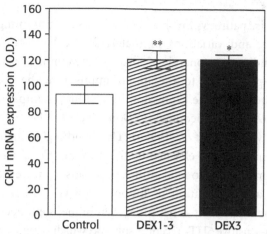

Figure 5.7   Administering dexamethasone prenatally increased CRH mRNA levels in the amygdala of adult rats. Adapted from Welberg *et al.* (2000)

hippocampus where it facilitates acetylcholine transmission. Intriguingly prenatal stress potentiates this action of CRH, though the molecular basis is obscure (Day *et al.*, 1998).

A direct relationship between brain corticosteroid receptor levels and anxiety-like behaviour is supported by the phenotype of cre-lox transgenic mice with selective loss of GR gene expression in the brain, which show markedly reduced anxiety (Tronche *et al.*, 1999). Dexamethasone exposure increases GR and MR gene expression in the amygdala, though the subnuclei involved depend upon timing of exposure (Welberg *et al.*, 2001). In such details will doubtless lie the understanding of the links between programming and phenotype.

How might such mechanistically distinct effects come about with glucocorticoid exposure at different times during development? It seems reasonable to propose that programming may only happen at critical times during organ development. Thus, glucocorticoid exposure in the last days of gestation in the rat can target CNS regions actively developing, such as the hippocampus, but not those yet to develop or those already in their final state. The long and complex pre- and postnatal ontogeny of the brain makes it a prime target for programming. The complex patterns of expression of the key candidate genes GR, MR and the 11β-HSDs in the brain may underlie this (Diaz *et al.*, 1998; Matthews, 1998). Whilst the details of brain ontogeny patterns are species specific, the broad impression of tissues protected from or allowing timed exposure to glucocorticoids appears a tenable interpretation of these exquisite patterns of gene expression. Clearly exogenous (or endogenous) steroids can only have developmental effects on specific target genes and systems during their individual ontogenic windows of susceptibility.

Neuronal pathways and mechanisms

In recent years, the precise pathways involved in HPA axis programming associated with neonatal handling and variations in maternal care have been dissected. Handling acts via ascending serotonergic (5-hydroxytryptamine, 5HT) pathways from the midbrain raphe nuclei to the hippocampus (Smythe *et al.*, 1994). Activation of 5HT induces GR gene expression in fetal hippocampal neurones in vitro (Mitchell *et al.*, 1990) and in neonatal (O'Donnell *et al.*, 1994) and adult hippocampal neurones in vivo (Yau *et al.*, 1997a). The 'handling' induction of 5HT requires thyroid hormones that are elevated by the stimulus. Consistent with this, administration of dexamethasone to fetal guinea pigs leads to an elevation of fetal thyroid hormone and an upregulation of hippocampal GR mRNA (Dean and Matthews, 1999). At the hippocampal neuronal membrane, some recent findings implicate the ketanserin-sensitive $5HT_7$ receptor subtype, which is regulated by glucocorticoids (Yau *et al.*, 1997b) and positively coupled to cAMP generation, in the handling effects (Meaney *et al.*, 2000). In vitro, 5HT stimulation of GR expression in hippocampal neurones is blocked by ketanserin and mimicked by cAMP analogues (Mitchell *et al.*, 1990; 1992). $5HT_7$ receptors appear to play a key role in this action (Laplante *et al.*, 2002). In vivo, handling also stimulates cAMP generation in the hippocampus (Diorio *et al.*, 1996). The next step appears to involve stimulation of cAMP associated and other transcription factors, most notably nerve growth factor-inducible factor A (NGFI-A) and activator protein 2 (AP-2) (Meaney *et al.*, 2000). NGFI-A and AP-2 may bind to the GR gene promoter (Encio and Detera-Wadleigh, 1991), though direct evidence for this is lacking. This pathway might also be involved in some *prenatal* programming paradigms affecting the HPA axis since last trimester dexamethasone exposure increases 5HT transporter expression in the rat brain (Fumagalli *et al.*, 1996; Slotkin *et al.*, 1996b), an effect predicted to reduce 5HT availability in the hippocampus and elsewhere. This may well induce a fall of GR and MR, the converse of postnatal handling.

The GR gene: a common programming target?

Expression of the GR gene is regulated in a complex tissue-specific manner. Although GR are expressed in all cells, their density and regulation vary considerably between tissues, and even within a tissue (Herman *et al.*, 1989). Transgenic mice with a reduction of 30–50% in tissue levels of GR have major neuroendocrine, metabolic and immunological abnormalities (Pepin *et al.*, 1992; King *et al.*, 1995). The level of expression of GR is thus critical for cell function. As discussed, there is much evidence to suggest that GR gene transcription can be programmed in a tissue-specific manner by perinatal events. The GR promoter is extremely complex, with multiple tissue-specific alternate untranslated first exons in rats (McCormick *et al.*, 2000) and mice (Cole *et al.*, 1995), most within a transcriptionally active 'CpG island'. All these mRNA species give rise to the same receptor protein, as only exons 2–9 encode the protein. The alternate untranslated first exons are spliced onto the common translated sequence beginning at exon 2. In the rat, two of the alternate exons are present in all tissues which have been studied; however, others are tissue specific (McCormick et al., 2000). This permits considerable complexity of tissue-specific variation in the control of GR expression and, potentially programming.

The tissue-specific first exon usage appears to be altered by perinatal environment manipulations (McCormick et al., 2000). Indeed, handling permanently programmes increased expression of only one of the six alternate first exons (exon 1_7) utilized in the hippocampus (McCormick et al., 2000). Exon 1_7 contains sites appropriate to bind the very third messenger/intermediate early gene transcription factors (AP-2, NGFI-A) induced by the neonatal manipulation (Meaney et al., 2000). In contrast, prenatal dexamethasone exposure, which increases hepatic GR expression, decreased the proportion of hepatic GR mRNA containing the predominant exon (exon 1_{10}), suggesting an increase in a minor exon 1 variant (McCormick et al., 2000). Such tissue specificity of promoter usage may help explain why prenatal dexamethasone programmes increased adult GR expression in the periportal zone of the liver and in the amygdala, but reduced GR expression in the hippocampus, and unchanged expression in many other brain regions and tissues.

Intriguingly, the apparent congruence between the effects of prenatal and postnatal environmental manipulations upon the adult HPA axis appears to reflect distinct underlying processes. Prenatal dexamethasone exposure permanently alters developing monoaminergic systems. Prenatal treatment decreases brain 5HT levels and advances the expression of the neuronal 5HT transporter which functions as a re-uptake site, removing 5HT from the synapse and thus attenuating its action, including in the hippocampus (Slotkin et al., 1996a; Muneoka et al., 1997). In the postnatal handling model, animals in the non-handled group have decreased hippocampal 5HT turnover. It appears that distinct mechanisms operating at different times of development can produce apparently similar permanent alterations in phenotype, in this case increased HPA axis activity.

The next crucial questions ask how discrete late prenatal/early postnatal events can permanently alter gene expression. Intriguing recent data have explored this in terms of chromatin. Some evidence is emerging for selective methylation/demethylation of specific promoters of the GR gene. Preliminary data suggest that the putative NGFI-A site around exon 1_7 is subject to differential and permanent methylation/demethylation in association with variations in maternal care (Weaver et al., 2002). Moreover, GR itself appears under some circumstances to mediate differential demethylation of target gene promoters, at least in liver-derived cells. The demethylation persists after steroid withdrawal. During development, such target promoter demethylation occurs before birth and may fine-tune the promoter to 'remember' regulatory events occurring during development (Thomassin *et al.*, 2001). This provocative novel mechanism of gene control by early life environmental events that persist throughout the lifespan remains to be confirmed in other systems.

Glucocorticoid programming in humans?

From the above, it is clear that prenatal exposure to excess glucocorticoids reduces birth weight in animal models and in humans. In animal models there are persisting effects on blood pressure, glucose tolerance and the HPA axis. Here we assess the possible relevance of such findings to human pathophysiology.

Glucocorticoid treatment during pregnancy reduces birth weight (French *et al.*, 1999; Bloom *et al.*, 2001), but there is a worrying dearth of evidence addressing the longer-term effects of prenatal glucocorticoid exposure. 11β-HSD-2 substrates such as cortisol and prednisolone would be anticipated to have little effect; however, glucocorticoids such as dexamethasone are commonly exploited because of their effect on the fetus. Substituted glucocorticoids such as dexamethasone and betamethasone, which are poor substrates for 11β-HSD-2, are most commonly used to treat fetuses at risk of preterm delivery, which may occur in up to 10% of pregnancies. There is no doubt that such synthetic glucocorticoids enhance lung maturation and reduce mortality in preterm infants (Crowley, 2000). Additionally, a single course of prenatal corticosteroid is associated with a significant reduction in the incidence of intraventricular haemorrhage and a trend towards less neurodevelopmental disability (Crowley, 2000). However, a recent survey of British obstetric departments showed that 98% were prescribing repeated courses of antenatal glucocorticoids (Brocklehurst *et al.*, 1999). Corticosteroid injections may be repeated four or more times in threatened preterm labour between 24 and 34 weeks of gestation; however, there is little evidence for the safety and efficacy of such a regime (Whitelaw and Thoresen, 2000). In addition, women at risk of bearing fetuses at risk of congenital adrenal hyperplasia often receive low-dose dexamethasone from the first trimester to suppress fetal adrenal androgen overproduction. Birth weight in such infants has been reported as normal (Forest *et al.*, 1993a; Mercado *et al.*, 1995a); however, it must be remembered that programming effects of antenatal glucocorticoids are seen in animal models in the absence of any reduction in birth weight (Moss *et al.*, 2001).

Recent overviews suggest that there is no evidence for additional benefit from repeated courses of glucocorticoid therapy in pregnancy (Kay *et al.*, 2000; Walfisch *et al.*, 2001), but that clear conclusions are prevented by the lack of prospective randomized-controlled trials and by variations in protocols employed (type of glucocorticoid, route and timing of administration, number of treatment courses). There remains considerable concern that a view which approximates, 'if some glucocorticoid is good, then more is better', is likely to be as erroneous for these steroids in perinatal medicine as it is in other therapeutic arenas (Seckl and Miller, 1997).

Antenatal glucocorticoid administration has also been linked with higher blood pressure in adolescence (Doyle *et al.*, 2000), although this study is complicated by the powerful effects of differential growth rates around puberty on blood pressure. A number of studies aimed at establishing the long-term neurological and developmental effects of antenatal glucocorticoid exposure have been complicated by the fact that most of the children studied were born before term and were therefore already at risk of delayed neurological development. In a group of 6-year-old children, antenatal glucocorticoid exposure was associated with subtle effects on neurological function, including reduced visual closure and visual memory (MacArthur *et al.*, 1982). Children exposed to dexamethasone, in early pregnancy because they were at risk of congenital adrenal hyperplasia, and who were born at term, showed increased emotionality, unsociability, avoidance and behavioural problems (Trautman *et al.*, 1995). These effects were seen in unaffected glucocorticoid-exposed offspring. Furthermore, a recent study has shown that multiple doses of antenatal glucocorticoids given to women at risk of preterm delivery were associated with reduced head circumference in the offspring (French *et al.*, 1999). There were also significant effects on behaviour; three or more courses of glucocorticoids were associated with an increased risk of externalizing behaviour problems, distractibility and inattention (French *et al.*, 1998).

As in other mammals, the human's HPA axis appears to be programmed by the early life environment. Higher plasma and urinary glucocorticoid levels are found in children and adults who were of lower birth weight (Clark *et al.*, 1996; Phillips *et al.*, 1998). This appears to occur in disparate populations (Phillips *et al.*, 2000) and may precede overt adult disease (Levitt *et al.*, 2000), at least in a socially disadvantaged South African population. Additionally, adult HPA responses to ACTH stimulation are exaggerated in those of low birth weight (Levitt *et al.*, 2000; Reynolds *et al.*, 2001), reflecting the stress axis biology elucidated in animal models. The HPA axis activation is associated with higher blood pressure, insulin resistance, glucose intolerance and hyperlipidaemia (Reynolds *et al.*, 2001). Finally, the human GR gene promoter has multiple alternate untranslated first exons (R. Reynolds and K. E. Chapman, unpublished observations), analogous to those found in the rat and mouse. Whether these are the subjects of early life regulation and the molecular mechanisms by which this is achieved remain to be determined.

Acknowledgements

Work in the authors' laboratory is funded by grants from the Wellcome Trust, the Scottish Hospitals Endowments Research Trust, the European Union and the British Heart Foundation.

REFERENCES

Albiston, A. L., Obeyesekere, V. R., Smith, R. E. and Krozowski, Z. S. (1994). Cloning and tissue distribution of the human 11β-hydroxysteroid dehydrogenase type 2 enzyme. *Mol. Cell. Endocrinol.*, **105**(2), R11–17.

Antonow-Schlorke, I., Schwab, M., Li, C. and Nathanielsz, P. W. (2003). Glucocorticoid exposure at the dose used clinically alters cytoskeletal proteins and presynaptic terminals in the fetal baboon brain. *J. Physiol. London*, **547**(1), 117–23.

Arai, Y. and Gorski, R. A. (1968). Critical exposure time for androgenization of the developing hypothalamus in the female rat. *Endocrinology*, **82**, 1010–14.

Baird, J., Osmond, C., MacGregor, A. *et al.* (2001). Testing the fetal origins hypothesis in twins: the Birmingham twin study. *Diabetologia*, **44**, 33–9.

Barker, D. J. P. (1991). *Fetal and Infant Origins of Adult Disease*, London: BMJ.

Barker, D. J. P., Osmond, C., Goldings, J., Kuh, D. and Wadsworth, M. E. J. (1989a). Growth in utero, blood pressure in childhood and adult life, and mortality from cardiovascular disease. *Br. Med. J.*, **298**, 564–7.

Barker, D. J. P., Winter, P. D., Osmond, C., Margetts, B. and Simmonds, S. J. (1989b). Weight in infancy and death from ischaemic heart disease. *Lancet*, **ii**, 577–80.

Barker, D. J. P., Bull, A. R., Osmond, C. and Simmonds, S. J. (1990). Fetal and placental size and risk of hypertension in adult life. *Br. Med. J.*, **301**, 259–63.

Barker, D. J. P., Gluckman, P. D., Godfrey, K. M. *et al.* (1993a). Fetal nutrition and cardiovascular disease in adult life. *Lancet*, **341**, 938–41.

Barker, D. J. P., Hales, C. N., Fall, C. H. D. *et al.* (1993b). Type 2 (non-insulin dependent) diabetes mellitus, hypertension and hyperlipidaemia (syndrome X): relation to reduced fetal growth. *Diabetologia*, **36**, 62–7.

Bavdekar, A., Yajnik, C. S., Fall, C. H. *et al.* (1999). Insulin resistance syndrome in 8-year-old Indian children: small at birth, big at 8 years, or both? *Diabetes*, **48**(12), 2422–9.

Beitens, I. Z., Bayard, F., Ances, I. G., Kowarski, A. and Migeon, C. J. (1973). The metabolic clearance rate, blood production, interconversion and transplacental passage of cortisol and cortisone in pregnancy near term. *Pediatr. Res.*, **7**, 509–19.

Benediktsson, R., Lindsay, R., Noble, J., Seckl, J. R. and Edwards, C. R. W. (1993). Glucocorticoid exposure in utero: a new model for adult hypertension. *Lancet*, **341**, 339–41.

Benediktsson, R., Brennand, J., Tibi, L. *et al.* (1995). Fetal osteocalcin levels are related to placental 11β-hydroxysteroid dehydrogenase activity. *Clin. Endocrinol.*, **42**, 551–5.

Benediktsson, R., Calder, A. A., Edwards, C. R. W. and Seckl, J. R. (1997). Placental 11β-hydroxysteroid dehydrogenase type 2 is the placental barrier to maternal glucocorticoids: ex vivo studies. *Clin. Endocrinol.*, **46**, 161–6.

Berry, L. M., Polk, D. H., Ikegami, M. *et al.* (1997). Preterm newborn lamb renal and cardiovascular responses after fetal or maternal antenatal betamethasone. *Am. J. Physiol. Regul. Integr. Comp. Physiol.*, **41**, R1972–9.

Bertram, C., Trowern, A. R., Copin, N., Jackson, A. A. and Whorwood, C. B. (2001). The maternal diet during pregnancy programs altered expression of the glucocorticoid receptor and type 2 11beta-hydroxysteroid dehydrogenase: potential molecular mechanisms underlying the programming of hypertension in utero. *Endocrinology*, **142**(7), 2841–53.

Bian, X. P., Seidler, F. J. and Slotkin, T. A. (1992). Promotional role for glucocorticoids in the development of intracellular signalling: enhanced cardiac and renal adenylate cyclase reactivity to β-adrenergic and non-adrenergic stimuli after low-dose fetal dexamethasone exposure. *J. Develop. Physiol.*, **17**, 289–97.

Bian, X. P., Seidler, F. J. and Slotkin, T. A. (1993). Fetal dexamethasone exposure interferes with establishment of cardiac noradrenergic innervation and sympathetic activity. *Teratology*, **47**, 109–17.

Blondeau, B., Lesage, J., Czernichow, P., Dupouy, J. P. and Breant, B. (2001). Glucocorticoids impair fetal beta-cell development in rats. *Am. J. Physiol. Endocrinol. Metab.*, **281**(3), E592–9.

Bloom, S. L., Sheffield, J. S., McIntire, D. D. and Leveno, K. J. (2001). Antenatal dexamethasone and decreased birth weight. *Obstet. Gynecol.*, **97**(4), 485–90.

Bohn, M. C. (1980). Granule cell genesis in the hippocampus of rats treated neonatally with hydrocortisone. *Neuroscience*, **5**, 2003–12.

Bohn, M. C. and Lauder, J. M. (1978). The effects of neonatal hydrocortisone on rat cerebellar development: an autoradiographic and light microscopic study. *Develop. Neurosci.*, **1**, 250–66.

Bohn, M. C. and Lauder, J. M. (1980). Cerebellar granule cell genesis in hydrocortisone-treated rat. *Develop. Neurosci.*, **3**, 81–9.

Bremner, J. D., Randall, P., Scott, T. M. *et al.* (1995). MRI-based measurement of hippocampal volume in patients with combat-related posttraumatic stress disorder [comment]. *Am. J. Psychiatr.*, **152**(7), 973–81.

Brocklehurst, P., Gates, S., McKenzie-McHarg, K., Alfirevic, Z. and Chamberlain, G. (1999). Are we prescribing multiple courses of antenatal corticosteroids? A survey of practice in the UK [comment]. *Br. J. Obstetr. Gynaecol.*, **106**(9), 977–9.

Brown, R. W., Diaz, R., Robson, A. C. *et al.* (1996a). The ontogeny of 11β-hydroxysteroid dehydrogenase type 2 and mineralocorticoid receptor gene expression reveal intricate control of glucocorticoid action in development. *Endocrinology*, **137**, 794–7.

Brown, R. W., Kotolevtsev, Y., Leckie, C. *et al.* (1996b). Isolation and cloning of human placental 11β-hydroxysteroid dehydrogenase-2 cDNA. *Biochem. J.*, **313**, 1007–17.

Canlon, B., Erichsen, S., Nemlander, E. *et al.* (2003). Alterations in the intrauterine environment by glucocorticoids modifies the development programme of the auditory system. *Eur. J. Neurosci.*, **17**(10), 2035–41.

Catalani, A., Marinelli, M., Scaccianoce, S. *et al.* (1993). Progeny of mothers drinking corticosterone during lactation has lower stress-induced corticosterone secretion and better cognitive performance. *Brain Res.*, **624**, 209–15.

Cetin, I., Morpurgo, P. S., Radaelli, T. *et al.* (2000). Fetal plasma leptin concentrations: relationship with different intrauterine growth patterns from 19 weeks to term. *Pediatr. Res.*, **48**(5), 646–51.

Chen, X., Lin, J., Hausman, D. B. *et al.* (2000). Alterations in fetal adipose tissue leptin expression correlate with the development of adipose tissue. *Biol. Neonate*, **78**(1), 41–7.

Clark, P. M., Hindmarsh, P. C., Shiell, A. W. *et al.* (1996). Size at birth and adrenocortical function in childhood. *Clin. Endocrinol.*, **45**(6), 721–6.

Cleasby, M. E., Kelly, P. A. T., Walker, B. R. and Seckl, J. R. (2003a). Programming of rat muscle and fat metabolism by in utero overexposure to glucocorticoids. *Endocrinology*, **144**(3), 999–1007.

Cleasby, M. E., Livingstone, D. E. W., Nyirenda, M. J., Seckl, J. R. and Walker, B. R. (2003b). Is programming of glucocorticoid receptor expression by prenatal dexamethasone in the rat secondary to metabolic derangement in adulthood? *Eur. J. Endocrinol.*, **148**(1), 129–38.

Cole, T. J. (1995). Cloning of the mouse 11beta-hydroxysteroid dehydrogenase type 2 gene: tissue specific expression and localization in distal convoluted tubules and collecting ducts of the kidney. *Endocrinology*, **136**, 4693–6.

Cole, T. J., Blendy, J. A., Monaghan, A. P. *et al.* (1995). Molecular genetic analysis of glucocorticoid signalling during mouse development. *Steroids*, **60**(1), 93–6.

Combs, T. P., Berg, A. H., Rajala, M. W. *et al.* (2003). Sexual differentiation, pregnancy, calorie restriction, and aging affect the adipocyte-specific secretory protein adiponectin. *Diabetes*, **52**, 268–76.

Cratty, M. S., Ward, H. E., Johnson, E. A., Azzaro, A. J. and Birkle, D. L. (1995). Prenatal stress increases corticotropin-releasing factor (CRF) content and release in rat amygdala minces. *Brain Res.*, **675**(1–2), 297–302.

Crowley, P. (2000). Prophylactic corticosteroids for preterm birth. *Cochrane Database of Systematic Reviews* (2): CD000065.

Curhan, G. C., Chertow, G. M., Willett, W. C. *et al.* (1996a). Birth-weight and adult hypertension and obesity in women. *Circulation*, **94**, 1310–15.

Curhan, G. C., Willett, W. C., Rimm, E. B. *et al.* (1996b). Birth weight and adult hypertension, diabetes mellitus, and obesity in US men. *Circulation*, **94**, 3246–50.

Dave-Sharma, S., Wilson, R. C., Harbison, M. D. *et al.* (1998). Extensive personal experience – examination of genotype and phenotype relationships in 14 patients with apparent mineralocorticoid excess. *J. Clin. Endocrinol. Metab.*, **83**, 2244–54.

Davis, E. C., Popper, P. and Gorski, R. A. (1996). The role of apoptosis in sexual differentiation of the rat sexually dimorphic nucleus of the preoptic area. *Brain Res.*, **734**(1–2), 10–18.

Day, J. C., Koehl, M., Deroche, V., Le Moal, M. and Maccari, S. (1998). Prenatal stress enhances stress- and corticotropin-releasing factor-induced stimulation of hippocampal acetylcholine release in adult rats. *J. Neurosci.*, **18**(5), 1886–92.

Dean, F. and Matthews, S. G. (1999). Maternal dexamethasone treatment in late gestation alters glucocorticoid and mineralocorticoid receptor mRNA in the fetal guinea pig brain. *Brain Res.*, **846**(2), 253–9.

Dean, F., Yu, C., Lingas, R. I. and Matthews, S. G. (2001). Prenatal glucocorticoid modifies hypothalamo–pituitary–adrenal regulation in prepubertal guinea pigs. *Neuroendocrinology*, **73**(3), 194–202.

Diaz, R., Ögren, S. O., Blum, M. and Fuxe, K. (1995). Prenatal corticosterone increases spontaneous and d-amphetamine induced locomotor activity and brain dopamine metabolism in prepubertal male and female rats. *Neuroscience*, **66**, 467–73.

Diaz, R., Fuxe, K. and Ogren, S. O. (1997). Prenatal corticosterone treatment induces long-term changes in spontaneous and apomorphine-mediated motor activity in male and female rats. *Neuroscience*, **81**, 129–40.

Diaz, R., Brown, R. W. and Seckl, J. R. (1998). Ontogeny of mRNAs encoding glucocorticoid and mineralocorticoid receptors and 11β-hydroxysteroid dehydrogenases in prenatal rat brain development reveal complex control of glucocorticoid action. *J. Neurosci.*, **18**, 2570–80.

Diorio, J., Francis, D., Walker, M., Steverman, A. and Meaney, M. J. (1996). Postnatal handling induces changes in the hippocampal expression of cyclic nucleotide-dependent response element binding proteins in the rat. *Soc. Neurosci. Abstr.*, **22**, 486–7.

Docherty, C., Kalmar-Nagy, J., Engelen, M. and Nathanielz, P. J. (2001). Effect of in vivo infusion of dexamethasone at 0.75 gestation on responses to endothelin-1 in isolated fetal ovine resistance arteries. *Am. J. Physiol.*, **281**, R261–8.

Dodic, M., May, C. N., Wintour, E. M. and Coghlan, J. P. (1998). An early prenatal exposure to excess glucocorticoid leads to hypertensive offspring in sheep. *Clin. Sci.*, **94**, 149–55.

Dodic, M., Peers, A., Coghlan, J. *et al.* (1999). Altered cardiovascular haemodynamics and baroreceptor – heart rate reflex in adult sheep after prenatal exposure to dexamethasone. *Clin. Sci.*, **97**, 103–9.

Dodic, M., Baird, R., Hantzis, V. *et al.* (2001). Organs/systems potentially involved in one model of programmed hypertension in sheep. *Clin. Exp. Pharmacol. Physiol.*, **28**(11), 952–6.

Dodic, M., Hantzis, V., Duncan, J. *et al.* (2002a). Programming effects of short prenatal exposure to cortisol. *FASEB J.*, **16**(9), 1017–26.

Dodic, M., Moritz, K., Koukoulas, I. and Wintour, E. M. (2002b). Programmed hypertension: kidney, brain or both? *Trend. Endocrinol. Metab.*, **13**(9), 403–8.

Dodic, M., Peers, A., Moritz, K., Hantzis, V. and Wintour, E. M. (2002c). No evidence for HPA reset in adult sheep with high blood pressure due to short prenatal exposure to dexamethasone. *Am. J. Physiol. Regul. Integr. Comp. Physiol.*, **282**(2), R343–50.

Doyle, L. W., Ford, G. W., Davis, N. M. and Callanan, C. (2000). Antenatal corticosteroid therapy and blood pressure at 14 years of age in preterm children. *Clin. Sci.*, **98**(2), 137–42.

Dunger, D., Ong, K., Huxtable, S. *et al.* (1998). Association of the INS VNTR with size at birth. *Nat. Genet.*, **19**, 1061–4036.

Dunlop, S. A., Archer, M. A., Quinlivan, J. A., Beazley, L. D. and Newnham, J. P. (1997). Repeated prenatal corticosteroids delay myelination in the ovine central nervous system. *J. Matern. Fetal Med.*, **6**(6), 309–13.

Dunn, A. J. and Berridge, C. W. (1990). Physiological and behavioral responses to corticotropin-releasing factor administration: is CRF a mediator of anxiety or stress responses? *Brain Res. – Brain Res. Rev.*, **15**(2), 71–100.

Duong, D. T., Waltner-Law, M. E., Sears, R., Sealy, L. and Granner, D. K. (2002). Insulin inhibits hepatocellular glucose production by utilizing liver-enriched transcriptional inhibitory protein to disrupt the association of CREB-binding protein and RNA polymerase II with the phosphoenolpyruvate carboxykinase gene promoter. *J. Biol. Chem.*, **277**(35), 32234–42.

Edwards, C. R. W., Benediktsson, R., Lindsay, R. and Seckl, J. R. (1993). Dysfunction of the placental glucocorticoid barrier: a link between the foetal environment and adult hypertension? *Lancet*, **341**, 355–7.

Encio, I. J. and Detera-Wadleigh, S. D. (1991). The genomic structure of the human glucocorticoid receptor. *J. Biol. Chem.*, **266**(11), 7182–8.

Fall, C. H. D., Osmond, C., Barker, D. J. P. *et al.* (1995). Fetal and infant growth and cardiovascular risk factors in women. *Br. Med. J.*, **310**, 428–32.

Feldman, S. and Weidenfeld, J. (1998). The excitatory effects of the amygdala on hypothalamo-pituitary-adrenocorticol responses are mediated by hypothalamic norepinephrine, serotonin, and CRF-41. *Brain Res. Bull.*, **45**, 389–93.

Forest, M. G., David, M. and Morel, Y. (1993). Prenatal diagnosis and treatment of 21-hydroxylase deficiency. *J. Steroid Biochem. Mol. Biol.*, **45**(1–3), 75–82.

Forhead, A. J., Thomas, L., Crabtree, J. *et al.* (2002). Plasma leptin concentration in fetal sheep during late gestation: ontogeny and effect of glucocorticoids. *Endocrinology*, **143**(4), 1166–73.

Forsen, T., Eriksson, J. G., Tuomilehto, J. *et al.* (1997). Mother's weight in pregnancy and coronary heart disease in a cohort of Finnish men: follow up study. *Br. Med. J.*, **315**, 837–40.

Frayling, T. M. and Hattersley, A. T. (2001). The role of genetic susceptibility in the association of low birth weight with type 2 diabetes. *Br. Med. Bull.*, **60**, 89–101.

Frayling, T. M., Hattersley, A. T., McCarthy, A. *et al.* (2002). A putative functional polymorphism in the IGF-I gene: association studies with type 2 diabetes, adult height, glucose tolerance, and fetal growth in U.K. populations. *Diabetes*, **51**(7), 2313–16.

French, N. P., Hagan, R., Evans, S., Godfrey, M. and Newnham, J. P. (1998). Repeated antenatal corticosteroids: behaviour outcomes in a regional population of very preterm infants. *Pediatr. Res.*, **43**, 214A (abstract no. 1252).

French, N. P., Hagan, R., Evans, S. F., Godfrey, M. and Newnham, J. P. (1999). Repeated antenatal corticosteroids: size at birth and subsequent development. *Am. J. Obstetr. Gynecol.*, **180**(1 Pt 1), 114–21.

Fumagalli, F., Jones, S. R., Caron, M. G., Seidler, F. J. and Slotkin, T. A. (1996). Expression of mRNA coding for the serotonin transporter in aged vs. young rat brain: differential effects of glucocorticoids. *Brain Res.*, **719**, 225–8.

Fuxe, K., Wikstrom, A.-C., Okret, S. *et al.* (1985). Mapping of glucocorticoid receptor immunoreactive neurons in the rat tel- and diencephalon using a monoclonal antibody against rat liver glucocorticoid receptor. *Endocrinology*, **117**, 1803–12.

Gale, C. R., Martyn, C. N., Kellingray, S., Eastell, R. and Cooper, C. (2001). Intrauterine programming of adult body composition. *J. Clin. Endocrinol. Metab.*, **86**(1), 267–72.

Gandelman, R. and Rosenthal, C. (1981). Deleterious effects of prenatal prednisolone exposure upon morphological and behavioral development of mice. *Teratology*, **24**(3), 293–301.

Garofano, A., Czernichow, P. and Breant, B. (1997). In utero undernutrition impairs rat beta-cell development. *Diabetologia*, **40**(10), 1231–4.

Garofano, A., Czernichow, P. and Breant, B. (1998). Beta-cell mass and proliferation following late fetal and early postnatal malnutrition in the rat. *Diabetologia*, **41**(9), 1114–20.

Gatford, K. L., Wintour, E. M., de Blasio, M. J., Owens, J. A. and Dodic, M. (2000). Differential timing for programming of glucose homoeostasis, sensitivity to insulin and blood pressure by in utero exposure to dexamethasone in sheep. *Clin. Sci.*, **98**, 553–60.

Geary, M., Herschkovitz, R., Pringle, P. J., Rodeck, C. H. and Hindmarsh, P. C. (1999). Ontogeny of serum leptin concentrations in the human. *Clin. Endocrinol.*, **51**(2), 189–92.

Goland, R. S., Jozak, S., Warren, W. B. *et al.* (1993). Elevated levels of umbilical cord plasma corticotropin-releasing hormone in growth-retarded fetuses. *J. Clin. Endocrinol. Metab.*, **77**, 1174–9.

Goland, R. S., Tropper, P. J., Warren, W. B. *et al.* (1995). Concentrations of corticotropin-releasing hormone in the umbilical cord blood of pregnancies complicated by preeclampsia. *Reprod. Fert. Develop.*, **7**, 1227–30.

Gould, E., Woolley, C. S., Cameron, H. A., Daniels, D. C. and McEwen, B. S. (1991a). Adrenal steroids regulate postnatal development in the rat dentate gyrus. II. Effects of glucocorticoids on cell birth. *J. Comp. Neurol.*, **313**, 486–93.

Gould, E., Woolley, C. S. and McEwen, B. S. (1991b). Adrenal steroids regulate postnatal development in the rat dentate gyrus. I. Effects of glucocorticoids on cell death. *J. Comp. Neurol.*, **313**, 479–85.

Gunberg, D. L. (1957). Some effects of exogenous hydrocortisone on pregnancy in the rat. *Anat. Res.*, **129**, 133–53.

Gustafsson, J.-A., Mode, A., Norstedt, G. and Skett, P. (1983). Sex steroid-induced changes in hepatic enzymes. *Annu. Rev. Physiol.*, **45**, 51–60.

Hattersley, A., Beards, F., Ballantyne, E. *et al.* (1998). Mutations in the glucokinase gene of the fetus result in reduced birth weight. *Nat. Genet.*, **19**, 268–70.

Hawkins, P., Steyn, C., McGarrigle, H. H. *et al.* (2000). Cardiovascular and hypothalamic–pituitary–adrenal axis development in late gestation fetal sheep and young lambs following modest maternal nutrient restriction in early gestation. *Reprod. Fert. Develop.*, **12**(7–8), 443–56.

Herman, J. P., Patel, P. D., Akil, H. and Watson, S. J. (1989). Localization and regulation of glucocorticoid and mineralocorticoid receptor messenger RNAs in the hippocampal formation of the rat. *Mol. Endocrinol.*, **3**(11), 1886–94.

Hill, D. J. and Duvillie, B. (2000). Pancreatic development and adult diabetes. *Pediatr. Res.*, **48**(3), 269–74.

Hoggard, N., Hunter, L., Lea, R. G., Trayhurn, P. and Mercer, J. G. (2000). Ontogeny of the expression of leptin and its receptor in the murine fetus and placenta. *Br. J. Nutr.*, **83**(3), 317–26.

Holmes, M. C., Welberg, L. A. and Seckl, J. R. (2002). Early life programming of the brain by glucocorticoids. *Fifth International Congress of Neuroendocrinology*, Bristol, UK. September: S57.

Holson, R. R., Gough, B., Sullivan, P., Badger, T. and Sheehan, D. M. (1995). Prenatal dexamethasone or stress but not ACTH or corticosterone alter sexual behavior in male rats. *Neurotoxicol. Teratol.*, **17**, 393–401.

Hsu, D., Chen, F., Takahashi, L. and Kalin, N. (1998). Rapid stress-induced elevations in corticotropin-releasing hormone mRNA in rat central amygdala nucleus and hypothalamic paraventricular nucleus: an *in situ* hybridization analysis. *Brain Res.*, **788**, 305–10.

Hu, E., Liang, P. and Spiegelman, B. M. (1996). AdipoQ is a novel adipose-specific gene dysregulated in obesity. *J. Biol. Chem.*, **271**(18), 10697–703.

Huang, W. L., Beazley, L. D., Quinlivan, J. A. *et al.* (1999). Effect of corticosteroids on brain growth in fetal sheep. *Obstetr. Gynecol.*, **94**(2), 213–18.

Huang, W. L., Harper, C. G., Evans, S. F., Newnham, J. P. and Dunlop, S. A. (2001a). Repeated prenatal corticosteroid administration delays astrocyte and capillary tight junction maturation in fetal sheep. *Int. J. Develop. Neurosci.*, **19**(5), 487–93.

Huang, W. L., Harper, C. G., Evans, S. F., Newnham, J. P. and Dunlop, S. A. (2001b). Repeated prenatal corticosteroid administration delays myelination of the corpus callosum in fetal sheep. *Int. J. Develop. Neurosci.*, **19**(4), 415–25.

Huxley, R. R., Shiell, A. W. and Law, C. M. (2000). The role of size at birth and postnatal catch-up growth in determining systolic blood pressure: a systematic review of the literature. *J. Hypertens.*, **18**(7), 815–31.

Huxley, R. R., Neil, A. and Collins, R. (2002). Unravelling the fetal origins hypothesis: is there really an inverse association between birthweight and subsequent blood pressure? *Lancet*, 360(9334), 659–65.

Ikegami, M., Jobe, A. H., Newnham J. *et al.* (1997). Repetitive prenatal glucocorticoids improve lung function and decrease growth in preterm lambs. *Am. J. Resp. Crit. Care Med.*, 156(1), 178–84.

Irving, R. J., Belton, N. R., Elton, R. A. and Walker, B. R. (2000). Adult cardiovascular risk factors in premature babies. *Lancet*, 355, 2135–6.

Jacobson, L. and Sapolsky, R. (1991). The role of the hippocampus in feedback regulation of the hypothalamic–pituitary–adrenal axis. *Endocr. Rev.*, 12, 118–34.

Jamieson, P. M., Chapman, K. E., Edwards, C. R. W. and Seckl, J. R. (1995). 11β-hydroxysteroid dehydrogenase is an exclusive 11β-reductase in primary cultured rat hepatocytes: effect of physicochemical and hormonal manipulations. *Endocrinology*, 136, 4754–61.

Jamieson, P. M., Chapman, K. E. and Seckl, J. R. (1999). Tissue- and temporal-specific regulation of 11β-hydroxysteroid dehydrogenase type 1 by glucocorticoids in vivo. *J. Steroid Biochem. Mol. Biol.*, 68, 245–50.

Jamieson, P. M., Chapman, K. E., Walker, B. R. and Seckl, J. R. (2000). 11β-hydroxysteroid dehydrogenase type 1 is a predominant 11β-reductase in the intact perfused rat liver. *J. Endocrinol.*, 165, 685–92.

Jaquet, D., Leger, J., Levy-Marchal, C., Oury, J. F. and Czernichow, P. (1998). Ontogeny of leptin in human fetuses and newborns: effect of intrauterine growth retardation on serum leptin concentrations. *J. Clin. Endocrinol. Metab.*, 83(4), 1243–6.

Jaquet, D., Tregouet, D. A., Godefroy, T. *et al.* (2002). Combined effects of genetic and environmental factors on insulin resistance associated with reduced fetal growth. *Diabetes*, 51(12), 3473–8.

Jensen, E. C., Gallaher, B. W., Breier, B. H. and Harding, J. E. (2002). The effect of a chronic maternal cortisol infusion on the late-gestation fetal sheep. *J. Endocrinol.*, 174(1), 27–36.

Kari, M. A., Hallman, M., Eronen, M. *et al.* (1994). Prenatal dexamethasone treatment in conjunction with rescue therapy of human surfactant: a randomized placebo-controlled multicenter study. *Pediatrics*, 93, 730–6.

Kay, H. H., Bird, I. M., Coe, C. L. and Dudley, D. J. (2000). Antenatal steroid treatment and adverse fetal effects: What is the evidence? *J. Soc. Gynecol. Invest.*, 7(5), 269–78.

Keightley, M.-C. and Fuller, P. J. (1994). Unique sequences in the guinea pig glucocorticoid receptor induce constitutive transactivation and decrease steroid sensitivity. *Mol. Endocrinol.*, 8, 431–9.

King, L. B., Vacchio, M. S., Dixon, K. *et al.* (1995). A targeted glucocorticoid receptor antisense transgene increases thymocyte apoptosis and alters thymocyte development. *Immunity*, 3(5), 647–56.

Kinnunen, A. K., Koenig, J. I. and Bilbe, G. (2003). Repeated variable prenatal stress alters pre- and postsynaptic gene expression in the rat frontal pole. *J. Neurochem.*, 86(3), 736–48.

Kitraki, E., Kittas, C. and Stylianopoulou, F. (1997). Glucocorticoid receptor gene expression during rat embryogenesis. An *in situ* hybridization study. *Differentiation*, 62, 21–31.

Klemcke, H. G. (1995). Placental metabolism of cortisol at mid- and late gestation in swine. *Biol. Reprod.*, 53, 1293–301.

Koenen, S. V., Mecenas, C. A., Smith, G. S., Jenkins, S. and Nathanielsz, P. W. (2002). Effects of maternal betamethasone administration on fetal and maternal blood pressure and heart rate in the baboon at 0.7 of gestation. *Am. J. Obstet. Gynecol.*, **186**(4), 812–17.

Koenig, J. I., Kirkpatrick, B. and Lee, P. (2002). Glucocorticoid hormones and early brain development in schizophrenia. *Neuropsychopharmacology*, **27**(2), 309–18.

Koistinen, H. A., Koivisto, V. A., Andersson, S. *et al.* (1997). Leptin concentration in cord blood correlates with intrauterine growth. *J. Clin. Endocrinol. Metab.*, **82**(10), 3328–30.

Korte, S. M. (2001). Corticosteroids in relation to fear, anxiety and psychopathology. *Neurosci. Biobehav. Rev.*, **25**(2), 117–42.

Kotelevtsev, Y., Holmes, M. C., Burchell, A. *et al.* (1997). 11β-hydroxysteroid dehydrogenase type 1 knockout mice show attenuated glucocorticoid inducible responses and resist hyperglycaemia on obesity or stress. *Proc. Natl. Acad. Sci. USA*, **94**, 14924–9.

Kotelevtsev, Y., Brown, R. W., Fleming, S. *et al.* (1999). Hypertension in mice lacking 11β-hydroxysteroid dehydrogenase type 2. *J. Clin. Invest.*, **103**, 683–9.

Langdown, M. L., Holness, M. J. and Sugden, M. C. (2001a). Early growth retardation induced by excessive exposure to glucocorticoids in utero selectively increases cardiac GLUT1 protein expression and Akt/protein kinase B activity in adulthood. *J. Endocrinol.*, **169**(1), 11–22.

Langdown, M. L., Smith, N. D., Sugden, M. C. and Holness, M. J. (2001b). Excessive glucocorticoid exposure during late intrauterine development modulates the expression of cardiac uncoupling proteins in adult hypertensive male offspring. *Pflug. Arch. Eur. J. Physiol.*, **442**(2), 248–55.

Langdown, M. L., Holness, M. J. and Sugden, M. C. (2003). Effects of prenatal glucocorticoid exposure on cardiac calreticulin and calsequestrin protein expression during early development and in adulthood. *Biochem. J.*, **371**, 61–9.

Langley-Evans, S. C. (1997). Hypertension induced by foetal exposure to a maternal low-protein diet, in the rat, is prevented by pharmacological blockade of maternal glucocorticoid synthesis. *J. Hypertens.*, **15**, 537–44.

Langley-Evans, S. C., Gardner, D. S. and Jackson, A. A. (1996a). Maternal protein restriction influences the programming of the rat hypothalamic–pituitary–adrenal axis. *J. Nutr.*, **126**, 1578–85.

Langley-Evans, S. C., Philips, G., Benediktsson, R. *et al.* (1996b). Maternal dietary protein restriction, placental glucocorticoid metabolism and the programming of hypertension. *Placenta*, **17**, 169–72.

Laplante, P., Diorio, J. and Meaney, M. J. (2002). Serotonin regulates hippocampal glucocorticoid receptor expression via a 5-HT7 receptor. *Brain Res. – Develop. Brain Res.* **139**, 199–203.

Law, C. M., Shiell, A. W., Newsome, C. A. *et al.* (2002). Fetal, infant, and childhood growth and adult blood pressure: a longitudinal study from birth to 22 years of age. *Circulation*, **105**(9), 1088–92.

Leon, D. A., Koupilova, I., Lithell, H. O. *et al.* (1996). Failure to realise growth potential in utero and adult obesity in relation to blood pressure in 50 year old Swedish men. *Br. Med. J.*, **312**, 401–6.

Lepercq, J., Challier, J. C., Guerre-Millo, M. *et al.* (2001). Prenatal leptin production: evidence that fetal adipose tissue produces leptin. *J. Clin. Endocrinol. Metab.*, **86**(6), 2409–13.

Lesage, J., Blondeau, B., Grino, M., Breant, B. and Dupouy, J. P. (2001). Maternal undernutrition during late gestation induces fetal overexposure to glucocorticoids and intrauterine growth retardation, and disturbs the hypothalamo–pituitary adrenal axis in the newborn rat. *Endocrinology*, **142**(5), 1692–702.

Levine, S. (1957). Infantile experience and resistance to physiological stress. *Science*, **126**, 405–6.

Levine, S. (1962). Plasma-free corticosteroid response to electric shock in rats stimulated in infancy. *Science*, **135**, 795–6.

Levine, R. S., Hennekens, C. H. and Jesse, M. J. (1994). Blood pressure in prospective population based cohort of newborn and infant twins. *Br. Med. J.*, **308**, 298–302.

Levitt, N., Lindsay, R. S., Holmes, M. C. and Seckl, J. R. (1996). Dexamethasone in the last week of pregnancy attenuates hippocampal glucocorticoid receptor gene expression and elevates blood pressure in the adult offspring in the rat. *Neuroendocrinology*, **64**, 412–18.

Levitt, N. S., Lambert, E. V., Woods, D. *et al.* (2000). Impaired glucose tolerance and elevated blood pressure in low birth weight, nonobese, young South African adults: early programming of cortisol axis. *J. Clin. Endocrinol. Metab.*, **85**(12), 4611–18.

Lindsay, R. S., Lindsay, R. M., Edwards, C. R. W. and Seckl, J. R. (1996a). Inhibition of 11β-hydroxysteroid dehydrogenase in pregnant rats and the programming of blood pressure in the offspring. *Hypertension*, **27**, 1200–4.

Lindsay, R. S., Lindsay, R. M., Waddell, B. and Seckl, J. R. (1996b). Programming of glucose tolerance in the rat: role of placental 11β-hydroxysteroid dehydrogenase. *Diabetologia*, **39**, 1299–305.

Lindsay, R. S., Funahashi, T., Hanson, R. L. *et al.* (2002). Adiponectin and development of type 2 diabetes in the Pima Indian population. *Lancet*, **360**(9326), 57–8.

Lindsay, R., Walker, J., Havel, P. *et al.* (2003). Adiponectin is present in cord blood but is unrelated to leptin and birth weight. *Diabetes Care*, **26**, 2244–8.

Lithell, H. O., McKeigue, P. M., Berglund, L. *et al.* (1996). Relation of size at birth to non-insulin dependent diabetes and insulin concentrations in men aged 50–60 years. *Br. Med. J.*, **312**, 406–10.

Liu, D., Diorio, J., Tannenbaum, B. *et al.* (1997). Maternal care, hippocampal glucocorticoid receptors, and hypothalamic–pituitary–adrenal responses to stress. *Science*, **277**, 1659–62.

Liu, L., Li, A. and Matthews, S. G. (2001). Maternal glucocorticoid treatment programs HPA regulation in adult offspring: sex-specific effects. *Am. J. Physiol. Endocrinol. Metab.*, **280**(5), E729–39.

Lopez-Bernal, A., Flint, A. P. F., Anderson, A. B. M. and Turnbull, A. C. (1980). 11β-hydroxysteroid dehydrogenase activity (E.C.1.1.1.146) in human placenta and decidua. *J. Steroid Biochem.*, **13**, 1081–7.

Lopez Bernal, A. and Craft, I. L. (1981). Corticosteroid metabolism in vitro by human placenta, foetal membranes and decidua in early and late gestation. *Placenta*, **2**, 279–85.

MacArthur, B. A., Howie, R. N., Dezoete, J. A. and Elkins, J. (1982). School progress and cognitive development of 6-year-old children whose mothers were treated antenatally with betamethasone. *Pediatrics*, **70**(1), 99–105.

Maccari, S., Piazza, P. V., Kabbaj, M. *et al.* (1995). Adoption reverses the long-term impairment in glucocorticoid feedback induced by prenatal stress. *J. Neurosci.*, **15**, 110–16.

Makino, S., Gold, P. W. and Schulkin, J. (1994). Effects of corticosterone on CRH mRNA and content in the central nucleus of the amygdala and the parvocellular region of the paraventricular nucleus of the hypothalamus. *Brain Research*, **640**, 105–112.

Matthews, S. G. (1998). Dynamic changes in glucocorticoid and mineralocorticoid receptor mRNA in the developing guinea pig brain. *Brain Res. – Develop. Brain Res.*, **107**(1), 123–32.

Matthews, S. G. (2000). Antenatal glucocorticoids and programming of the developing CNS. *Pediatr. Res.*, **47**(3), 291–300.

Matthews, S. G. (2002). Early programming of the hypothalamo–pituitary–adrenal axis. *Trend. Endocrinol. Metab.*, **130**, 373–80.

McCormick, C. M., Smythe, J. W., Sharma, S. and Meaney, M. J. (1995). Sex-specific effects of prenatal stress on hypothalamic–pituitary–adrenal responses to stress and brain glucocorticoid receptor density in adult rats. *Develop. Brain Res.*, **84**, 55–61.

McCormick, J. A., Lyons, V., Jacobson, M. D. *et al.* (2000). 5′-heterogeneity of glucocorticoid receptor messenger RNA is tissue specific: differential regulation of variant transcripts by early-life events. *Mol. Endocrinol.*, **14**(4), 506–17.

McTernan, C. L., Draper, N., Nicholson, H. *et al.* (2001). Reduced placental 11 beta-hydroxysteroid dehydrogenase type 2 mRNA levels in human pregnancies complicated by intrauterine growth restriction: an analysis of possible mechanisms. *J. Clin. Endocrinol. Metab.*, **86**(10), 4979–83.

Meaney, M. J., Aitken, D. H., van Berkel, C., Bhatnagar, S. and Sapolsky, R. M. (1988). Effect of neonatal handling on age-related impairments associated with the hippocampus. *Science*, **239**, 766–8.

Meaney, M. J., Aitken, D. H., Viau, V., Sharma, S. and Sarrieau, A. (1989). Neonatal handling alters adrenocortical negative feedback sensitivity and hippocampal type II glucocorticoid receptor binding in the rat. *Neuroendocrinology*, **50**, 597–604.

Meaney, M. J., Aitken, D. H., Sharma, S. and Viau, V. (1992). Basal ACTH, corticosterone and corticosterone-binding globulin levels over the diurnal cycle, and hippocampal corticosteroid receptors in young and aged, handled and non-handled rats. *Neuroendocrinology*, **55**, 204–13.

Meaney, M. J., Diorio, J., Francis, D. *et al.* (1996). Early environmental regulation of forebrain glucocorticoid receptor gene expression: implications for adrenocortical responses to stress. *Develop. Neurosci.*, **18**, 49–72.

Meaney, M. J., Diorio, J., Francis, D. *et al.* (2000). Postnatal handling increases the expression of cAMP-inducible transcription factors in the rat hippocampus: the effects of thyroid hormones and serotonin. *J. Neurosci.*, **20**(10), 3926–35.

Mercado, A. B., Wilson, R. C., Cheng, K. C., Wei, J. Q. and New, M. I. (1995a). Prenatal treatment and diagnosis of congenital adrenal hyperplasia owing to steroid 21-hydroxylase deficiency. *J. Clin. Endocrinol. Metab.*, **80**(7), 2014–20.

Mercado, A. B., Wilson, R. C., Cheng, K. C., Wei, J. Q. and New, M. I. (1995b). Prenatal treatment and diagnosis of congential adrenal hyperlasia owing to 21-hydroxylase deficiency. *J. Clin. Endocrinol. Metab.*, **80**, 2014–20.

Meyer, J. S. (1983). Early adrenalectomy stimulates subsequent growth and development of the rat brain. *Exp. Neurol.*, **82**, 432–46.

Mitchell, J. B., Rowe, W., Boksa, P. and Meaney, M. J. (1990). Serotonin regulates type II corticosteroid receptor binding in hippocampal cell cultures. *J. Neurosci.*, **10**(6), 1745–52.

Mitchell, J. B., Betito, K., Rowe, W., Boksa, P. and Meaney, M. J. (1992). Serotonergic regulation of type II corticosteroid receptor binding in hippocampal cell cultures: evidence for the importance of serotonin-induced changes in cAMP levels. *Neuroscience*, **48**(3), 631–9.

Molnar, J., Nijland, M. J. M., Howe, D. C. and Nathanielsz, P. W. (2002). Evidence for microvascular dysfunction after prenatal dexamethasone at 0.7, 0.75, and 0.8 gestation in sheep. *Am. J. Physiol. Regul. Integr. Comp. Physiol.*, **283**(3), R561–7.

Molnar, J., Howe, D. C., Nijland, M. J. M. and Nathanielsz, P. W. (2003). Prenatal dexamethasone leads to both endothelial dysfunction and vasodilatory compensation in sheep. *J. Physiol. London*, **547**(1), 61–6.

Moore, V. M., Miller, A. G., Boulton, T. J. C. *et al.* (1996). Placental weight, birth measurements, and blood pressure at age 8 years. *Arch. Dis. Child.*, **74**, 538–41.

Moritz, K. M., Johnson, K., Douglas-Denton, R., Wintour, E. M. and Dodic, M. (2002). Maternal glucocorticoid treatment programs alterations in the renin–angiotensin system of the ovine fetal kidney. *Endocrinology*, **143**(11), 4455–63.

Moss, T. J., Sloboda, D. M., Gurrin, L. C. *et al.* (2001). Programming effects in sheep of prenatal growth restriction and glucocorticoid exposure. *Am. J. Physiol. Regul. Integr. Comp. Physiol.*, **281**(3), R960–70.

Mostyn, A., Keisler, D. H., Webb, R., Stephenson, T. and Symonds, M. E. (2001). The role of leptin in the transition from fetus to neonate. *Proc. Nutr. Soc.*, **60**(2), 187–94.

Mostyn, A., Pearce, S., Budge, H. *et al.* (2003). Influence of cortisol on adipose tissue development in the fetal sheep during late gestation. *J. Endocrinol.*, **176**, 23–30.

Muneoka, K., Mikuni, M., Ogawa, T. *et al.* (1997). Prenatal dexamethasone exposure alters brain monoamine metabolism and adrenocortical response in rat offspring. *Am. J. Physiol.*, **273**(5 Pt 2), R1669–75.

Murphy, V. E., Zakar, T., Smith, R. *et al.* (2002). Reduced 11beta-hydroxysteroid dehydrogenase type 2 activity is associated with decreased birth weight centile in pregnancies complicated by asthma. *J. Clin. Endocrinol. Metab.*, **87**(4), 1660–8.

Newnham, J. P. and Moss, T. J. (2001). Antenatal glucocorticoids and growth: single versus multiple doses in animal and human studies. *Semin. Neonatol.*, **6**(4), 285–92.

Newnham, J. P., Evans, S. F., Godfrey, M. *et al.* (1999). Maternal, but not fetal, administration of corticosteroids restricts fetal growth. *J. Matern. Fetal Med.*, **8**(3), 81–7.

Nyirenda, M. J., Lindsay, R. S., Kenyon, C. J., Burchell, A. and Seckl, J. R. (1998). Glucocorticoid exposure in late gestation permanently programmes rat hepatic phosphoenolpyruvate carboxykinase and glucocorticoid receptor expression and causes glucose intolerance in adult offspring. *J. Clin. Invest.*, **101**, 2174–81.

Nyirenda, M. J., Welberg, L. A. M. and Seckl, J. R. (2001). Programming hyperglycaemia in the rat through prenatal exposure to glucocorticoids – fetal effect or maternal influence? *J. Endocrinol.*, **170**(3), 653–60.

O'Donnell, D., Larocque, S., Seckl, J. R. and Meaney, M. J. (1994). Postnatal handling alters glucocorticoid, but not mineralocorticoid messenger RNA expression in the hippocampus of adult rats. *Brain Res. – Mol. Brain Res.*, **26**(1–2), 242–8.

Ong, K. K., Ahmed, M. L., Sherriff, A. *et al.* (1999). Cord blood leptin is associated with size at birth and predicts infancy weight gain in humans. ALSPAC Study Team, Avon Longitudinal Study of Pregnancy and Childhood. *J. Clin. Endocrinol. Metab.*, **84**(3), 1145–8.

Ortiz, L. A., Quan, A., Weinberg, A. and Baum, M. (2001). Effect of prenatal dexamethasone on rat renal development. *Kidney Int.*, **59**(5), 1663–9.

Osmond, C., Barker, D. J. P., Winter, P. D., Fall, C. H. D. and Simmonds, S. J. (1993). Early growth and death from cardiovascular disease in women. *Br. Med. J.*, **307**, 1524–7.

Pepin, M. C., Pothier, F. and Barden, N. (1992). Impaired type II glucocorticoid-receptor function in mice bearing antisense RNA transgene. *Nature*, **355**(6362), 725–8.

Phillips, D. I., Barker, D. J., Fall, C. H. *et al.* (1998). Elevated plasma cortisol concentrations: a link between low birth weight and the insulin resistance syndrome? *J. Clin. Endocrinol. Metab.*, **83**(3), 757–60.

Phillips, D. I., Walker, B. R., Reynolds, R. M. *et al.* (2000). Low birth weight predicts elevated plasma cortisol concentrations in adults from 3 populations. *Hypertension*, **35**(6), 1301–6.

Reinisch, J. M., Simon, N. G. and Karwo, W. G. *et al.* (1978). Prenatal exposure to prednisone in humans and animals retards intra-uterine growth. *Science*, **202**, 436–8.

Reul, J. M. H. M. and de Kloet, E. R. (1985). Two receptor systems for corticosterone in rat brain: microdissection and differential occupation. *Endocrinology*, **117**, 2505–11.

Reynolds, R. M., Walker, B. R., Syddall, H. E. *et al.* (2001). Altered control of cortisol secretion in adult men with low birth weight and cardiovascular risk factors. *J. Clin. Endocrinol. Metab.*, **86**(1), 245–50.

RichEdwards, J. W., Stampfer, M. J., Manson, J. E. *et al.* (1997). Birth weight and risk of cardiovascular disease in a cohort of women followed up since 1976. *Br. Med. J.*, **315**, 396–400.

Robson, A. C., Leckie, C., Seckl, J. R. and Holmes, M. C. (1998). Expression of 11β-hydroxysteroid dehydrogenase type 2 in the postnatal and adult rat brain. *Mol. Brain Res.*, **61**, 1–10.

Rogerson, F. M., Kayes, K. and White, P. C. (1996). No correlation in human placenta between activity or mRNA for the K (type 2) isozyme of 11β-hydroxysteroid dehydrogenase and fetal or placental weight. *Tenth International Congress of Endocrinology Abstracts* (P1–231), 193.

Rogerson, F. M., Kayes, K. M. and White, P. C. (1997). Variation in placental type 2 11beta-hydroxysteroid dehydrogenase activity is not related to birth weight or placental weight. *Mol. Cell. Endocrinol.*, **128**, 103–9.

Rosella, G., Zajac, J. D., Kaczmarczyk, S. J., Andrikopoulos, S. and Proietto, J. (1993). Impaired suppression of gluconeogenesis induced by overexpression of a noninsulin-responsive phospho-enolpyruvate carboxykinase gene. *Mol. Endocrinol.*, **7**(11), 1456–62.

Saegusa, H., Nakagawa, Y., Liu, Y. J. and Ohzeki, T. (1999). Influence of placental 11 beta-hydroxysteroid dehydrogenase (11 beta-HSD) inhibition on glucose metabolism and 11 beta-HSD regulation in adult offspring of rats. *Metab. Clin. Exp.*, **48**(12), 1584–8.

Sapolsky, R. M. (1999). Glucocorticoids, stress, and their adverse neurological effects: relevance to aging. *Exp. Gerontol.*, **34**(6), 721–32.

Schubring, C., Kiess, W., Englaro, P. *et al.* (1997). Levels of leptin in maternal serum, amniotic fluid, and arterial and venous cord blood: relation to neonatal and placental weight. *J. Clin. Endocrinol. Metab.*, **82**(5), 1480–3.

Seckl, J. R. (1994). Glucocorticoids and small babies. *Quart. J. Med.*, **87**, 259–62.

Seckl, J. R. (1998). Physiologic programming of the fetus. *Clin. Perinatol.*, **25**, 939–64.

Seckl, J. R. and Miller, W. L. (1997). How safe is long-term prenatal glucocorticoid treatment? *J. Am. Med. Assoc.*, **277**, 1077–9.

Seckl, J. R. and Walker, B. R. (2001). 11β-hydroxysteroid dehydrogenase type 1: a tissue-specific amplifier of glucocorticoid action. *Endocrinology*, **142**, 1371–6.

Seckl, J. R., Dickson, K. L., Yates, C. and Fink, G. (1991). Distribution of glucocorticoid and min-cralocorticoid receptor messenger RNA expression in human postmortem hippocampus. *Brain Res.*, **561**, 332–7.

Shams, M., Kilby, M. D., Somerset, D. A. *et al.* (1998). 11beta hydroxysteroid dehydrogenase type 2 in human pregnancy and reduced expression in intrauterine growth retardation. *Hum. Reprod.*, **13**, 799–804.

Sheline, Y. I., Wang, P. W., Gado, M. H., Csernansky, J. G. and Vannier, M. W. (1996). Hippocampal atrophy in recurrent major depression. *Proc. Natl. Acad. Sci. USA*, **93**, 3908–13.

Shen, C.-N., Seckl, J., Slack, J. and Tosh, D. (2003). Glucocorticoids suppress beta cell development and induce hepatic metaplasia in embryonic pancreas. *Biochem. J.*, **375**, 41–50.

Simerly, R. B. (2002). Wired for reproduction: organization and development of sexually dimorphic circuits in the mammalian forebrain. *Annu. Rev. Neurosci.*, **25**, 507–36.

Slieker, L. J., Sloop, K. W., Surface, P. L. *et al.* (1996). Regulation of expression of ob mRNA and protein by glucocorticoids and cAMP. *J. Biol. Chem.*, **271**(10), 5301–4.

Sloboda, D. M., Moss, T. J., Gurrin, L. C., Newnham, J. P. and Challis, J. R. (2002a). The effect of prenatal betamethasone administration on postnatal ovine hypothalamic–pituitary–adrenal function. *J. Endocrinol.*, **172**(1), 71–81.

Sloboda, D. M., Newnham, J. P. and Challis, J. R. G. (2002b). Repeated maternal glucocorticoid administration and the developing liver in fetal sheep. *J. Endocrinol.*, **175**, 535–43.

Slotkin, T. A., Barnes, G. A., McCook, E. C. and Seidler, F. J. (1996a). Programming of brainstem serotonin transporter development by prenatal glucocorticoids. *Brain Res. – Develop. Brain Res.*, **93**(1–2), 155–61.

Slotkin, T. A., Barnes, G. A., McCook, E. C. and Seidler, F. J. (1996b). Programming of brainstem serotonin transporter development by prenatal glucocorticoids. *Develop. Brain Res.*, **93**, 155–61.

Smith, J. T. and Waddell, B. J. (2002). Leptin receptor expression in the rat placenta: changes in Ob-Ra, Ob-Rb, and Ob-Re with gestational age and suppression by glucocorticoids. *Biol. Reprod.*, **67**(4), 1204–10.

Smythe, J. W., Rowe, W. B. and Meaney, M. J. (1994). Neonatal handling alters serotonin (5-HT) turnover and 5-HT2 receptor binding in selected brain regions: relationship to the handling effect on glucocorticoid receptor expression. *Brain Res. – Develop. Brain Res.*, **80**(1–2), 183–9.

Stein, M. B., Koverola, C., Hanna, C., Torchia, M. G. and McClarty, B. (1997). Hippocampal volume in women victimized by childhood sexual abuse. *Psychol. Med.*, **27**(4), 951–9.

Stewart, P. M., Corrie, J. E. T., Shackleton, C. H. L. and Edwards, C. R. W. (1988). Syndrome of apparent mineralocorticoid excess: a defect in the cortisol–cortisone shuttle. *J. Clin. Invest.*, **82**, 340–9.

Stewart, P. M., Murry, B. A. and Mason, J. I. (1994). Type 2 11β-hydroxysteroid dehydrogenase in human fetal tissues. *J. Clin. Endocrinol. Metab.*, **78**, 1529–32.

Stewart, P. M., Rogerson, F. M. and Mason, J. I. (1995). Type 2 11β-hydroxysteroid dehydrogenase messenger RNA and activity in human placenta and fetal membranes: its relationship to birth weight and putative role in fetal steroidogenesis. *J. Clin. Endocrinol. Metab.*, **80**, 885–90.

Stocker, C., O'Dowd, J., Morton, N. *et al.* (2004). Modulation of susceptibility to weight gain and insulin resistance in low birthweight rats by treatment of their mothers with leptin during pregnancy and lactation. *Int. J. Obesity*, **28**, 129–36.

Sugden, M. C., Langdown, M. L., Munns, M. J. and Holness, M. J. (2001). Maternal glucocorticoid treatment modulates placental leptin and leptin receptor expression and materno-fetal leptin physiology during late pregnancy, and elicits hypertension associated with hyperlepti-naemia in the early-growth-retarded adult offspring. *Eur. J. Endocrinol.*, **145**(4), 529–39.

Sun, K., Yang, K. and Challis, J. R. G. (1997). Differential expression of 11beta-hydroxysteroid dehydrogenase types 1 and 2 in human placenta and fetal membranes. *J. Clin. Endocrinol. Metab.*, **82**, 300–5.

Tangalakis, K., Lumbers, E. R., Moritz, K. M., Towstoless, M. K. and Wintour, E. M. (1992). Effect of cortisol on blood pressure and vascular reactivity in the ovine fetus. *Exp. Physiol.*, **77**, 709–17.

Thomas, L., Wallace, J. M., Aitken, R. P. *et al.* (2001). Circulating leptin during ovine pregnancy in relation to maternal nutrition, body composition and pregnancy outcome. *J. Endocrinol.*, **169**(3), 465–76.

Thomassin, H., Flavin, M., Espinas, M. L. and Grange, T. (2001). Glucocorticoid-induced DNA demethylation and gene memory during development. *EMBO J.*, **20**(8), 1974–83.

Trautman, P. D., Meyer-Bahlburg, H. F., Postelnek, J. and New, M. I. (1995). Effects of early pre-natal dexamethasone on the cognitive and behavioral development of young children: results of a pilot study. *Psychoneuroendocrinology*, **20**(4), 439–49.

Tronche, F., Kellendonk, C., Kretz, O. *et al.* (1999). Disruption of the glucocorticoid receptor gene in the nervous system results in reduced anxiety. *Nat. Genet.*, **23**, 99–103.

Uno, H., Lohmiller, L., Thieme, C. *et al.* (1990). Brain damage induced by prenatal exposure to dexamethasone in fetal rhesus macaques. I. hippocampus. *Develop. Brain Res.*, **53**, 157–67.

Uno, H., Eisele, S., Sakai, A. *et al.* (1994). Neurotoxicity of glucocorticoids in the primate brain. *Horm. Behav.*, **28**, 336–48.

Vaessen, N., Heutink, P., Janssen, J. A. *et al.* (2001). A polymorphism in the gene for IGF-I: func-tional properties and risk for type 2 diabetes and myocardial infarction. *Diabetes*, **50**(3), 637–42.

Valera, A., Pujol, A., Pelegrin, M. and Bosch, F. (1994). Transgenic mice overexpressing phospho-enolpyruvate carboxykinase develop non-insulin-dependent diabetes mellitus. *Proc. Natl. Acad. Sci. USA*, **91**(19), 9151–4.

Venihaki, M. A., Carrigan, P., Dikkes. *et al.* (2000). Circadian rise in maternal glucocorticoid pre-vents pulmonary dysplasia in fetal mice with adrenal insufficiency. *Proc. Natl. Acad. Sci. USA*, **97**, 7336–41.

Voice, M., Seckl, J. R., Edwards, C. R. W. and Chapman, K. E. (1996). 11β-hydroxysteroid dehy-drogenase type 1 expression in 2S-FAZA hepatoma cells is hormonally-regulated: a model for the study of hepatic corticosteroid metabolism. *Biochem. J.*, **317**, 621–5.

Walfisch, A., Hallak, M. and Mazor, M. (2001). Multiple courses of antenatal steroids: risks and benefits. *Obstetr. Gynecol.*, **98**(3), 491–7.

Ward, R. M. (1994). Pharmacologic enhancement of fetal lung maturation. *Clin. Perinatol.*, **21**, 523–42.

Weaver, I. C. G., Szyf, M. and Meaney, M. J. (2002). From maternal care to gene expression: DNA methylation and the maternal programming of stress responses. *Endocr. Res.*, **28**(4), 699.

Weinstock, M. (2001). Alterations induced by gestational stress in brain morphology and behav-iour of the offspring. *Prog. Neurobiol.*, **65**, 427–51.

Weinstock, M., Matlina, E., Maor, G. I., Rosen, H. and McEwen, B. S. (1992). Prenatal stress selectively alters the reactivity of the hypothalamic–pituitary adrenal system in the female rat. *Brain Res.*, **595**, 195–200.

Welberg, L. A. M. and Seckl, J. R. (2001). Prenatal stress, glucocorticoids and the programming of the brain. *J. Neuroendocrinol.*, **13**, 113–28.

Welberg, L. A. M., Seckl, J. R. and Holmes, M. C. (2000). Inhibition of 11β-hydroxysteroid dehydrogenase, the feto-placental barrier to maternal glucocorticoids, permanently programs amygdala glucocorticoid receptor mRNA expression and anxiety-like behavior in the offspring. *Eur. J. Neurosci.*, **12**, 1047–54.

Welberg, L. A. M., Seckl, J. R. and Holmes, M. C. (2001). Prenatal glucocorticoid programming of brain corticosteroid receptors and corticotrophin-releasing hormone: possible implications for behaviour. *Neuroscience*, **104**, 71–9.

Weyer, C., Funahashi, T., Tanaka, S. *et al.* (2001). Hypoadiponectinemia in obesity and type 2 diabetes: close association with insulin resistance and hyperinsulinemia. *J. Clin. Endocrinol. Metab.*, **86**(5), 1930–5.

White, P. C., Mune, T. and Agarwal, A. K. (1997). 11beta-hydroxysteroid dehydrogenase and the syndrome of apparent mineralocorticoid excess. *Endocr. Rev.*, **18**, 135–56.

Whitelaw, A. and Thoresen, M. (2000). Antenatal steroids and the developing brain. *Arch. Dis. Child. Fetal Neonatal Edn.*, **83**(2), F154–7.

Whorwood, C. B., Franklyn, J. A., Sheppard, M. C. and Stewart, P. M. (1991). Tissue localization of 11β-hydroxysteroid dehydrogenase and its relationship to the glucocorticoid receptor. *J. Steroid Biochem. Mol. Biol.*, **41**, 21–8.

Whorwood, C. B., Firth, K. M., Budge, H. and Symonds, M. E. (2001). Maternal undernutrition during early to midgestation programs tissue-specific alterations in the expression of the glucocorticoid receptor, 11 beta-hydroxysteroid dehydrogenase isoforms, and type 1 angiotensin II receptor in neonatal sheep. *Endocrinology*, **142**(7), 2854–64.

Yajnik, C. S., Fall, C. H. D., Vaidya, U. *et al.* (1995). Fetal growth and glucose and insulin metabolism in four-year-old Indian children. *Diabetic Med.*, **12**, 330–6.

Yang, K., Matthews, S. G. and Challis, J. R. G. (1995). Developmental and glucocorticoid regulation of pituitary 11beta-hydroxysteroid dehydrogenase 1 gene expression in the ovine fetus and lamb. *J. Mol. Endocrinol.*, **14**, 109–16.

Yau, J. L., Noble, J. and Seckl, J. R. (1997a). Site-specific regulation of corticosteroid and serotonin receptor subtype gene expression in the rat hippocampus following 3,4-methylenedioxymethamphetamine: role of corticosterone and serotonin. *Neuroscience*, **78**(1), 111–21.

Yau, J. L. W., Noble, J., Widdowson, J. and Seckl, J. R. (1997b). Impact of adrenalectomy on 5-HT6 and 5-HT7 receptor gene expression in the rat hippocampus. *Mol. Brain Res.*, **45**, 182–6.

Yuen, B. S., McMillen, I. C., Symonds, M. E. and Owens, P. C. (1999). Abundance of leptin mRNA in fetal adipose tissue is related to fetal body weight. *J. Endocrinol.*, **163**(3), R11–4.

6

Prenatal stress and stress physiology influences human fetal and infant development

Elysia Poggi Davis[1], Calvin J. Hobel[2], Curt A. Sandman[3], Laura Glynn[3] and Pathik D. Wadhwa[4]

[1] Department of Psychiatry and Human Behavior, University of California, Irvine, California, USA
[2] Department of Obstetrics and Gynecology, Cedars Sinai Medical Center, Los Angeles, California, USA
[3] Department of Psychiatry and Human Behavior, University of California, Irvine, California, USA
[4] Departments of Psychiatry and Human Behavior, and Obstetrics and Gynecology, University of California, Irvine, California, USA

Prenatal stress has been proposed as a risk factor that may have developmental consequences persisting throughout the lifespan. Exposing rodents to stress during pregnancy has consequences for brain development, stress regulation, learning, emotionality (increased anxiety), and social behavior (increased withdrawal) of the offspring (Weinstock, 2001; Chapillon et al., 2002). Additionally, non-human primates who experience stress during pregnancy have offspring with enhanced behavioral reactivity to stressors later in life (Clarke et al., 1994), lowered levels of motor behavior (Schneider, 1992), compromised neuromotor responses (Schneider and Coe, 1993), irritable temperament (Schneider et al., 1992), and attentional problems (Schneider et al., 1999).

Many researchers have focused on the hypothalamic–pituitary–adrenocortical (HPA) axis, one of the body's major stress systems, as a mechanism that may mediate these effects (Ward and Phillips, 2001; Welberg and Seckl, 2001). The HPA axis activity is regulated by the release of hypothalamic corticotropin-releasing hormone (CRH) that stimulates the biosynthesis and release of adrenocorticotropin hormone (ACTH) and β-endorphin (βE) from the anterior pituitary. The release of ACTH triggers the biosynthesis and release of glucocorticoids (cortisol in primates and corticosterone in rodents) from the adrenal cortex. Glucocorticoids are released into the

Corresponding author: Pathik D. Wadhwa, MD, PhD., Behavioral Perinatology Research Program, University of California, Irvine, 3117 Gillespie Neuroscience Research Facility, Irvine, CA 92697. Tel: (949) 824-8238, Fax: (949) 824-8218, E-mail: pwadhwa@uci.edu

Preparation of this manuscript was supported, in part, by US PHS (NIH) grants HD-33506 and HD-41696 to P.D.W.

general circulation and have effects on nearly every organ and tissue in the body (Munck *et al.*, 1984). Consequences of glucocorticoid release include energy mobilization and immunosuppression (Chrousos and Gold, 1992). Glucocorticoids easily pass through the blood–brain barrier (Zarrow *et al.*, 1970). There are receptors for glucocorticoids throughout the central nervous system (CNS) (de Kloet *et al.*, 1998; Sanchez *et al.*, 2000). Glucocorticoids regulate their own release by negative feedback actions at the hypothalamus and pituitary inhibiting the release of CRH and ACTH. Glucocorticoids additionally act on extrahypothalamic sites including the hippocampus and frontal cortex further activating negative feedback regulation of CRH production in the hypothalamus (Jacobson and Sapolsky, 1991; Sanchez *et al.*, 2000). In contrast glucocorticoids increase CRH production in extrahypothalamic brain regions, such as the central nucleus of the amygdala (Swanson and Simmons, 1989; Makino *et al.*, 1994; Watts and Sanchez-Watts, 1995).

The HPA axis is particularly sensitive to early experiences. In rat pups, manipulations, such as daily handling or maternal deprivation produce lifelong changes in stress reactivity, fearful behavior, and cognitive functioning (Levine, 1957; Meaney *et al.*, 1988; Liu *et al.*, 1997). Rodent models further suggest that prenatal stress has an impact that persists through adulthood. The offspring of stressed dams display prolonged glucocorticoid responses to stress indicating that exposure to stress in utero may impair negative feedback mechanisms (Weinstock *et al.*, 1992; Henry *et al.*, 1994; Herman and Cullinan, 1997). The offspring of rodents stressed during pregnancy also display an increase in behavioral signs of anxiety (Takahashi *et al.*, 1992; Vallee *et al.*, 1997). Alterations of CRH regulation in the amygdala is a proposed mechanism for this effect. The amygdala is considered to be the structure where fear-inducing sensory and autonomic input and behavioral output converge. Prenatally stressed rats display an increase in amygdala CRH (Cratty *et al.*, 1995). Thus, elevations in amygdala CRH, resulting from prenatal stress, may contribute to the increase in HPA axis reactivity and anxiety seen in these animals. Cognitive functions are also impaired in prenatally stressed animals. This may be particularly true for functions that are dependant on the hippocampus, a structure that is vulnerable to elevations in glucocorticoids (Takahashi, 1998; McEwen, 1999). In sum, these studies suggest that prenatal stress has lasting implications for CNS development and function.

Animal studies have offered valuable insights into physiological mechanisms that may be involved in mediating the effects of stressful maternal and intrauterine environments on the developing organism. However, the generalizability of these findings from animals to humans is limited by the existence of inter-species differences in physiology and the developmental time-line. The timing of maturation of the HPA axis relative to birth is highly species-specific and is closely linked to landmarks of brain development (Dobbing and Sands, 1979). In animals that give birth to precocious offspring (sheep, guinea pigs, primates), maximal brain growth and a large proportion of neuroendocrine maturation takes place in utero. By contrast, in species that give birth to non-precocious offspring (rats, rabbits, mice), much of neuroendocrine development occurs in the postnatal period (Dent et al., 2000). A second major difference is that anthropoid primates are the only species known to produce placental CRH during pregnancy.

The placenta expresses the genes for CRH (hCRHmRNA) and the preprotein for ACTH and βE (pro-opiomelanocortin, POMC). Placental CRH is identical to hypothalamic CRH in structure, immunoreactivity, and bioactivity (Petraglia et al., 1996). There is, however, one crucial difference in the regulation of hypothalamic and placental CRH. In contrast to the negative control on hypothalamic CRH, glucocorticoids stimulate the expression of hCRHmRNA in the placenta creating a positive feedback loop that is similar to the central nucleus of the amygdala (Schulkin, 1999). Placental CRH is released into the maternal and fetal circulation, establishing a positive feedback loop that allows for the simultaneous increase of CRH, ACTH, and cortisol in the maternal and fetal compartments over the course of gestation (Petraglia et al., 1996; King et al., 2001).

The HPA–placental axis is a mechanism by which the environment shapes fetal development. The activity of the HPA–placental axis is regulated by characteristics of the maternal and intrauterine environment. Maternal cortisol, which crosses the placenta, increases with maternal stress (Wadhwa et al., 1996). Furthermore, in vitro and in vivo studies have demonstrated that placental CRH output is modulated in a positive, dose–response manner by the major biological effectors of stress, including cortisol (Korebrits et al., 1998; Marinoni et al., 1998). During pregnancy CRH levels were positively correlated with ACTH and βE (Wadhwa et al., 1997). These findings support the premise that in human pregnancy placental CRH activity is modulated by maternal pituitary adrenal hormones. Both placental CRH and cortisol in turn may influence fetal development. Placental CRH is involved in the physiology of normal parturition and elevated CRH concentrations are associated with an increased risk for spontaneous preterm birth (McLean et al., 1995; Hobel et al., 1999a; Erickson et al., 2001; Holzman et al., 2001; Inder et al., 2001; Moawad et al., 2002). It has been proposed that the activity of the maternal–HPA–placental axis during pregnancy programs the development of the offspring's HPA axis (Ward and Phillips, 2001; Matthews, 2002). Additionally, placental CRH and cortisol may contribute to the organization of the fetal CNS (Sandman et al., 1997a; Florio and Petraglia, 2001). Few studies have considered the consequences of prenatal stress on human fetal behavior and fewer still have assessed the effects of maternal stress on the continuum between the fetus and the infant. We will discuss a neurobiological model of prenatal stress that proposes the developmental consequences of maternal psychosocial stress are mediated, in part, via maternal–placental–fetal neuroendocrine mechanisms.

Methodological approaches

We have assessed the consequences of maternal stress during pregnancy on neuro-endocrine processes and fetal and infant development using a range of techniques. Primarily, we have employed longitudinal population-based cohort studies with a combined sample of approximately 750 women with singleton, intrauterine pregnancies. Women were recruited at various time points in pregnancy starting in the late first or second trimester of gestation and followed through delivery into the early postpartum period. Participants were heterogeneous in terms of sociodemographic and ethnic characteristics. Furthermore, based on conventional measures of obstetric risk we have included approximately equal numbers of subjects at low- and high-risk for adverse perinatal outcomes. In these studies standardized and validated interviews and questionnaires were administered at multiple time points over gestation to assess:

(a) *maternal psychosocial constructs* including various forms of prenatal stress, social support, personality characteristics, and attitudes towards pregnancy;
(b) *maternal behaviors* including diet and nutrition, physical activity, and smoking, alcohol, and drug use;
(c) *sociodemographic characteristics* including age, marital status, various indicators of socioeconomic status, and race/ethnicity.

Maternal and cord blood samples were collected during gestation and at delivery for bioassays of stress hormones, including ACTH, βE, cortisol and placental CRH. Obstetric and birth outcomes were abstracted from the medical records. All pregnancies are dated by best obstetric estimate using last menstrual period and early ultrasonographic confirmation. In a sub sample of 156 pregnancies, we have performed fetal assessments in the early third trimester of gestation, including fetal biometry, doppler flow velocimetry of the uteroplacental circulation, and an experimental challenge paradigm to quantify indices of fetal arousal, reactivity, learning and habituation, assessed by fetal heart rate (FHR) responses to a series of vibroacoustic (VA) stimuli. To examine direct effects of glucocorticoids on fetal and infant HPA axis development, a sample of infants whose mother did or did not receive synthetic glucocorticoids during their pregnancy were recruited. In this population cortisol levels at baseline and in response to stress were assessed.

Research findings
Maternal stress during pregnancy and birth outcomes

Disruption of reproductive function in mammals is a well-known consequence of stress. Results from experimental approaches in animal models support a causal role for prenatal stress as a developmental teratogen (Weinstock, 2001). In humans, studies examining the influence of maternal stress during pregnancy have focused primarily on length of gestation and fetal growth/size at birth, the two primary indicators of newborn health. Using women's self report of stress during pregnancy we have found that maternal psychosocial processes significantly influence both length of gestation and fetal growth and that this influence is independent of the effects of other established sociodemographic and obstetric risk factors (Wadhwa *et al.*, 1993; Rini *et al.*, 1999; Feldman *et al.*, 2000). Maternal stress has differential effects depending on its timing during pregnancy. From a prospective investigation of stress and stress physiology in pregnancy, 40 pregnant women were identified who had experienced a 6.8 magnitude earthquake during pregnancy or shortly after delivery. The participants lived, on average, 50 miles from the epicenter of the earthquake and were physically unaffected by the damage produced. The effect of exposure to the earthquake was linearly moderated by the stage in gestation of its occurrence. Women who experienced the earthquake earlier in their pregnancy had a significantly shorter gestational length than those who experienced it later in gestation (see Figure 6.1). This study supports the notion that the timing of stress in pregnancy may be an important factor in determining its impact on the length of human gestation (Glynn *et al.*, 2001).

Our results are consistent with several population-based epidemiological studies that have suggested that high levels of maternal psychosocial stress are independently associated with a significant increase in the risk for prematurity and that effects are observed across the entire range of the outcome distribution (Hedegaard *et al.*, 1993; Pritchard and Teo, 1994; Copper *et al.*, 1996; Hedegaard *et al.*, 1996; Misra *et al.*, 2001). Additionally, the effect size of maternal psychosocial processes in pregnancy on prematurity-related outcomes is comparable to that of most other obstetric risk factors suggesting that these processes warrant the same degree of consideration.

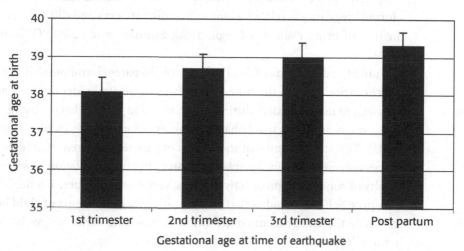

Figure 6.1   Stress during the first trimester of pregnancy significantly predicts shorter gestational length. Adapted from Glynn *et al.* (2001)

Maternal stress during pregnancy and infant developmental outcomes

Maternal psychological state during pregnancy seems to influence birth outcome in terms of length of gestation and fetal growth. The influence of maternal experiences during pregnancy on the development of the fetal CNS and the implications for infant development has largely been neglected in human research. Existing research considering the effects of prenatal experience on postnatal development in humans is often limited by a failure to control for the effects of birth outcome. For example, infants born prematurely or small for gestational age (GA) are at risk for a wide variety of developmental problems (Peterson *et al.*, 2003). It is necessary to consider these factors to examine the independent influence of prenatal stress physiology on postnatal development.

Recent studies suggest that maternal anxiety, stress and depression during pregnancy, shape the fetal behavioral patterns (DiPietro *et al.*, 2002; Monk *et al.*, 2003) and predict higher cortisol and norepinephrine and lower Brazelton scores in the newborn (Jones *et al.*, 1998; Lundy *et al.*, 1999). To examine whether this influence continued into infancy we conducted preliminary studies to prospectively assess the relationship between maternal stress during pregnancy and indices of infant behavioral development. Forty-seven mother–infant pairs were assessed during pregnancy and at 6 weeks after delivery. All infants in this sample were full term at birth. Questionnaires were administered to mothers to assess pre- and postnatal maternal anxiety and infant temperament. Infant fussiness was associated with higher levels of maternal anxiety during the third trimester even after controlling for postpartum maternal affect, intrapartum compromise, infant sex and birth weight (Davis *et al.*, 2003). These data are consistent with the few prospective studies present in the literature illustrating that maternal stress, anxiety, and depression during pregnancy is related to emotional disturbances and difficult temperament in the offspring (Van den Bergh, 1990; Susman *et al.*, 2001; O'Connor *et al.*, 2002a, b).

Subjective description of child behavior by the parent is confounded by the parent's psychological state at the time of reporting. One study identified an association between maternal anxiety during pregnancy and child behavior using a prospective design and objective behavioral observations of the child (Huizink *et al.*, 2002). This study found that the infants of mothers who reported higher levels of anxiety during pregnancy displayed poorer attention regulation. Owing to the difficulty of conducting prospective studies, very few exist. There is a need for further prospective human studies that employ objective assessments of child behavior to elucidate the independent contribution of postnatal maternal psychological state on development.

To differentiate the effects of prenatal and postnatal maternal psychological state, maternal anxiety and depression were assessed prospectively. Infant behavioral reactivity was assessed at 4 months using a standardized laboratory-based behavioral assessment protocol (i.e. the Harvard Infant Behavioral Reactivity Protocol, Kagan and Snidman, 1991). In this paradigm infant motor and cry reactivity to a series of visual and auditory challenges were assessed. Maternal anxiety and depression during the third trimester of pregnancy, but not postpartum were associated with the development of individual differences in infants' behavioral regulation. The offspring of mothers who were higher in anxiety and depression during pregnancy displayed greater behavioral reactivity to novelty. Notably, this association remained after controlling for postpartum maternal psychological state indicating that prenatal experiences were responsible for this association (Davis et al., 2004a). The selective effects of prenatal experiences on behavioral reactivity supports the hypothesis that the prenatal environment exerts programming effects on the fetus with consequences for infant behavior (Barker, 2002). These data support a model that prenatal maternal stress has an independent effect not only on regulation of length of gestation but also on development of the fetus and thus the infant.

Placental CRH and fetal growth and premature birth

The maternal–HPA axis is one mechanism that has been proposed to mediate the effects of maternal stress during pregnancy on birth outcome and the development of the fetus. During pregnancy maternal ACTH and cortisol increases in response to stress in ways that are similar to the non-pregnant state (Wadhwa et al., 1996). Via this pathway, maternal stress can modulate placental CRH production. Placental CRH is involved in the physiology of parturition as well as fetal cellular differentiation, growth, and maturation (Challis et al., 2001; Smith, 2001; Hillhouse and Grammatopoulos, 2002). We have conducted several studies to examine the role of CRH in regulation of timing of delivery and fetal growth. The first study involved a sample of 63 women with singleton, intrauterine pregnancies. Maternal plasma was collected at 28–30 weeks gestation, and placental CRH concentrations were determined by radioimmuno assay. Results indicated that maternal (placental) CRH levels at 28–30 weeks gestation significantly and negatively predicted gestational length after adjusting for antepartum risk. Moreover, subjects who delivered prematurely (prior to 37 weeks gestation) had significantly higher CRH levels in the early third trimester than those who delivered at term (Wadhwa et al., 1998).

To explore further the associations between CRH and gestational length and to examine effects of CRH on fetal growth, 245 women with singleton, intrauterine pregnancies were recruited. Maternal plasma CRH was assessed at 32–33 weeks gestation. It was found that elevated CRH was related to both risk of preterm birth and fetal growth restriction. After adjusting for effects of established risk factors women with elevated CRH were approximately 3 times more likely to deliver

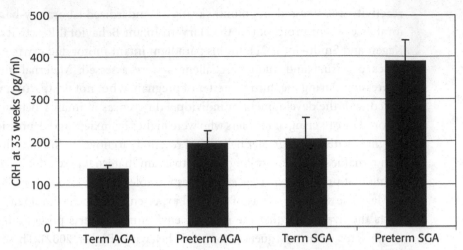

Figure 6.2   Infants born preterm or SGA more likely to be exposed to high levels of CRH during the third trimester of pregnancy. Adapted from Wadhwa *et al.* (2004). SGA: small for their gestational age; AGA: appropriate for gestational age

preterm and/or have an infant that was small for GA (see Figure 6.2; Wadhwa *et al.*, 2004). The results of this study suggest that placental CRH plays a role in the physiology of parturition as well as in processes related to fetal growth.

These studies suggest that increased activity by the placental–HPA axis during the third trimester predicts premature labor. The question remains as to whether increased placental CRH earlier in pregnancy might also predict length of gestation. To address this issue CRH was assessed in 524 women at 18–20, 28–30, and 35–36 weeks gestation. Eighteen women with spontaneous premature labor were compared to 18 women who delivered at term. Patients who delivered prematurely had higher levels of CRH at all three measurement time points (Hobel *et al.*, 1999a). Furthermore, women who delivered prematurely had lower levels of CRH-binding protein, which inactivates CRH (Hobel *et al.*, 1999a). Thus, maternal CRH was elevated as early as 18–20 weeks GA in woman who subsequently delivered prematurely.

Neuroendocrine function during pregnancy and human fetal CNS development

It has been proposed that the HPA–placental axis is a conduit for the effects of environmental stress on the fetus. Research with animals indicates that during prenatal development the hormones of the HPA axis have programming effects on the developing CNS (Matthews, 2000; Welberg and Seckl, 2001). The influence of the maternal and intrauterine environment on the developing human fetal brain is poorly understood. This is in part, because the assessment and quantification of human fetal brain development presents theoretical and methodological challenges.

To quantify and examine the influence of the fetal environment on its brain development we have utilized a habituation–dishabituation paradigm that assesses the ability of the fetus to learn information. By 32 weeks gestation the fetus habituates and dishabituates to external stimulation (Sandman *et al.*, 1997b). Faster fetal habituation has been associated with advancing GA (Shalev *et al.*, 1990) consistent with maturation of the CNS. We examined the effect of maternal–placental CRH on habituation processes. Thirty-three pregnant women were assessed between 30 and 32 weeks gestation. Fetal heart rate and uterine contractions were assessed by placing transducers on the maternal abdomen. A total of 41 trials of vibroacoustic (VA) stimuli were presented over a 45-min period. The first series of 15 VA (63 dB, 300 Hz) stimuli (S1) was presented on the maternal abdomen. On the 16th trial S2, the dishabituating VA stimuli (68 dB, 400 Hz, novel in frequency and intensity) was presented. The original VA stimuli (S1) was then presented for trials 17–31. As a control the final 10 stimuli were presented to the mother's thigh. The fetuses of mothers with highly elevated CRH levels did not respond significantly to the presence of the novel stimulus (Sandman *et al.*, 1999). These data provide preliminary evidence that abnormally elevated levels of placental CRH may play a role in impaired neurodevelopment, as assessed by the degree of dishabituation (Sandman *et al.*, 1999).

In addition to the effects of placental CRH on fetal CNS development described above, maternal pituitary and adrenal hormones may also shape fetal development. The influence of circulating maternal ACTH and βE levels with measures of fetal responses to challenge was determined in a sample of 132 women at 31–32 weeks gestation. Fetal responses were measured by measuring heart rate (HR) habituation to a series of repeated VA stimuli. Individual differences in habituation were determined by computing the number of consecutive HR responses that were greater than the standard deviation of the HR during a control (non-stimulated) period. There was no significant relation between absolute levels of ACTH, βE and fetal HR responses to challenge. However an index of POMC disregulation, the degree of uncoupling between ACTH and βE, was significantly related to fetal responses such that fetal exposure to relatively high levels of the maternal opiate, βE, relative to ACTH, was associated with a significantly lower rate of habituation (see Figure 6.3; Sandman *et al.*, 2003).

Our findings are consistent with those of longitudinal investigations of the functional development of the human fetal CNS over the course of gestation, that have suggested chronic maternal psychologic distress is significantly related to measures of fetal neurobehavioral maturation and reactivity (DiPietro *et al.*, 1996; DiPietro *et al.*, 2000; Monk *et al.*, 2000; DiPietro *et al.*, 2002; Monk *et al.*, 2003).

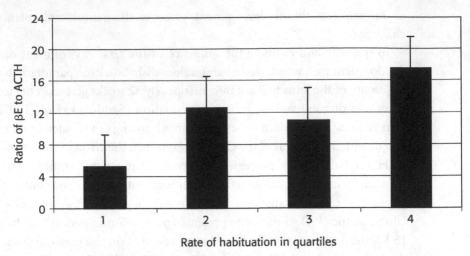

Figure 6.3   Fetal exposure to relatively high levels of the maternal opiate, βE, relative to ACTH, is associated with a significantly lower rate of habituation. Adapted from Sandman *et al.* (2003)

The continuity of development from prenatal to postnatal development requires further exploration.

Endocrine hormones during pregnancy and human infant development

Demonstration of an impact of maternal and placental hormones on fetal CNS functioning illustrates the importance of exploring the implications of fetal experiences on development in infancy and childhood. In rodents, primates and other species it has been shown that stimulation of the HPA axis or exposure to elevated glucocorticoids impairs brain development and HPA axis functioning in the offspring. There is transplacental passage of glucocorticoids to the fetus (Matthews *et al.*, 2002). Animals exposed to prenatal elevations in glucocorticoids display impairments in brain development and increased reactivity to stress (Takahashi, 1998; Matthews *et al.*, 2002; Antonow-Schlorke *et al.*, 2003).

One method for examining the effects of HPA axis hormone disregulation on human infant development involves examination of the effects of administration of synthetic glucocorticoids to women during pregnancy. Antenatal glucocorticoid administration is a standard of care for women at risk of premature delivery and has been shown to reduce mortality and respiratory distress among preterm infants born at less than 34 weeks gestation. However, studies with humans have demonstrated that antenatal glucocorticoid exposure is associated with reduced birth weight (Banks *et al.*, 1999; French *et al.*, 1999) and head circumference

(French *et al.*, 1999; Abbasi *et al.*, 2000). Additionally prenatal glucocorticoid treatment effects postnatal HPA axis regulation in the offspring. Baseline cortisol levels are suppressed for 2–7 days after prenatal corticosteroid treatment and subsequently return to normal levels (Wittekind *et al.*, 1993; Parker *et al.*, 1996; Kauppila *et al.*, 1978; Ballard *et al.*, 1980; Dorr *et al.*, 1989). These data suggest that prenatal exposure to elevated levels of glucocorticoids may have implications for infant development. The effect on the HPA axis response to stress has not, however, been assessed.

One of the sequelae of prenatal exposure to elevated glucocorticoids noted in the animal literature is disregulation of the HPA axis response to stress (Matthews, 2002). We thus examined the effects of prenatal glucocorticoid treatment on the cortisol response to stress during the first postnatal week in human infants born at 33–34 weeks with and without prenatal glucocorticoid treatment. Infants in the glucocorticoid group were on average 12 days post antenatal glucocorticoid treatment. Consistent with previous research demonstrating that baseline cortisol is suppressed only for the first 2–7 days after prenatal treatment, these two groups of infants did not differ in their resting baseline cortisol levels. Infants who were exposed to antenatal glucocorticoid, however, failed to mount a cortisol response to a painful stimulus, a heel-stick blood draw (see Figure 6.4). In contrast, premature infants who did not receive prenatal glucocorticoid treatment displayed an increase in cortisol in response to the heel-stick stressor (Davis *et al.*, 2004b). This cortisol response, also displayed by full term infants, is considered appropriate and

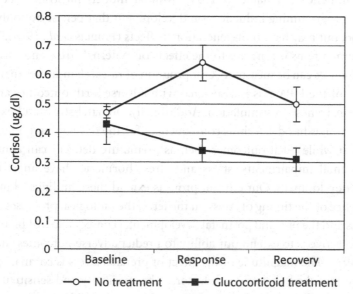

Figure 6.4   The cortisol response to a painful event is suppressed in infants with antenatal betamethasone treatment. Adapted from Davis *et al.* (2004b)

supports adaptation to challenge (Gunnar, 1992). This study suggests that even after baseline cortisol levels have returned to normal levels the ability to respond to stress appears disregulated. This finding is consistent with data indicating that infants exposed to antenatal glucocorticoids displayed a suppressed response to the CRH stimulation test (Ng *et al.*, 2002).

Prenatal exposure to glucocorticoids seems to have a lasting effect on regulation of physiologic stress responses in the newborn. Furthermore, as groups were similar in GA at birth and prenatal history, prenatal glucocorticoid exposure appears to have a direct effect on postnatal stress physiology. We are currently conducting longitudinal studies to examine whether this disregulation of the HPA axis response to stress persists throughout infancy and early childhood.

Conclusions and future directions

Development is an epigenetic process by which, each developing organism plays an active role in its own construction. This dynamic process is affected by systems that are present during embryonic and fetal life to acquire information about the nature of the environment, and to use this information to guide development. Due to the rapid development that takes place during the prenatal period the fetus may be especially vulnerable to both organizing and disorganizing influences. These influences on the fetus have been described as programming, a process by which a stimulus or insult during a critical developmental period has a long-lasting or permanent influence (Nathanielsz, 1999). Animal models illustrate that maternal stress has programming influences on development that persist not only through adulthood, but may have transgenerational effects (Francis *et al.*, 1999).

The human fetus is sensitive to the effects of maternal stress and furthermore, these influences can be measured. Our program of research indicates that maternal activation of the HPA axis is associated with adverse birth outcomes and altered fetal responsiveness to stimulation. Additionally, prenatal stress and exposure to stress hormones has deleterious consequences for the developing infant. We have shown that while birth outcomes such as premature delivery can contribute to developmental impairments, stress and stress hormones have an independent effect on development. Our current projects extend these findings to understand the influence of the timing of stress on the fetus, the biological processes associated with stress and the pre- and postnatal developmental consequences of prenatal stress.

One objective is to extend our ability to predict adverse outcomes such as premature birth. The magnitude of the effect of prenatal stress is comparable to that of other established obstetric risk factors. The specificity and sensitivity of these measures as predictors of adverse outcome(s) in any individual pregnancy is modest. For example, low levels of placental CRH in pregnancy are a good negative predictor of preterm birth but high levels are a poor positive predictor. This may suggest that parameters such as stress and placental CRH should be considered in conjunction with other risk factors.

In addition to the maternal–placental–fetal neuroendocrine processes discussed above, host (maternal and/or fetal) proinflammatory immune responses produced by intrauterine or reproductive tract infection have been implicated in adverse fetal outcomes, especially extreme prematurity (<30 weeks gestation) and white matter brain damage (Romero *et al.*, 2001). Although psychosocial stress is a well-established contributor to the risk of infection and its pathophysiological consequences (Cohen *et al.*, 1999) and the endocrine and immune systems are known to extensively regulate and counter-regulate one another (McEwen *et al.*, 1997; Shanks and Lightman, 2001; Elenkov and Chrousos, 2002), very little empirical work has been done to date to examine these interactions in the context of stress in pregnancy and fetal development. Thus, one of our current, ongoing studies is designed to examine psychoneuroendocrine–immune interactions in human pregnancy, to explore the hypothesis that maternal psychosocial stress and neuroendocrine stress responses may play a role in determining susceptibility to the development of reproductive tract infection and its pathophysiological consequences. We suggest this is a critical future direction for this work as the effect of either of these processes on a biological outcome of interest is modulated by the state/context of the other.

Returning to the concept of an epigenetic framework of development, it appears that embryonic and fetal developmental processes ultimately represent the dynamic interplay between two sets of information systems, fetal and maternal deoxyribonucleic acid (DNA) and the fetal and maternal environments. Genetic predispositions may make some pregnancies more vulnerable to environmental influences. We are not aware of any studies to date that have systematically examined the physiological genomics of maternal and fetal stress-related neuroendocrine systems and pathways in human pregnancy, and suggest this is yet another important future avenue for this line of research.

In conclusion, there is a compelling need to arrive at a better understanding of the determinants of individual differences in psychoneuroendocrine processes that underlie health and disease. The study of the interplay between biological and behavioral processes in fetal life, using a dynamic systems approach, holds great promise for our efforts to arrive at this understanding.

REFERENCES

Abbasi, S., Hirsch, D., Davis, J. *et al.* (2000). Effect of single versus multiple courses of antenatal corticosteroids on maternal and neonatal outcome. *Am. J. Obstet. Gynecol.*, **182**(5), 1243–9.

Antonow-Schlorke, I., Schwab, M., Li, C. and Nathanielsz, P. W. (2003). Glucocorticoid exposure at the dose used clinically alters cytoskeletal proteins and presynaptic terminals in the fetal baboon brain. *J. Physiol.*, **547**(1), 117–23.

Ballard, P. L., Gluckman, P. D., Liggens, G. C., Kaplan, S. K. and Grumbach, M. M. (1980). Steroid and growth hormone levels in premature infants after prenatal betamethasone therapy to prevent respiratory distress syndrome. *Pediatr. Res.*, **14**, 122–7.

Banks, B. A., Cnaan, A., Morgan, M. A. *et al.* (1999). Multiple courses of antenatal corticosteroids and outcome of premature neonates. *Am. J. Obstet. Gynecol.*, **181**(3), 709–17.

Barker, D. J. (2002). Fetal programming of coronary heart disease. *Trend Endocrinol. Metabolis.*, **13**(9), 364–8.

Challis, J. R., Sloboda, D., Matthews, S. G. *et al.* (2001). The fetal placental hypothalamic–pituitary–adrenal (HPA) axis, parturition and postnatal health. *Mol. Cell. Endocrinol.*, **185**(1–2), 135–44.

Chapillon, P., Patin, V., Roy, V., Vincent, A. and Caston, J. (2002). Effects of pre- and postnatal stimulation on developmental, emotional, and cognitive aspects in rodents: a review. *Develop. Psychobiol.*, **41**(4), 373–87.

Chrousos, G. P. and Gold, P. W. (1992). The concept of stress and stress system disorders. *J. Am. Med. Assoc.*, **267**(9), 1244–52.

Clarke, A. S., Wittwer, D. J., Abbott, D. H. and Schneider, M. L. (1994). Long-term effects of prenatal stress on HPA activity in juvenile rhesus monkeys. *Develop. Psychobiol.*, **27**(5), 257–69.

Cohen, S., Doyle, W. J. and Skoner, D. P. (1999). Psychological stress, cytokine production, and severity of upper respiratory illness. *Psychosom. Med.*, **61**(2), 175–80.

Copper, R. L., Goldenberg, R. L., Elder, N. *et al.* (1996). The preterm prediction study: maternal stress is associated with spontaneous preterm birth at less than thirty-five weeks' gestation. *Am. J. Obstet. Gynecol.*, **175**, 1286–92.

Cratty, M. S., Ward, H. E., Johnson, E. A., Azzaro, A. J. and Birkle, D. L. (1995). Prenatal stress increases corticotropin-releasing factor (CRF) content and release in rat amygdala minces. *Brain Res.*, **675**(1–2), 297–302.

Davis, E. P., Snidman, N., Wadhwa, P. D. *et al.* (2003). The impact of maternal psychological state during pregnancy on infant temperament. *Develop. Psychobiol.*, **43**(3), 252.

Davis, E. P., Snidman, N., Wadhwa, P. D. *et al.* (2004a). Prenatal maternal anxiety and depression predict behavioral reactivity in infancy. *Infancy*, **6**(3), 319–31.

Davis, E. P., Townsend, E. L., Gunnar, M. R. *et al.* (2004b). Effects of prenatal corticosteroid exposure on regulation of stress physiology in healthy premature infants. *Psychoneuroendocrinology*, **29**, 1028–36.

de Kloet, R., Vreugdenhil, E., Oitzl, M. S. and Joels, A. (1998). Brain corticosteroid receptor balance in health and disease. *Endocr. Rev.*, **19**(3), 269–301.

Dent, G. W., Smith, M. A. and Levine, S. (2000). Rapid induction of corticotropin-releasing hormone gene transcription in the paraventricular nucleus of the developing rat. *Endocrinology*, **141**(5), 1593–8.

DiPietro, J. A., Hodgson, D. M., Costigan, K. A. and Johnson, T. R. (1996). Fetal antecedents of infant temperament. *Child Develop.*, **67**(5), 2568–83.

DiPietro, J. A., Costigan, K. A., Pressman, E. K. and Doussard-Roosevel, J. A. (2000). Antenatal origins of individual differences in heart rate. *Develop. Psychobiol.*, **37**(4), 221–8.

DiPietro, J. A., Hilton, S. C., Hawkins, M., Costigan, K. A. and Pressman, E. K. (2002). Maternal stress and affect influence fetal neurobehavioral development. *Develop. Psychol.*, **38**(5), 659–68.

Dobbing, J. and Sands, J. (1979). Comparative aspects of the brain growth spurt. *Early Hum. Develop.*, **3**(1), 79–83.

Dorr, H. G., Heller, A., Versmold, H. T. *et al.* (1989). Longitudinal study of progestins, mineralo-corticoids, and glucocorticoids throughout human pregnancy. *J. Clin. Endocrinol. Metabolis.*, **68**(5), 863–868.

Elenkov, I. J. and Chrousos, G. P. (2002). Stress hormones, proinflammatory and antiinflamma-tory cytokines, and autoimmunity. *Ann. New York Acad. Sci.*, **966**, 290–303.

Erickson, K., Thorsen, P., Chrousos, G. *et al.* (2001). Preterm birth: associated neuroendocrine, medical and behavioral risk factors. *J. Clin. Endocrinol. Metabolis.*, **86**(6), 2544–52.

Feldman, P. J., Dunkel Schetter, C., Sandman, C. A. and Wadhwa, P. D. (2000). Maternal social sup-port predicts birth weight and fetal growth in human pregnancy. *Psychosom. Med.*, **62**, 715–25.

Florio, P. and Petraglia, F. (2001). Human placental corticotropin releasing factor (CRF) in the adaptive response to pregnancy. *Stress*, **4**, 247–61.

Francis, D., Diorio, J., Liu, D. and Meaney, M. J. (1999). Nongenomic transmission across gener-ations of maternal behavior and stress responses in the rat. *Science*, **286**(5442), 1155–8.

French, N., Hagan, R., Evans, S. F., Godfrey, M. and Newnham, J. (1999). Repeated antenatal cor-ticosteroids: size at birth and subsequent development. *Am. J. Obstet. Gynecol.*, **180**, 114–21.

Glynn, L., Wadhwa, P. D., Dunkel Schetter, C. and Sandman, C. A. (2001). When stress happens matters: the effects of earthquake timing on stress responsivity in pregnancy. *Am. J. Obstet. Gynecol.*, **184**, 637–42.

Gunnar, M. R. (1992). Reactivity of the hypothalamic–pituitary–adrenocortical system to stressors in normal infants and children. *Pediatrics*, **90**(3), 491–7.

Hedegaard, M., Henriksen, T. B., Sabroe, S. and Secher, N. J. (1993). Psychological distress in pregnancy and preterm delivery. *Brit. Med. J.*, **307**, 234–9.

Hedegaard, M., Henriksen, T. B., Secher, N. J., Hatch, M. C. and Sabroe, S. (1996). Do stressful life events affect duration of gestation and risk of preterm delivery? *Epidemiology*, **7**(4), 339–45.

Henry, C., Kabbaj, M., Simon, H., LeMoal, M. and Maccari, S. (1994). Prenatal stress increases the hypothalamio–pituitary–adrenal axis response in young and adult rats. *J. Neuroendocrinol.*, **6**(3), 341–5.

Herman, J. P. and Cullinan, W. E. (1997). Neurocircuitry of stress: central control of the hypo-thalamio–pituitary–adrenocortical axis. *Trend. Neurosci.*, **20**(2), 78–84.

Hillhouse, E. W. and Grammatopoulos, D. K. (2002). Role of stress peptides during human pregnancy and labor. *Reproduction*, **124**(3), 323–9.

Hobel, C. J., Dunkel-Schetter, C., Roesch, S. C., Castro, L. C. and Arora, C. P. (1999). Maternal plasma corticotropin-releasing hormone associated with stress at 20 weeks gestation in preg-nancies ending in preterm delivery. *Am. J. Obstet. Gynecol.*, **180**(1 Pt 3), 257–63.

Holzman, C., Jetton, J., Siler-Khodr, T., Fisher, R. and Rip, T. (2001). Second trimester corticotropin-releasing hormone levels in relation to preterm delivery and ethnicity. *Obstet. Gynecol.*, **97**, 657–63.

Huizink, A. C., De Medina, P. G., Mulder, E. J., Visser, G. H. and Buitelaar, J. K. (2002). Psychological measures of prenatal stress as predictors of infant temperament. *J. Am. Acad. Child and Adolescent Psychiat.*, **41**(9), 1078–85.

Inder, W. J., Prickett, T. C., Ellis, M. J. *et al.* (2001). The utility of plasma CRH as a predictor of preterm delivery. *J. Clin. Endocrinol. Metabolis.*, **86**(12), 5706–10.

Jacobson, L. and Sapolsky, R. (1991). The role of the hippocampus in feedback regulation of the hypothalamic pituitary adrenocortical axis. *Endocr. Rev.*, **12**(2), 118–34.

Jones, N. A., Field, T., Fox, N. A. *et al.* (1998). Newborns of mothers with depressive symptoms are physiologically less developed. *Infant Behav. Develop.*, **21**(3), 537–41.

Kagan, J. and Snidman, N. (1991). Temperamental factors in human development. *Am. Psychol.*, **46**, 856–62.

Kauppila, A., Koivisto, M., Pukka, M. and Tuimala, R. (1978). Umbilical cord and neonatal cortisol levels. Effect of gestational and neonatal factors. *Obstet. Gynecol.*, **52**(6), 666–72.

King, B. R., Smith, R. and Nicholson, R. C. (2001). The regulation of human corticotrophin-releasing hormone gene expression in the placenta. *Peptides*, **22**(11), 1941–7.

Korebrits, C., Yu, D. H., Ramirez, M. M. *et al.* (1998). Antenatal glucocorticoid administration increases corticotrophin-releasing hormone in maternal plasma. *Brit. J. Obstet. Gynecol.*, **105**(5), 556–61.

Levine, S. (1957). Infantile experience and resistance to physiological stress. *Science*, **126**, 405–6.

Liu, D., Diorio, J., Tannenbaum, B. *et al.* (1997). Maternal care, hippocampal glucocorticoid receptors, and hypothalamic–pituitary–adrenal responses to stress. *Science*, **277**, 1659–62.

Lundy, B. L., Jones, N. A., Field, T. *et al.* (1999). Prenatal depression effects on neonates. *Infant Behav. Develop.*, **22**(1), 119–29.

Makino, S., Gold, P. W. and Scchulkin, J. (1994). Effects of corticosterone on CRH mRNA and content in the central nucleus and the parvocellular region of the paraventricular nucleus of the hypothalamus. *Brain Res.*, **640**, 105–12.

Marinoni, E., Korebrits, C., Di Lorio, R., Cosmi, E. V. and Challis, J. R. (1998). Effect of betamethasone in vivo on placental corticotropin-releasing hormone in human pregnancy. *Am. J. Obstet. Gynecol.*, **178**(4), 770–8.

Matthews, S. G. (2000). Antenatal glucocorticoids and programming of the developing CNS. *Pediatr. Res.*, **47**(3), 291–300.

Matthews, S. G. (2002). Early programming of the hypothalamo–pituitary–adrenal axis. *Trend. Endocrinol. Metab.*, **13**(9), 373–80.

Matthews, S. G., Owen, D., Benjamin, S. and Andrews, M. H. (2002). Glucocorticoids, hypothalamo–pituitary–adrenal (HPA) development, and life after birth. *Endocr. Res.*, **28**(4), 709–18.

McEwen, B. S. (1999). Stress and hippocampal plasticity. *Annu. Rev. Neurosci.*, **22**, 105–22.

McEwen, B. S., Biron, C. A., Brunson, K. W. *et al.* (1997). The role of adrenocorticoids as modulators of immune function in health and disease: neural, endocrine, and immune interactions. *Brain Res. Rev.*, **23**(1–2), 79–133.

McLean, M., Bisits, A., Davies, J. *et al.* (1995). A placental clock controlling the length of human pregnancy. *Nat. Med.*, **1**, 460–3.

Meaney, M. J., Aitken, D. H., Van Berkel, C., Bhatnagar, S. and Sapolsky, R. M. (1988). Effect of neonatal handling on age-related impairments associated with the hippocampus. *Science*, **239**, 766–8.

Misra, D. P., O'campo, P. and Strobino, D. (2001). Testing a sociomedical model for preterm delivery. *Pediatr. Perinatol. Epidemiol.*, **15**, 110–22.

Moawad, A. H., Goldenberg, R. L., Mercer, B. *et al.* (2002). The preterm prediction study: the value of serum alkaline phosphatase, alpha-fetoprotein, plasma corticotropin-releasing hormone, and other serum markers for the prediction of spontaneous preterm birth. *Am. J. Obstet. Gynecol.*, **186**(5), 990–6.

Monk, C., Fifer, W. P., Myers, M. M. *et al.* (2000). Maternal stress responses and anxiety during pregnancy: effects on fetal heart rate. *Develop. Psychobiol.*, **36**(1), 67–77.

Monk, C., Myers, M. M., Sloan, R. P., Ellman, L. M. and Fifer, W. P. (2003). Effects of women's stress-elicited physiological activity and chronic anxiety on fetal heart rate. *J. Develop. Behav. Pediatr.*, **24**(1), 32–8.

Munck, A., Guyre, P. M. and Holbrook, N. J. (1984). Physiological functions of glucocorticoids in stress and their relation to pharmacological actions. *Endocr. Rev.*, **5**(1), 25–44.

Nathanielsz, P. W. (1999). *Life in the Womb: The Origin of Health and Disease*. Ithaca, New York: Promethean Press.

Ng, P. C., Lam, C. W., Lee, C. H. *et al.* (2002). Reference range and factors affecting the human corticotropin-releasing hormone test in preterm, very low birth weight infants. *J. Clin. Endocrinol. Metabolis.*, **87**(10), 4621–8.

O'Connor, T. G., Heron, J. and Glover, V. (2002a). Antenatal anxiety predicts child behavioral/emotional problems independently of postnatal depression. *J. Am. Acad. Child Adolescent Psychiat.*, **41**(12), 1470–7.

O'Connor, T. G., Heron, J., Golding, J., Beveridge, M. and Glover, V. (2002b). Maternal antenatal anxiety and children's behavioural/emotional problems at 4 years: report from the Avon longitudinal study of parents and children. *Brit. J. Psychiat.*, **180**, 502–8.

Parker, C. R. J., Atkinson, M. W., Owen, J. and Andrews, W. W. (1996). Dynamics of the fetal adrenal, cholesterol, and apolipoprotein B responses to antenatal betamethasone therapy. *Am. J. Obstet. Gynecol.*, **174**(2), 562–5.

Peterson, B. S., Anderson, A. W., Ehrenkranz, R. *et al.* (2003). Regional brain volumes and their later neurodevelopmental correlates in term and preterm infants. *Pediatrics*, **111**(5), 939–48.

Petraglia, F., Florio, P., Nappi, C. and Genazzani, A. R. (1996). Peptide signaling in human placenta and membranes: autocrine, paracrine, and endocrine mechanisms. *Endocr. Rev.*, **17**, 156–86.

Pritchard, C. W. and Teo, P. Y. (1994). Preterm birth, low birthweight and the stressfulness of the household role for pregnant women. *Soc. Sci. Med.*, **38**, 89–96.

Rini, C. K., Dunkel Schetter, C., Wadhwa, P. D. and Sandman, C. A. (1999). Psychological adaptation and birth outcomes: the role of personal resources, stress and sociocultural context during pregnancy. *Health Psychol.*, **18**, 333–45.

Romero, R., Gomez, R., Chaiworapongsa, T. *et al.* (2001). The role of infection in preterm labour and delivery. *Pediatr. Perinatal Epidemiol.*, **15**(S2), 41–56.

Sanchez, M. M., Young, L. J., Plotsky, P. M. and Insel, T. R. (2000). Distribution of corticosteroid receptors in the rhesus brain: relative absence of glucocorticoid receptors in the hippocampal formation. *J. Neurosci.*, **20**(12), 4657–68.

Sandman, C. A., Wadhwa, P. D., Chicz-DeMet, A., Dunkel-Schetter, C. and Porto, M. (1997a). Maternal stress, HPA activity, and fetal/infant outcome. *Ann. New York Acad. Sci.*, **814**, 266–75.

Sandman, C. A., Wadhwa, P. D., Hetrick, W., Porto, M. and Peeke, H. V. S. (1997b). Human fetal heart rate dishabituation at thirty-two weeks gestation. *Child Develop.*, **68**, 1031–40.

Sandman, C. A., Wadhwa, P. D., Chicz-DeMet, A., Garite, T. J. and Porto, M. (1999). Maternal corticotropin-releasing hormone (CRH) influences heart rate reactivity to challenge in human pregnancy. *Develop. Psychobiol.*, **34**(3), 163–73.

Sandman, C., A., Glynn, L., Wadhwa, P. D. *et al.* (2003). Maternal hypothalamic–pituitary–adrenal disregulation during the third trimester influences human fetal responses. *Develop. Neurosci.*, **25**, 41–9.

Schneider, M. L. (1992). Prenatal stress exposure alters postnatal behavioral expression under conditions of novelty challenge in rhesus monkey infants. *Develop. Psychobiol.*, **25**(7), 529–40.

Schneider, M. L. and Coe, C. L. (1993). Repeated social stress during pregnancy impairs neuro-motor development of the primate infant. *J. Develop. Behav. Pediatr.*, **14**, 81–7.

Schneider, M. L., Coe, C. L. and Lubach, G. R. (1992). Endocrine activation mimics the adverse effects of prenatal stress on the neuromotor development of the infant primate. *Develop. Psychobiol.*, **25**(6), 427–39.

Schneider, M. L., Roughton, E. C., Koehler, A. J. and Lubach, G. R. (1999). Growth and development following prenatal stress exposure in primates: an examination of ontogenetic vulnerability. *Child Develop.*, **70**(2), 263–74.

Schulkin, J. (1999). CRH in allostatic overload. *J. Endocrinol.*, **161**, 349–56.

Shalev, E., Benett, M. J., Megory, E., Wallace, R. M. and Zuckerman, H. (1990). Fetal habituation to sound stimulus in various behavioral states. *Gynecol. Obstet. Invest.*, **29**, 115–17.

Shanks, N. and Lightman, S. L. (2001). The maternal–neuronatal neuro-immune interface: are there long-term implications for inflammatory or stress-related disease? *J. Clin. Invest.*, **108**(11), 1567–73.

Smith, R. (2001). *The Endocrinology of Parturition.* Newcastle, Australia: Karger.

Susman, E. J., Schmeelk, K. H., Ponirakis, A. and Gariepy, J. L. (2001). Maternal prenatal, post-partum, and concurrent stressors and temperament in 3-year-olds: a person and variable analysis. *Develop. Psychopathol.*, **13**(3), 629–52.

Swanson L. W., Simmons, D. M. (1989). Differential steroid hormone and neural influences on peptide mRNA levels in corticotropin-releasing hormone cells of the paraventricular: a hybridization histochemical study in the rat. *J. Comp. Neurol.*, **285**, 413–35.

Takahashi, L. K. (1998). Prenatal stress: consequences of glucocorticoids on hippocampal development and function. *Int. J. Develop. Neurosci.*, **16**(3), 199–207.

Takahashi, L. K., Turner, J. G. and Kalin, N. H. (1992). Prenatal stress alters brain catecholaminergic activity and potentiates stress-induced behavior in adult rats. *Brain Res.*, **514**, 131–7.

Vallee, M., Mayo, W., Dellu, F. *et al.* (1997). Prenatal stress induces high anxiety and postnatal handling induces low anxiety in adult offspring: correlation with stress-induced corticosterone injection. *J. Neurosci.*, **17**, 2626–36.

Van den Bergh, B. (1990). The influence of maternal emotion during pregnancy on fetal and neonatal behavior. *Pre- Peri-natal Psychol.*, **5**(2), 119–30.

Wadhwa, P. D., Sandman, C. A., Porto, M., Dunkel Schetter, C. and Garite, T. J. (1993). The association between prenatal stress and infant birth weight and gestational age at birth: a prospective investigation. *Am. J. Obstet. Gynecol.*, **169**, 858–65.

Wadhwa, P. D., Dunkel Schetter, C., Chicz-DeMet, A., Porto, M. and Sandman, C. A. (1996). Prenatal psychosocial factors and the neuroendocrine axis in human pregnancy. *Psychosom. Med.*, **58**, 432–46.

Wadhwa, P. D., Sandman, C. A., Chicz-DeMet, A. and Porto, M. (1997). Placental CRH modulates maternal pituitary–adrenal function in human pregnancy. *Ann. New York Acad. Sci.*, **814**, 276–81.

Wadhwa, P. D., Porto, M., Garite, T. J., Chicz-DeMet, A. and Sandman, C. A. (1998). Maternal corticotropin-releasing hormone levels in the third trimester predict length of gestation in human pregnancy. *Am. J. Obstet. Gynecol.*, **179**, 1079–85.

Wadhwa, P. D., Garite, T. J., Porto, M. *et al.* (2004). Placental corticotropin-releasing hormone (CRH), Spontaneous preterm birth and fetal growth restriction: a prospective investigation. *Am. J. Obstet. Gynecol*, **191**, 1063–9.

Ward, A. M. V. and Phillips, D. J. W. (2001). Fetal programming of stress responses. *Stress*, **4**, 263–71.

Watts, A. G., Sanchez-Watts, G. (1995). Region specific regulation of neuropeptide mRNAs in rat limbic forebrain neurones by aldosterone and corticosterone. *J. Physiol.*, **484**, 721–36.

Weinstock, M. (2001). Alterations induced by gestational stress in brain morphology and behaviour of the offspring. *Prog. Neurobiol.*, **65**, 427–51.

Weinstock, M., Matlina, E., Maor, G. I., Rosen, H. and McEwen, B. S. (1992). Prenatal stress selectively alters the reactivity of the hypothalamic–pituitary adrenal system in the female rat. *Brain Res.*, **595**, 195–200.

Welberg, L. A. and Seckl, J. (2001). Prenatal stress, glucocorticoids and the programming of the brain. *J. Neuroendocrinol.*, **191, 1063–106913**, 113–28.

Wittekind, C. A., Arnold, J. D., Leslie, G. I., Luttrell, B. and Jones, M. P. (1993). Longitudinal study of plasma ACTH and cortisol in very low birth weight infants in the first 8 weeks of life. *Early Hum. Develop.*, **33**(3), 191–200.

Zarrow, M. X., Philpott, J. E. and Denenberg, V. H. (1970). Passage of 14-C-4 Corticosterone from the rat mother to the fetus and neonate. *Nature*, **226**, 1058–9.

7

Glucocorticoids and the ups and downs of neuropeptide gene expression

Alan G. Watts

The NIBS-Neuroscience Program and Department of Biological Sciences, University of Southern California, Los Angeles, California, CA, USA

Introduction

Neuropeptides, such as corticotropin-releasing hormone (CRH) are critical molecules that act as neuromodulators throughout the central nervous system. They are implicated in controlling a wide range of behavioral, autonomic, and neuroendocrine functions. Glucocorticoids are important hormones that have profound effects on many aspects of neuronal function, including the regulation of neuropeptide biosynthesis. Elevated levels of maternal and fetal glucocorticoids play important roles in the normal progression of pregnancy and fetal growth; however, they also have been implicated in many pathologies of pregnancy and fetal development (see Chapters 3–6). Their role in regulating neuropeptides, both in fetal and maternal brain, has been suggested as a causal link in their effects on pregnancy and fetal development.

The proposed effects of glucocorticoids on the maternal–placental–fetal axis are based on epidemiological evidence and experimental manipulations in animal models. The mechanisms by which glucocorticoids regulate neuropeptide storage, release, and gene expression, however, are not completely understood. A clearer understanding of these processes is necessary to generate and test meaningful hypotheses about how these mechanisms are controlled. Recent findings indicate that glucocorticoids have variable effects on CRH regulation depending on cell type, and intra- and extracellular factors.

Perhaps the most familiar example of glucocorticoid actions on neuropeptide gene expression is its inhibitory actions on CRH and arginine vasopressin (AVP) genes in neuroendocrine neurons of the hypothalamic paraventricular nucleus (PVH). Despite the apparent simplicity of this particular effect and its importance for controlling glucocorticoid secretion from the adrenal cortex, its cellular basis is undoubtedly complex and remains unclear. What is known, however, is that glucocorticoids have very different effects on CRH gene expression in other cells.

For example, CRH messenger ribonucleic acid (mRNA) expression is upregulated by glucocorticoids in the central nucleus of the amygdala and in the human placenta. This means that the effects of these steroids are dependent on the particular cellular environment in which the CRH gene is expressed.

This chapter will review our current understanding of how glucocorticoids regulate the expression of the genes that encode these important neural signals. The regulation of the CRH gene provides a model for considering cell-specific glucocorticoid regulation of other neuropeptides.

Glucocorticoids and their interaction with neuropeptide gene expression

For many years the influence of glucocorticoids has been recognized as a critical feature that inhibits the output signals of the brain and anterior pituitary (see Yates and Maran, 1974; Dallman *et al.*, 1987; Sapolsky *et al.*, 2000, for reviews). More recently, the way corticosterone regulates the expression of genes encoding the adrenocorticotropic hormone (ACTH) secretogogues CRH and AVP has been taken as an exemplar for how end-organ hormones contribute to the molecular mechanisms ultimately controlling the activity within the system.

CRH and AVP are synthesized in neurons located in the medial parvicellular (mp) (neuroendocrine) part of the PVH. They are released in a stimulus-dependent manner into the hypophysial portal vasculature from terminals in the median eminence (ME). Many studies during the last 15 years have documented powerful inhibitory actions of glucocorticoids on the synthesis, storage, and release of CRH and AVP in the PVHmp and ME (see Swanson and Simmons, 1989; Whitnall, 1993; Watts, 1996, for reviews). For the most part, however, this inhibition has been considered simply as a gene-targeted negative-feedback servo-mechanism embedded within the larger and more complex regulatory mechanisms operating within the hypothalamus–pituitary–adrenal (HPA) axis (Figure 7.1). But despite the obvious importance for glucocorticoid feedback on PVHmp gene expression to the functioning of the HPA axis, the mechanisms responsible for directing this apparently simple event remain frustratingly elusive.

Principles of negative feedback

Ever since the pioneering work of Moore and Price (1932), and Hohlweg and Junkmann (1932), the axiom that steroid hormones constitute negative-feedback signals has been a central tenet of endocrine physiology. Rudimentary closed-loop feedback of the type originally developed in the 1930s for target-organ regulation of the pituitary has remained a popular model for explaining neuroendocrine mechanisms of homeostasis, despite the fact that the level of sophistication with

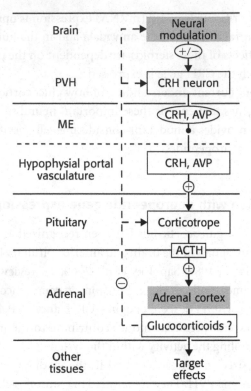

Figure 7.1   A schematic view of the HPA axis. CRH neurons in the neuroendocrine PVH nucleus release CRH and AVP into the hypophysial portal vasculature to stimulate ACTH release from anterior pituitary corticotropes. ACTH in turn stimulates cells in the zona fasciculata of the adrenal cortex to release glucocorticoids, which have multiple functions throughout the body. They also exert regulatory influences upon the actions of corticotropes, CRH neurons, and a variety of neural circuits

which control theory could be applied to endocrinology in general (e.g. Hoskins, 1949) was raised over 50 years ago by the publication of *Cybernetics* (Weiner, 1948). The concepts derived from control theory were extensively applied by Yates's group throughout the 1960s to explain how HPA secretory activity was regulated by corticosterone (e.g. Yates and Maran, 1974).

The classic closed-loop feedback model posits that neuroendocrine secretogogue peptides and their mRNAs, together with circulating hormone concentrations are all maintained between upper- and lower-limit values by comparator-generated error signals derived from the difference between set-point and actual values (Figure 7.2(a)). As other influences – for example, a stressor, in the case of the HPA axis – move variable values outside these limits, negative-feedback signals from the target generate the appropriate responses to return variables back between the

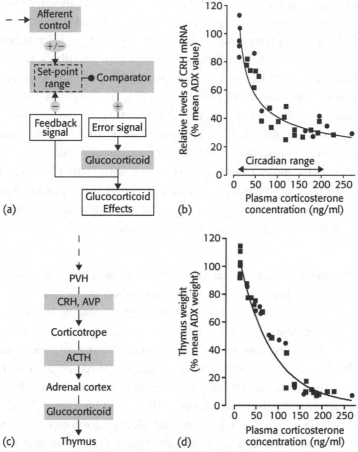

Figure 7.2   (a) The organization of a closed-loop feedback loop. The level of a target variable is
maintained between a set-point range by a 'push–pull' mechanism consisting of the drive
from a variety of neural afferents and the negative-feedback influence of glucocorticoid. A
hypothetical comparator system then generates an error signal in the form of CRH and
AVP to adjust glucocorticoid levels. Although widely used to explain the way
glucocorticoids regulate the activity of CRH neurons and corticotropes, this simple system
cannot explain the complex influence of corticosterone on CRH neurons in the
paraventricular nucleus. (b) The relationship between CRH mRNA levels in the
paraventricular nucleus and circulating corticosterone in adrenalectomized (ADX) male
rats with various doses of exogenously applied corticosterone. Note that CRH mRNA is
most sensitive to circulating corticosterone within the range of concentrations found
across the circadian day. Data adapted from Watts and Sanchez-Watts (1995a). (c) The
organization of an open-loop feedback system. Unlike the closed-loop system depicted in
(a), there is no influence from final target, the thymus, to the control mechanisms in the
brain. (d) The well-documented relationship between thymus weight and circulating
corticosterone. Data adapted from Watts and Sanchez-Watts (1995a)

set-point limits (Figure 7.2(a)). For the HPA axis, the negative-feedback action of corticosterone is regarded as the major inhibitory signal that acts to reduce the value of all the appropriate variables (gene expression, peptide levels, and secretory rates) within the system. In reality, however, negative-feedback loops offer little more than the application of a simple 'push–pull' principle to neuroendocrine control. Although this model offers reasonable explanations for simple reflex neuroendocrine mechanisms (e.g. the AVP secretory response to hemorrhage or elevated plasma osmolality), it fails to account satisfactorily for those complex synthetic and secretory features of HPA neuroendocrinology that have a more anticipatory nature. Examples of anticipatory events within the HPA axis include the daily variations in glucocorticoid secretion timed by the suprachiasmatic nucleus (SCH) that precede activity and feeding, or the conditioning or habituating effects of repeated stimuli on the glucocorticoid responses.

How is glucocorticoid inhibition manifest on ACTH secretogogue gene expression?

This question has been most commonly addressed using unstressed adrenalectomized (ADX) rats maintained with ad lib food/water/saline, and given a regimen of constant exogenous corticosterone for 5–7 days. Experiments of this type generate the simple inverse $\log_{10}$ function between circulating corticosterone and CRH mRNA levels in the PVHmp (Watts and Sanchez-Watts, 1995a) that has formed the basis of the classic 'negative-feedback' model of gene control (Figure 7.2(b)). For comparison with this closed-loop feedback model, Figure 7.2(d) shows the familiar inverse relationship between circulating corticosterone and thymus weight. This is an open-loop arrangement (Figure 7.2(c)) because, in contrast to the closed-loop feedback actions of corticosterone on the CRH neuron, there is no target-derived negative-feedback signal from the thymus to the HPA axis.

In male rats the inverse relationship between circulating corticosterone and CRH mRNA levels has the greatest dynamic range between corticosterone concentrations of 10 to about 150 ng/ml (Figure 7.2(b)), which is that found during the normal daily variations (Swanson and Simmons, 1989; Watts and Sanchez-Watts, 1995a; Watts et al., 2004). Virtually no further reduction in CRH mRNA occurs if concentrations increase beyond 200 ng/ml. Although a comparable dose–response curve has not been obtained for AVP mRNA in the PVHmp, AVP gene products are apparently even more sensitive to circulating corticosterone than CRH; only very low circulating levels are required to reduce mRNA to undetectable levels.

Cell specificity

At this point it is important to note that corticosterone regulates CRH gene expression in a cell-specific manner. Although glucocorticoids are sometimes thought of as downregulating CRH gene expression in the brain, in fact the only cell type where this actually occurs is the CRH neuroendocrine motor neuron in the PVHmp. In every other cell type that synthesizes CRH, glucocorticoids either upregulate gene expression or have no effect whatsoever (Beyer *et al.*, 1988; Swanson and Simmons, 1989; Frim *et al.*, 1990; Makino *et al.*, 1994; Watts and Sanchez-Watts, 1995a). An interesting comparison in this regard is the neurons in the lateral part of the central nucleus of the amygdala (CEAl). Here, corticosterone concentrations over the daily range increase CRH mRNA in a manner that is virtually the inverse of that seen in the PVHmp (Figure 7.3; Watts and Sanchez-Watts, 1995a). These data emphasize that rather than a fixed component of the CRH gene regulation determining how glucocorticoids function, variations in the local cellular environment, including intracellular factors (e.g. signal transduction pathways) together with extracellular factors (e.g. the nature of afferent inputs) play major roles in determining how glucocorticoids interact with the CRH gene.

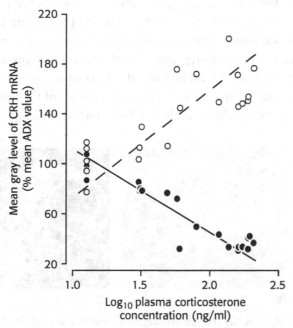

o Central nucleus of the amygdala   • Paraventricular nucleus

Figure 7.3   CRH mRNA levels in the paraventricular nucleus (solid circles, solid line) and lateral part of the central nucleus of the amygdala (open circles, dashed line) from adrenalectomized male rats with various doses of exogenously applied corticosterone. Note that corticosterone has very different effects on the accumulation rates of CRH mRNA depending on the cell type examined. (Data adapted from Watts and Sanchez-Watts 1995a)

How do glucocorticoids regulate CRH gene expression?

The PVH

The rat PVH is the classic example of a hypothalamic motor nucleus that controls many different neuroendocrine, autonomic, and behavioral actions. Before we discuss what we know of the mechanisms engaged by glucocorticoids to regulate CRH gene expression in the PVH, it is worth briefly describing the overall organization of this complex cell group. I will do this by first describing the PVH in terms of its different structural compartments, and then describe CRH neuroendocrine motor neurons in terms of their functional compartments to provide the backdrop for considering in more detail how glucocorticoids regulate CRH and AVP gene expression in these neurons.

Structural compartmentalization of the PVH

In keeping with its diverse functional roles, the PVH contains a number of structurally distinct compartments. These are most easily seen in the rat, where there is clear spatial segregation between compartments (Swanson and Kuypers, 1980), but is less obvious in other species. Based upon its efferent projections, the PVH is divisible into at least two major structural compartments: neuroendocrine motor neurons that project to the neurohypophysis, and parvicellular pre-autonomic neurons that project to the hindbrain and spinal cord (Figure 7.4). Each of these major compartments can be further subdivided, first in terms of their projections, and then again by way of the different chemical phenotypes that represent great

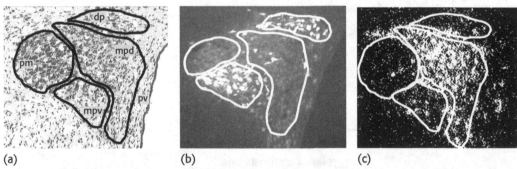

(a)   (b)   (c)

Figure 7.4   The organization of the rat PVH. (a) The *cytoarchitectonics* shows a Nissl stained coronal section through PVH. The majority of CRH neuroendocrine neurons are located in the dorsal part of the mp (mpd) PVH. Also shown are the posterior magnocellular (pm), the periventricular (pv), and dorsal parvicellular (dp) and ventral parts of the mp (mpv) PVH both of which project to the hindbrain and spinal cord. (b) The *efferents* show neurons retrogradely labeled after injections of two fluorescent tracers into the vasculature (dark cells in the pm, mpd, and pv), and the cervical spinal cord (white cells in the dp and mpv). (c) The *CRH mRNA* shows the in situ hybridization signal from CRH mRNA in the mpd

potential for diverse neural signaling. In this way, the neuroendocrine compartment consists of oxytocin and AVP-containing magnocellular motor neurons that project to the posterior pituitary, together with six different types of parvicellular motor neurons that project to the ME and control hormone secretion from the anterior pituitary.

Subdividing parvicellular pre-autonomic neurons in terms of their efferent projections is more complex because they project to a variety of targets in the midbrain, hindbrain, and spinal cord. One significant difference, however, is whether they project to the dorsal vagal complex or to the spinal cord (Swanson and Kuypers, 1980). Parvicellular pre-autonomic neurons contain a variety of neuropeptides, including oxytocin, AVP, enkephalin, dynorphin, and CRH (Hallbeck *et al.*, 2001). It is worth noting that most PVH neurons also appear to be glutamatergic (Herman *et al.*, 2002). Depending on the physiological status of the animal, CRH is synthesized in all the major structural compartments of the rat PVH (Swanson 1991; Watts, 1992; 1996) and importantly, that corticosterone influences the expression of the CRH gene in these PVH cell types in quite different ways (Swanson and Simmons, 1989).

Functional compartmentalization of the CRH neuroendocrine motor neuron

Corticosterone can affect the activity of the HPA axis at many different levels ranging from how the CRH gene is transcribed to secretion rates of ACTH. Similarly, the actions of corticosterone are likely to alter the function of CRH neuroendocrine neurons at a variety of different levels. This complexity means that particular attention has to be directed towards the behavior of dependent variables as interpreted within the context of CRH gene control.

One way to deal with a system as complex as the CRH neuron is to partition it into functional compartments and then examine how these compartments interact. Figure 7.5 illustrates one such schema for the CRH neuron (designated by the gray box), which can help constrain the interpretational models derived from the behavior of particular dependent variables. Although it is somewhat arbitrary as to where one compartment ends and another starts, this model allows us to place the cellular processes occurring in each compartment within a wider context of the whole neuron.

The first compartment in this model (numbered 1 in Figure 7.5) consists of the afferent sets that project to CRH neurons and control their activity. The structural organization of these afferents is considered later in this section. In the second compartment (numbered 2 in Figure 7.5) afferent sets interact with CRH neurons using appropriate sets of receptors and signal transduction pathways. In this manner, the effects of stress, energy metabolism or indeed of any other physiological process are ultimately mediated by the actions of neurotransmitters and

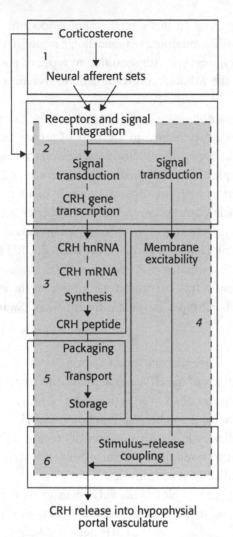

Figure 7.5   A schematic to show six possible functional compartments within a CRH neuroendocrine neuron in the PVH. It shows that neural afferents regulate two principal processes: *membrane excitability*, which controls peptide release, and *peptide synthesis*. Corticosterone can regulate both processes either by modulating the activity of neural afferents, or more directly by way of transmitter receptors, signal transduction pathways, or gene transcription

circulating factors at this functional level. These factors are continually integrated by CRH neurons to generate their ongoing activity patterns. Signal integration and signal transduction mechanisms then control two fundamental processes:

(1) CRH synthesis (*Compartment 3*).
(2) Membrane excitability (*Compartment 4*).

The third compartment contains the machinery in the endoplasmic reticulum and Golgi complex that controls the translation of CRH mRNA into CRH peptide. The fourth compartment controls membrane excitability by way of the neuron's specific complement of ion channels, and so ultimately controls firing rate and subsequent release of CRH from terminals in the ME (*Compartment 6*). Processes in the fifth compartment package peptide into vesicles and transport them along axons for storage in neuroendocrine terminals in the ME for release. And the sixth compartment contains the stimulus–release coupling mechanisms that release peptide from terminals in the ME into the hypophysial vasculature in an activity-dependent manner.

Of course, the final component that we have to consider in this schema is corticosterone, although the effects of corticosterone upon overall HPA function have been extensively documented (e.g. Dallman *et al.*, 1987; Jones and Gillham, 1988), the specific mechanisms by which it controls CRH neuronal function remain unclear. As corticosterone can control a wide range of cellular processes, it is possible that it can indirectly regulate mechanisms in all six compartments of the CRH neuron. However, its direct actions within CRH neurons will be limited to effects on receptors, signal transduction cascades, and genes (Figure 7.5; Brann *et al.*, 1995; Burke *et al.*, 1997; Reichardt *et al.*, 1998; Kovács *et al.*, 2000). We will consider the specifics of these mechanisms later.

Figure 7.5 shows that two processes are targeted by processes that control the activity of CRH neurons: (a) changes in membrane excitability (potential) and (b) CRH heteronuclear (hn) RNA levels. However, each contributes quite differently to CRH neuronal function: CRH hnRNA is an initial component in the path leading to peptide biosynthesis; membrane excitability is critical for stimulus–release coupling that controls CRH release at the neuroendocrine terminal. In broader terms, membrane excitability can be seen as controlling the *immediate* response of CRH neurons to a stimulus; while changes in the expression of the CRH gene – or indeed any other gene – can be seen as an *adaptive* response.

Again, it is worth remembering that there is great cell specificity about how genes and their products are controlled. For example, the way corticosterone regulates the CRH gene in the PVH is very different from the way this regulation occurs in the CEAl (Watts and Sanchez-Watts, 1995a), the cerebral cortex, the human placenta, or in vitro cell lines. This cell specificity emphasizes that where possible, we should use in vivo models to examine regulatory mechanisms, and when focusing on one cell type, we should use care if we infer mechanisms using results derived from others (e.g. Dumont *et al.*, 2002; King *et al.*, 2002).

Multiple levels of interaction

As we have discussed, glucocorticoids can stimulate, repress or have no effect on CRH gene expression in the brain depending on the cell type examined (Beyer *et al.*,

1988; Swanson and Simmons, 1989; Frim *et al.*, 1990; Watts and Sanchez-Watts, 1995a). This shows that we cannot look solely to the CRH gene to explain gluco- corticoid effects on CRH gene expression. Indeed, a great deal of evidence points to the fact that the cellular actions of glucocorticoid are highly complex and utilize mechanisms other than direct gene interactions (Beato *et al.*, 1995; Brann *et al.*, 1995). In this way, there must be multiple levels at which glucocorticoids can act, and this next section considers four possible levels of glucocorticoid interaction with CRH control mechanisms: gene, cell, neural network, and time domains.

Actions on the gene

The inhibitory actions of glucocorticoids on CRH gene expression in the PVH appear to be effected by glucocorticoid receptor (GR) rather than a mineralocor- ticoid receptor (MR)-dependent mechanisms (Watts, 1996; Reichardt *et al.*, 1998), and a functional GR is an absolute requirement for glucocorticoid inhibition of CRH gene expression in the PVH (Reichardt *et al.*, 1998; Kretz *et al.*, 1999). With this in mind, the most direct way that glucocorticoids can control CRH gene expression is to affect the rate of transcription through direct interactions between the ligand-activated GR and GR-control elements on the CRH gene. Although some studies suggest that the CRH gene does not contain a consensus glucocorti- coid-regulatory element (GRE), there is evidence that regions of the CRH gene will bind glucocorticoids. Malkoski and co-workers have identified a negative- glucocorticoid-response element that mediates glucocorticoid repression of cyclic adenosine monophosphate (cAMP)-stimulated but not basal CRH gene expres- sion in transfected AtT20 cells (Malkoski *et al.*, 1997; Malkoski and Dorin, 1999). Furthermore, King *et al.* (2002) have recently used transfected AtT20 cells to iden- tify a second cAMP-response element (CRE) on the CRH gene that is distinct from the consensus CRE. They conclude that different regions of the CRH gene confer the inhibitory and stimulatory actions of glucocorticoids.

However, it remains to be determined whether these mechanisms actually oper- ate in the neuroendocrine PVH in vivo. Indeed evidence for a direct action of the ligand-activated GR binding to the CRH gene in the PVH is currently inconclusive. The fact that corticosterone applied directly to the PVH in vivo appears to have lit- tle effect on CRH mRNA levels in ADX rats (Kovács and Mezey, 1987) is consistent with more indirect actions. Furthermore, some intriguing evidence suggests that glucocorticoid downregulation of CRH gene expression in the PVH in vivo may not in fact involve DNA binding at all. Thus, mutant mice that have a GR incapable of binding to DNA ($GR^{dim/dim}$) have normal CRH peptide levels in the ME (Reichardt *et al.*, 1998). In contrast, proopiomelanocortin (POMC) gene expres- sion in these same mice is markedly upregulated showing that DNA binding is required for the GR regulation of this particular gene.

Cell: actions on mechanisms

Receptor mechanisms

CRH neurons express a host of transmitter (gamma amino butyric acid (GABA), glutamate, monoamine) and peptide receptors (Whitnall, 1993; Herman et al., 2002). In turn, corticosterone can modify receptor function in the PVH (Figure 7.5), for example angiotensin receptors (Aguilera et al., 1995; Shelat et al., 1998), neuropeptide Y (NPY) receptors (Akabayashi et al., 1994), and adrenoreceptors (Jhanwar-Uniyal and Leibowitz, 1986; Day et al., 1999).

Signal transduction mechanisms

There is strong evidence that glucocorticoids can downregulate CRH gene expression by modifying those signal transduction mechanisms that directly control transcription (Figure 7.5). Currently the best-defined direct transcriptional regulator of the CRH gene is cAMP, which regulates transcription in many cell types using the CRE-binding protein (CREB). The CRH gene contains a functional CRE, and CRH gene transcription in vitro is increased by agents, such as forskolin, that increase cAMP using protein kinase (PK) A, rather than PKC-associated mechanisms (Majzoub et al., 1993). Much evidence suggests that unlike many other transcription factors that act by binding to a DNA promoter sequence, CREB is usually constitutively bound to the appropriate promoter of the target gene. However, CREB does not apparently bind constituently to the CRH gene, but is phosphorylated to form pCREB by a stimulus-initiated PKA-dependent cascade. Only then does pCREB bind to a CREB-binding protein (CBP) to interact with the CRE on the CRH gene so that the pCREB/CBP/CRE complex initiates CRH gene transcription (Wolfl et al., 1999).

Glucocorticoids can repress the stimulatory actions of cAMP and CREB on CRH gene expression in vitro (Majzoub et al., 1993; Guardiola-Diaz et al., 1996; Malkoski et al., 1997). But the fact that in these same systems glucocorticoid has no effect on the unstimulated rates of CRH gene transcription suggests that the actions of glucocorticoid requires some form of coincidence between the receptor activation and the appropriate signal transduction pathway to exert its effects.

Direct in vivo evidence for the transcriptional activation of the CRH gene by way of a pCREB-dependent mechanism, or indeed any other signal transduction mechanism, remains scant. However, data do suggest that the activation of signaling molecules and CRH gene expression can occur very rapidly following appropriate stimulation. In one experiment, Kovacs and Sawchenko (1996a) used a pulse-chase design to show that a brief episode of ether anesthesia triggers a cascade of cellular events beginning within 5 min of the stressor with the concurrent accumulation of immunocytochemically detectable pCREB and the CRH primary transcript; increases in CRH mRNA levels and AVP hnRNA followed later.

Increases in other signaling processes are similarly rapid. For example, Khan and Watts (2004) showed that intravenous 2-deoxyglucose (2-DG) elevates CRH gene transcription together with the phosphorylation of the mitogen-activated protein (MAP) kinases, Erk 1/2, within 10 min in CRH neurons. Similar increases in Erk 1/2 phosphorylation are seen after local norepinephrine injections into the region of the PVH (Khan and Watts, 2003) suggesting that these signaling kinases can act as intermediaries between catecholaminergic inputs and CRH gene expression following 2-DG. Although little work has been performed in vivo to determine how glucocorticoids interact with CREB and MAP kinase signaling systems, evidence shows that the GR agonist dexamethasone modulates stress-induced accumulation of pCREB in CRH neurons (Legradi *et al.*, 1997).

Network

Evidence presented in the previous two sections (Gene and Cell) strongly support the notion that the inhibitory actions of glucocorticoid on CRH gene expression in the PVH are complex. If this is the case then we also need to look outside the PVH for answers and examine potential mechanisms that operate at the network level. In this section I will briefly discuss a model of the afferent inputs to CRH neuro-endocrine neurons, and then use this as a framework to examine glucocorticoid actions.

Efferent organization

Afferent control processes involve a range of neural and hormonal components that operate with bewildering complexity. To provide a framework for understanding the functional organization of CRH neuronal-control processes, for experimental design, and for interpreting data, we consider that a hierarchically ordered model of neural and corticosterone-dependent-control processes is a useful working hypothesis (Figure 7.6). This model is based on the accepted notion that CRH neuroendocrine neurons are motor neurons, since they control the activity of non-neuronal cells outside the brain: that is, corticotropes. Hierarchical models have long proved useful for explaining neural control of the somatic motor system, and it seems reasonable to use this type of organization as a framework for exploring the neural control of CRH gene expression, at least as a first approximation (Schneider and Watts, 2002; Watts and Swanson, 2002). The advantages of this approach is that it provides a useful and manageable way for organizing afferent inputs, and also encourages us to think about the different control mechanisms in a more integrative way, rather than considering each as being an isolated system.

   To do this we have taken those neural systems known to control CRH neural function and divided them into two broad categories: *Level 1* neurons make synaptic

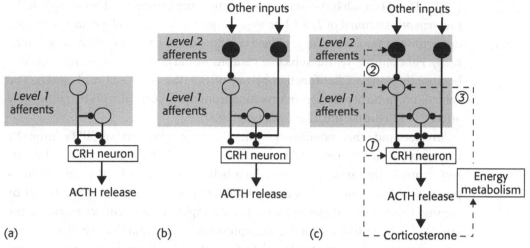

Figure 7.6   The neural afferents controlling the activity of CRH neurons can be categorized hierarchically. (a) Level 1 neurons, either individually or as part of a more complex network, synapse directly upon CRH neurons; (b) while Level 2 neurons control CRH neurons indirectly by way of Level 1 neurons and (c) glucocorticoids can regulate CRH neuronal activity using both hierarchical levels

contact with CRH neurons and control their function directly (Figure 7.6(a)). These can be considered analogous to pre-motor neurons in the somatic motor system. Examples include NPY/GABAergic neurons in the arcuate nucleus (Schneider and Watts, 2002), and local glutamatergic neurons (Herman *et al.*, 2002). Catecholaminergic inputs that originate in the hindbrain and encode interosensory information and provide important regulatory control of CRH gene expression (Swanson and Sawchenko, 1983; Ritter *et al.*, 2003) also fall into this category.

It is important to note that *Level 1* afferents are not organized as a parallel array of independently acting inputs. Interactions between them will form networks that allow for a more sophisticated level of control. Figure 7.6(a) illustrates a simple example, where one set of afferents collateralizes with another either at its cell body or at its terminal; interactions between catecholaminergic inputs to the paraventricular and the dorsomedial nucleus of the hypothalamus (PVH and DMH, respectively) (Thompson and Swanson, 1998) are probably arranged in this manner.

Level 2 neurons influence CRH neuronal function indirectly by altering the signaling properties of *Level 1* neurons. These interactions may occur outside the PVH – for example, hypothalamic projections into the DMH (Thompson and Swanson, 1998); amygdalar projections to the bed nucleus of the stria terminalis

(BST) (Dong *et al.*, 2001) – or they may occur more proximally, for example at the pre-synaptic terminal of *Level 1* neurons (Figure 7.6(b)). *Level 2* neurons provide opportunities for a wide range of neural influences to control CRH function indirectly. For example, ventral subicular neurons would be considered *Level 2* neurons because they affect CRH function by way of the BST (Cullinan *et al.*, 1993). The subiculum, in turn, processes information from many cortical areas that ultimately affect CRH neuronal function (Swanson, 2000).

Stressors and other modulatory influences are going to control CRH neurons by engaging distinct 'afferent sets'. Each set will consist of arrays of *Levels 1* and *2* control neurons, the constituency of which being determined by the sensory composition of the stimulus. Sets encoding different stimuli may contain distinct or common individual afferent groups. For example, the afferent set encoding the effects of dehydration on CRH gene expression will contain both similar and distinct afferents to the sets encoding the effects of hypovolemia or starvation (Watts, 1996; Watts and Sanchez-Watts, 2002).

Importantly, this arrangement also offers a useful framework for thinking about the way glucocorticoids affect CRH neuronal function. We suggest that there are at least three spatial domains in which corticosterone can operate (Figure 7.6(c)):

(1) Direct actions on CRH neurons (as just discussed in the *Gene* and *Cell* sections).
(2) Actions by way of corticosterone-sensitive afferents.
(3) Corticosterone-sensitive physiological processes, whose effects on CRH neurons are then mediated by way of neural afferents, of which its effects on energy metabolism are an example (Laugero *et al.*, 2001).

Time domains

In a classic review Keller-Wood and Dallman (1984) discussed the importance of different time domains (short-term, intermediate, and long-term) when considering how glucocorticoids regulate ACTH release. They also noted that each of these domains involved different mechanisms ranging from actions on the corticotrope to alterations on the neural systems that regulated secretogogue release. There is evidence to suggest that similar time-domains are important when considering glucocorticoids actions on gene expression.

A basic property of the way corticosterone regulates the overall level of CRH gene transcription is the time required for transcription to respond to changes in circulating corticosterone. Evidence suggests that the time frames for its actions on AVP and CRH gene expression are very different. Using intra-peritoneal (i.p.) bolus injections of supra-physiological doses of corticosterone, Ma *et al.* (1997)

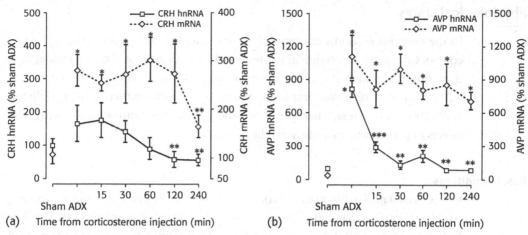

Figure 7.7   Supra-physiological doses of corticosterone acutely injected suppress CRH and AVP gene expression in the PVH with different time scales. AVP gene expression is downregulated more rapidly than CRH. Data from Ma *et al.* (1997)

showed that reductions in AVP hnRNA occurred within minutes, while CRH hnRNA was much less responsive (Figure 7.7). These data suggest that corticosterone uses different mechanisms to control CRH and AVP gene expression. However, this type of experiment makes it very difficult to determine the actions of corticosterone, since the i.p. injection itself acts as a stressor. This means that the administered corticosterone is acting in non-basal (i.e. stressed) conditions and that other factors will make interpretation difficult. Due to these problems determining exactly how long physiological levels of corticosterone take to alter CRH gene expression in unstressed animals remains unclear, but the consensus is that it is slow and of the order of hours. Certainly if circulating corticosterone shifts above or below the circadian mean for a significant period (during chronic stress or following adrenalectomy with or without exogenous corticosterone treatment) resultant changes in CRH gene expression take at least 12 h to become measurable (Swanson and Simmons, 1989; Ma and Aguilera, 1999). Considered together, these data suggest that one component responsible for the sluggish response of CRH gene expression to changes in circulating corticosterone is mediated by mechanisms that modify either the rate of increase or decline in CRH gene transcription, depending on whether corticosterone is decreasing or increasing across the day (Watts *et al.*, 2004). The fact that the time when transcriptional activation/decline occurs is constrained within daily time windows implies that CRH gene expression is, like ACTH secretion (Akana *et al.*, 1986), differentially sensitive to corticosterone across a 24-h period.

Physiological states

In the previous section I examined four domains in which glucocorticoids act to control CRH gene expression in neuroendocrine neurons. I will now consider how this control is manifest during two major physiological states: basal conditions, when glucocorticoids exert important regulatory actions on metabolism (Dallman *et al.*, 2000); and stress, when glucocorticoid secretion is stimulated to control the effects of perturbations away from the basal state.

Basal conditions

It has been known for many years that in most mammals, including humans, ACTH and glucocorticoid secretion rates are not constant throughout the day. Both hormones exhibit daily variations where maximum secretion occurs around the time that maximum activity begins and minimum secretion around the time that general activity slows (see Watts *et al.*, 2004, for references).

To drive this daily secretory rhythm, signals from the circadian clock in the SCH schedule CRH and, to lesser extent, AVP release from neuroendocrine terminals. In turn, releasable pools of CRH and AVP in neuroendocrine terminals are sustained by synthetic mechanisms in the PVHmp, a critical component of which involves transcribing primary (hn) RNA transcripts from their cognate genes. Considering the interaction between glucocorticoids and CRH and AVP gene expression we discussed earlier, the question arises whether this relationship is manifest across the day in the absence of stress? Is ACTH secretogogue synthesis maintained by continuous low-level transcription, or are there significant episodes of CRH or AVP gene transcription?

We recently showed that in intact rats there is a prominent increase in CRH hnRNA levels that occurs at night when rats are most active (Figure 7.8). This strongly suggests that, like the secretory components of the HPA axis, CRH gene transcription is not constant across a 24-h period, but increases and decreases in a simple rhythm (Watts *et al.*, 2004). Interestingly, the rate of CRH gene transcription is completely out of phase with ACTH secretion (Figure 7.8), suggesting that separate mechanisms control secretogogue gene transcription and release at the ME, and these mechanisms are only loosely coupled. I will return to this point in a later section.

In this same study we showed that the fluctuating levels of circulating corticosterone normally seen across the day are not required for daily rhythm of CRH gene expression. However, varying levels of circulating corticosterone do have a significant effect on the overall level of CRH gene transcription (Figure 7.9). In the absence of stress the overall level of transcription is significantly higher in ADX rats with no corticosterone replacement compared to intact animals (Watts *et al.*,

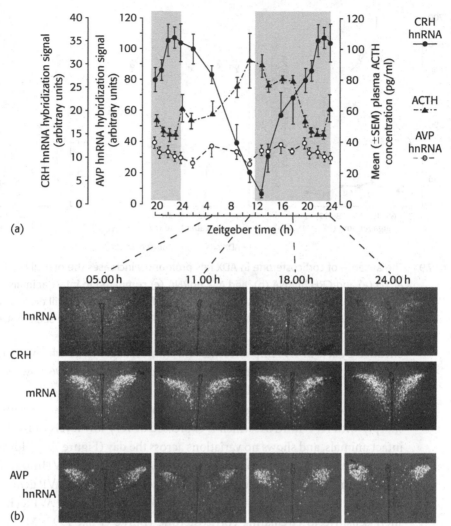

Figure 7.8   (a) CRH gene transcription (as indexed by CRH hnRNA levels) exhibits a marked daily variation in intact animals. In contrast AVP gene transcription shows no change over the day. Maximum CRH hnRNA levels are seen around the time of lights on, while the lowest levels are around the time of lights off. The time of lights off is shown by the gray boxes. Also note that the pattern of CRH gene transcription is completely out of phase with ACTH secretion, suggesting that CRH gene transcription and release are uncoupled in the absence of stress and (b) Corresponding photomicrographs at selected times of the day are shown. Data adapted from Watts *et al.* (2004)

2004). Thus, the amount of CRH hnRNA present at both the nadir and peak of the cycle is a crucial target of corticosterone's long-term actions on CRH synthesis in the PVHmp. It is likely that different mechanisms determine the values of each of these parameters, which in turn involve the integration of neural information

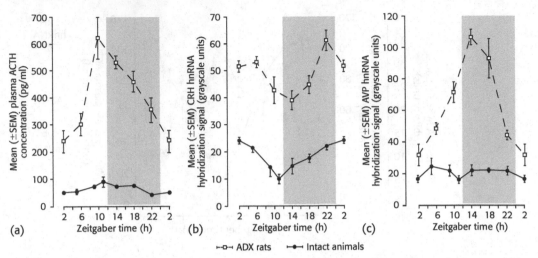

Figure 7.9   The absence of corticosterone in ADX rats profoundly increases the overall level of plasma ACTH (a) and CRH hnRNA (b), and AVP hnRNA (c) compared to intact animals. However, significant daily variations in plasma ACTH (a) and CRH hnRNA (b) still occur in both intact and ADX rats, whereas a daily rhythm of AVP hnRNA (c) is only seen in ADX rats

encoded by sets of PVHmp afferents and humoral agents, of which corticosterone is the most important (Lightman and Harbuz, 1993; Watts, 1996; Sawchenko *et al.*, 2000; Watts and Sanchez-Watts, 2002).

The pattern of fluctuating CRH hnRNA levels we see in intact animals contrasts sharply with AVP hnRNA, which is expressed at very low levels in the PVHmp of intact animals, and shows no variations across the day (Figure 7.8). However, there are significant daily variations of AVP hnRNA levels in the PVHmp of ADX animals (Figure 7.9). Given that the actions of corticosterone on AVP gene expression are rapid and involve direct actions on the gene, and that the AVP gene is exquisitely sensitive to circulating corticosterone (Burke *et al.*, 1997; Ma *et al.*, 1997; Kovács *et al.*, 2000; Watts and Sanchez-Watts, 2002), it would seem that the amounts of corticosterone circulating in intact rats during the latter part of the light period and early dark period are sufficient to suppress completely the mechanism that drives AVP gene expression. This suggests that, unlike CRH gene transcription, the dynamics of circulating corticosterone in intact animals are important for blunting daily variations in AVP gene transcription. The constant and very low levels of AVP hnRNA we see throughout the day is consistent with studies using Brattleboro rats (Ixart *et al.*, 1982), CRH knockout mice (Muglia *et al.*, 1997), and CRH immunoneutralization (Ixart *et al.*, 1985) showing that diurnal corticosterone release in intact animals is driven almost exclusively by CRH release.

Given that corticosterone alone cannot account for the daily variations of CRH and AVP hnRNA, a major component in the integrative process that controls CRH and AVP gene expression in CRH neurons must be the large group of afferent sets encoding the extero- and interosensory information. Considering the fact that changes in corticosterone secretion are not sufficient to drive these nocturnal transcriptional episodes, it would seem likely that at least one of these afferent sets plays a significant role in activating gene transcription during the dark phase. Currently, the detailed architecture of the afferent systems responsible for shaping CRH neuroendocrine function across the day in the absence of stress is poorly understood. However, the circadian timing system controlled by the SCH should be considered as one potential controller of CRH and AVP gene activation in these circumstances. The SCH provides the principal timing signal for daily surges of plasma ACTH and corticosterone (Moore and Eichler, 1972; Szafarczyk et al., 1979; Cascio et al., 1987; Buijs et al., 1993a; 1998).

Some SCH efferents clearly innervate the PVHmp, but these are more sparse than those that innervate other nearby targets (Vrang et al. 1995a, b; Watts et al., 1987; Leak and Moore, 2001) particularly the DMH, which heavily innervates the PVHmp and is heavily implicated in influencing circadian corticosterone output (Watts et al., 1987; Buijs et al., 1993b; 1998; Vrang et al., 1995a, b; Kalsbeek et al., 1996; Thompson et al., 1996; Leak and Moore, 2001; Chou et al., 2003). The exact nature of the afferent set controlled by the SCH remains to be established.

Stress

Like the daily variations associated with feeding and the responses to negative energy balance, the physiological consequences of the HPA motor response to stress are in many respects more anticipatory than reactive events. Although ACTH and corticosterone secretion are obviously triggered by the stressor, they are not motor responses that act to remove the immediate consequences of the stress, as occurs with reactive homeostatic motor events. The target actions of increased circulating corticosterone (mediated in part by its interactions with leptin, insulin, and the thyroid hormones) anticipate the possibility that the stressor will lead to a debilitating sequence of events, particularly the catabolic effects of negative energy balance (see also Sapolsky et al., 2000). In comparison, the more reflex homeostatic motor components of the stress response are exemplified by the consequences of sympathetic activation that counteract the immediate effects of the stress; for example, hypotension or hypoglycemia are stress-derived effects that can be rapidly negated by reactive sympathetic responses (e.g. vasoconstriction, increased heart rate, hyperglycemia) that have evolutionarily ancient homologs (Watts, 2000).

To provide the framework for examining the regulatory actions of glucocorticoids on PVH neuroendocrine peptide gene expression during stress, we should consider two issues within this context. First, what precisely is the function of increased CRH and AVP (because of its importance to ACTH secretion during stress) gene expression in neuroendocrine CRH neurons during the ACTH response to stress? The most likely answer is that rather than impacting ongoing stress events, stress-associated augmentation of mRNA levels are recuperative mechanisms that provide the peptide synthetic mechanisms of the neuroendocrine neuron with the ability to sustain future secretory activity. Second, what is the temporal organization of the gene-regulatory response to stress? This sequence is obviously quite complex, and is best considered when broken down into phases, each of which is likely to be differentially regulated by corticosterone in a manner that may not necessarily operate with an inhibitory action.

Constrained by this perspective, I will now evaluate glucocorticoid action on CRH and AVP gene expression within the context of four components of the HPA secretory response to stress:

(1) How the preceding corticosterone environment affects the onset of gene expression (*Initiation*).
(2) The duration of gene activation (*Dynamics*).
(3) Which genes are activated (*Which genes?*).
(4) Corticosterone's ongoing actions on secretogogue gene expression during the secretory response itself (*Negative feedback*).

To approach these questions we have taken advantage of a viscerosensory stressor (sustained hypovolemia) that has four qualities useful for data interpretation that are not found with many other commonly used stressors. First, its sensory transduction and physiological mechanisms are very well understood; second, its physiological onset can be determined accurately; and third, because this occurs some time after the stress of handling and injection, any effects resulting from the stressor are easily distinguished from these initial non-specific effects; and finally, its intensity increases linearly for up to 4 h (Tanimura *et al.*, 1998).

Initiation

Two questions concerning the initiation of gene transcription can be addressed using sustained hypovolemia. First, how do the processes in the CRH neuron that initiate secretogogue gene transcription temporally interact with those that control secretogogue release? Second, are these interactions dependent on corticosterone? Answers to these questions should provide clues about the nature of the intracellular mechanisms that link peptide synthesis to those that control peptide release at the neuroendocrine terminal in the ME.

We have shown that ACTH secretogogue release from neuroendocrine terminals in the ME during the early part sustained hypovolemia can occur in the absence of an accompanying episode of CRH or AVP gene transcription (Figures 7.10–7.12).

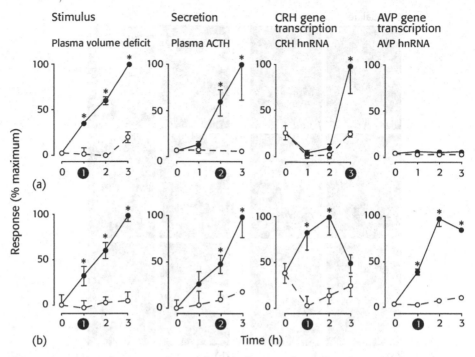

Figure 7.10   The presence of corticosterone has profound effects on the ability of sustained hypovolemic stress to initiate and sustain CRH gene transcription. (a) in intact animals sustained hypovolemia activates CRH gene transcription 3 h after stress onset; (b) but this occurs earlier and transiently in ADX animals. Note that both the development of the stimulus (as measured plasma volume deficit) and the secretory response of the CRH neuron (as measured by ACTH release) are unaffected by the presence or absence of corticosterone. Finally, AVP gene expression only occurs in the absence of corticosterone. Black circled times on the X-axes indicated when a significant effect is first detected. Data adapted from Tanimura *et al.* (1998) and Tanimura and Watts (2000). Open circles, injected corticosterone; solid circles, sustained hypovolemia; * indicates $p < 0.05$

This result shows clearly that the mechanisms responsible for gene transcription are dissociable from those initiating activity-dependent secretogogue release. Secretogogue gene transcription is activated only if release is maintained for a significantly longer period as the stressor increases in intensity (Tanimura *et al.*, 1998). Importantly, these data show that increased gene transcription does not invariably accompany an ongoing secretory event, and emphasize that the cellular events that activate gene expression are very likely different from those responsible for secretion. However, secretogogue release and ACTH secretogogue gene transcription both occur together in the absence of corticosterone during sustained hypovolemia (Tanimura and Watts, 2000).

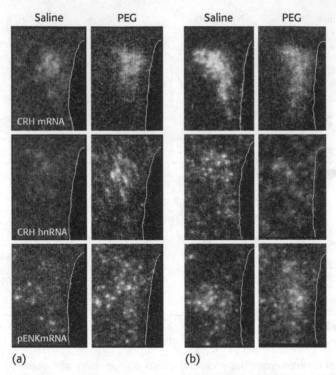

Figure 7.11   Photomicrographs showing CRH mRNA, CRH hnRNA, and proenkephalin (pENK) mRNA in situ hybridization signals in the PVH of (a) intact and (b) ADX animals 5 h after a subcutaneous saline or polyethylene glycol (PEG) injection. Note that the absence of corticosterone is associated with a lower CRH mRNA and hnRNA response to PEG compared to the saline controls. However, the pENK mRNA response remains intact. Data from Tanimura and Watts (1998)

Dynamics of transcriptional activation

What effect does corticosterone have on determining the dynamics of CRH gene activation during sustained hypovolemia? In intact animals CRH gene transcription occurs (as evidenced by measuring CRH hnRNA levels in the PVHmp) only when a certain stress intensity threshold is reached (Figure 7.12; Tanimura et al., 1998). Once this happens, transcription is then maintained in the presence of elevated plasma corticosterone for up to 5 h. However, in two experiments we have demonstrated that the detailed dynamics of this response are critically dependent upon the corticosterone environment to which the CRH neuron has been exposed before the stressor occurs.

First, we examined the effect of manipulating preceding circulating corticosterone concentrations on the magnitude of the CRH mRNA response 5 h into the stress, when the CRH mRNA response to the stressor is at its greatest (Tanimura

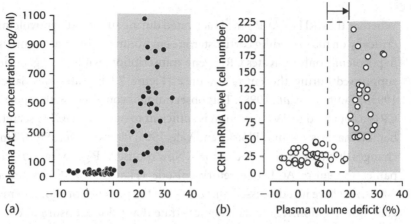

Figure 7.12 The relationship between stimulus intensity (percent of plasma volume deficit) and the response of (a) ACTH secretion and (b) CRH hnRNA following injections of polyethylene glycol (PEG) to intact animals. Note that ACTH secretion is activated at a lower stimulus intensity than is CRH gene transcription suggesting that the mechanisms controlling these two process can be uncoupled. Data adapted from Tanimura *et al.* (1998)

and Watts, 1998). In ADX animals with no corticosterone replacement, we found that instead of increasing CRH transcription and mRNA levels, these were actually lower at this time in stressed animals than in the unstressed controls. The magnitude of CRH gene response to stress returned to that seen in intact animals when preceding plasma corticosterone were clamped at levels seen in intact animals. However, the magnitude of the CRH mRNA response was enhanced compared to intact animals, when plasma corticosterone levels were clamped at levels lower than those required to normalize thymus weights. Activation of the pre-proenkephalin gene (which is also increased by this stressor) was unaffected by these manipulations of corticosterone. In a second experiment, we looked in more detail at how the absence of corticosterone affected the temporal response of CRH gene expression to stress (Tanimura and Watts, 2000). We found that the reason for the reversal seen at 5 h in ADX animals was not because they could not initiate CRH gene transcription, but because an initial and, compared to that in intact animals, premature transcriptional episode could not be maintained (Figure 7.10). Collectively, these data show that corticosterone has a profound effect on directing how the CRH gene responds to the stressor, and that at very low plasma concentrations, corticosterone acts as a facilitatory agent that supports CRH gene transcription in the face of a sustained stressor. Where this facilitatory action occurs is unknown, but could target anywhere from the afferent sets encoding hypovolemia to mechanisms in the CRH neuron itself.

Which genes?

Whether the CRH or AVP gene is activated during sustained hypovolemia depends critically on the preceding corticosterone environment. In intact animals sustained hypovolemia only activates CRH gene transcription, while AVP gene activation is suppressed during the entire response (Figure 7.10; Watts and Sanchez-Watts, 1995b; Tanimura et al., 1998). This observation is consistent with reports that show CRH as opposed to AVP secretion is sufficient to maintain ACTH secretion during hemodynamic stressors (Plotsky and Vale, 1984; Plotsky et al., 1985). This situation changes dramatically in ADX animals. Now robust AVP gene transcription accompanies the entire ACTH secretory episode (Figure 7.10; Tanimura and Watts, 2000). As I have just discussed, this occurs in the presence of short premature CRH gene transcription. These data demonstrate that prior exposure to corticosterone has a profound effect on which signal transduction pathway (CRH or AVP) is selected during stress.

Since the AVP gene contains a GRE and that corticosterone interacts with signal transduction pathways (Beato et al., 1995), at least part of these effects of corticosterone likely occurs within the neuron itself. But because the type of stressor (and therefore the afferent input) is critical in determining whether the AVP gene is activated in PVHmp neurons, corticosterone may also have actions on afferent pathways to determine when and which genes are activated (Itoi et al., 1999). Thus, in contrast to hemodynamic stressors, some other stressors are followed by increases in AVP hnRNA and mRNA (Herman, 1995; Kovács and Sawchenko, 1996a, b; Ma et al., 1997; Kovács et al., 2000). Since the preceding corticosterone environment is likely to be quite similar for all these stressors (i.e. all these studies used intact animals), differential afferent activation would seem to be at least partly responsible for why AVP gene activation is much more apparent with some stressors (e.g. restraint) than with others (hemodynamic stressors). Again these data support the hypothesis that selective secretogogue gene activation is mediated by the interaction of PVHmp afferents and corticosterone (Figure 7.6).

Negative feedback

Does a closed-loop negative-feedback signal from corticosterone operate during stress? One way to address this issue is to examine the dynamics of CRH gene expression during the prolonged secretion of corticosterone that occurs during sustained hypovolemia. If corticosterone provides a negative-feedback signal during stress, one would expect to see CRH hnRNA and mRNA levels fall in response to this elevated secretion. Does this occur? Two sets of observations suggest that in fact a negative-feedback signal does act on gene expression during stress, but it is not within a rapid (i.e. tens of minutes) time-frame. First, CRH mRNA levels do eventually fall under these circumstances, as would be consistent with closed-loop negative-feedback action (Tanimura *et al.*, 1998). However, the fact that this reduction is not accompanied by a concurrent fall in CRH hnRNA levels suggests that under these circumstances one effect of corticosterone is to decrease CRH mRNA half-life (Ma *et al.*, 2001). Second, CRH gene transcription is maintained during sustained hypovolemic stress for at least 3 h despite the presence of very high circulating levels of plasma corticosterone (Tanimura *et al.*, 1998). Similarly, Ma *et al.* (1997) showed that CRH gene transcription was not reduced by a supra-physiological bolus injection of corticosterone in ADX animals for at least 2 h. These studies provide no evidence for rapid negative-feedback regulation of the type that restrains ACTH secretion during certain stressors (Keller-Wood and Dallman, 1984), and emphasize that the mechanisms operating to regulate stressor-induced CRH gene expression are different from those that regulate stressor-induced ACTH secretogogue release.

What about the AVP gene? It is clear that in CRH neuroendocrine neurons, the AVP gene is regulated very differently from the CRH gene (Kovács and Sawchenko, 1996a, b; Kovács *et al.*, 2000; Kovacs, 1998; Ma *et al.*, 1997; Tanimura and Watts, 1998; 2000; Ma and Aguilera, 1999). Consistent with this notion is the fact that corticosterone produces a much more rapid negative-feedback signal on AVP gene expression than on CRH gene expression. Thus, a bolus injection of corticosterone takes less than 15 min to reduce AVP hnRNA levels compared to the 2 h required for CRH hnRNA (Figure 7.7; Ma *et al.*, 1997). In the presence of corticosterone, an AVP gene response to acute stress is much more difficult to evoke than CRH (Darlington *et al.*, 1992; Watts and Sanchez-Watts, 1995b; Kovács and Sawchenko, 1996a, b; Kovács *et al.*, 2000); only when corticosterone is removed before the stressor do we see significant AVP transcription (Figure 7.10; Kovacs, 1998; Tanimura and Watts, 2000), which in this case is concurrent with increased secretion (Figure 7.10).

Summary

Glucocorticoids are important regulators of neuropeptides. The original idea of glucocorticoids functioning as a negative-feedback-response molecule, restraining neuropeptide release and gene expression has given way to a more flexible, context-oriented understanding of regulation. The 'familiar' downregulation of CRH gene expression by glucocorticoids is actually only seen in cells in the mp part of the PVHmp. In other cell types glucocorticoids can either upregulate CRH gene expression or have no effect.

Even within the PVH, the effects of glucocorticoids on CRH cells depend on whether the cells are under basal or stimulated conditions. At low (basal) levels, corticosterone acts to facilitate CRH gene transcription in rat PVH. Although an absence of corticosterone results in an inability to restrain the vasopressin response in concordance with the negative-feedback model, in contrast it also results in an inability to sustain the CRH response.

Glucocorticoids can act directly or indirectly on CRH producing and releasing cells. There are multiple levels of interactions between glucocorticoids and CRH; cellular actions of glucocorticoids are highly complex and include more than direct gene interactions. CRH synthesis (translation of CRH mRNA into CRH peptide) and CRH release (membrane excitability) are different processes that can be either coupled or uncoupled. CRH release can be thought of as the immediate response to a stimulus; CRH synthesis a more long term, adaptive response. Although CRH transcription is eventually reduced in the presence of elevated glucocorticoids, it is not a rapid effect. CRH transcription can be maintained for hours. Mechanisms that regulate CRH gene expression are different from those that regulate CRH release.

Recent findings from human research and a large body of experimental evidence from animal models support the hypothesis that excessive maternal glucocorticoid (either endogenous or exogenous) can have organizational effects on the fetus that have long-term consequences. These effects can have social, behavioral, and temperament consequences that might be linked to alterations in the regulation of CRH or other neuropeptides in the brain (see Chapter 8). Understanding the different mechanisms by which glucocorticoids can regulate neuropeptides, such as CRH, enhances our ability to devise and test hypotheses regarding the regulation of neural function.

Acknowledgements

Work in the author's laboratory is supported by NS29728 and MH66168 from the National Institutes of Health.

REFERENCES

Aguilera, G., Kiss, A. and Luo, X. (1995). Increased expression of type 1 angiotensin II receptors in the hypothalamic paraventricular nucleus following stress and glucocorticoid administration. *J. Neuroendocrinol.*, **7**, 775–83.

Akana, S. F., Cascio, C. S., Du, J. Z., Levin, N. and Dallman, M. F. (1986). Reset of feedback in the adrenocortical system: an apparent shift in sensitivity of adrenocorticotropin to inhibition by corticosterone between morning and evening. *Endocrinology*, **119**, 2325–32.

Akabayashi, A., Watanabe, Y., Wahlestedt, C. *et al.* (1994). Hypothalamic neuropeptide Y, its gene expression and receptor activity: relation to circulating corticosterone in adrenalectomized rats. *Brain Res.*, **665**, 201–12.

Beato, M., Herrlich, P. and Schutz, G. (1995). Steroid hormone receptors: many actors in search of a plot. *Cell*, **83**, 851–7.

Beyer, H. S., Matta, S. G. and Sharp, B. M. (1988). Regulation of messenger ribonucleic acid for corticotropin-releasing factor in the paraventricular nucleus and other brain sites in the rat. *Endocrinology*, **123**, 2117–23.

Brann, D. W., Hendry, L. B. and Mahesh, V. B. (1995). Emerging diversities in the mechanism of action of steroid hormones. *J. Steroid Biochem. Mol. Biol.*, **52**, 113–33.

Buijs, R. M., Kalsbeek, A., van der Woude, T. P., van Heerikhuize, J. J. and Shinn, S. (1993a). Suprachiasmatic nucleus lesion increases corticosterone secretion. *Am. J. Physiol.*, **264**, R1186–92.

Buijs, R. M., Markman, M., Nunes-Cardoso, B., Hou, Y. X. and Shinn, S. (1993b). Projections of the suprachiasmatic nucleus to stress-related areas in the rat hypothalamus: a light and electron microscopic study. *J. Comp. Neurol.*, **335**, 42–54.

Buijs, R. M., Hermes, M. H. and Kalsbeek, A. (1998). The suprachiasmatic nucleus–paraventricular nucleus interactions: a bridge to the neuroendocrine and autonomic nervous system. *Prog. Brain Res.*, **119**, 365–82.

Burke, Z. D., Ho, M. Y., Morgan, H. *et al.* (1997). Repression of vasopressin gene expression by glucocorticoids in transgenic mice: evidence of a direct mechanism mediated by proximal 5′ flanking sequence. *Neuroscience*, **78**, 1177–85.

Cascio, C. S., Shinsako, J. and Dallman, M. F. (1987). The suprachiasmatic nuclei stimulate evening ACTH secretion in the rat. *Brain Res.*, **423**, 173–8.

Chou, T. C., Scammell, T. E., Gooley, J. J. *et al.* (2003). Critical role of dorsomedial hypothalamic nucleus in a wide range of behavioral circadian rhythms. *J. Neurosci.*, **23**, 10691–702.

Cullinan, W. E., Herman, J. P. and Watson, S. J. (1993). Ventral subicular interaction with the hypothalamic paraventricular nucleus: evidence for a relay in the bed nucleus of the stria terminalis. *J. Comp. Neurol.*, **332**, 1–20.

Dallman, M. F., Akana, S. F., Cascio, C. S. *et al.* (1987). Regulation of ACTH secretion: variations on a theme of B. *Recent Prog. Horm. Res.*, **43**, 113–73.

Dallman, M. F., Akana, S. F., Bhatnagar, S., Bell, M. E. and Strack, A. M. (2000). Bottomed out: metabolic significance of the circadian trough in glucocorticoid concentrations. *Int. J. Obes. Relat. Metab. Disord.*, **24**(Suppl 2), S40–6.

Darlington, D. N., Barraclough, C. A. and Gann, D. S. (1992). Hypotensive hemorrhage elevates corticotropin-releasing hormone messenger ribonucleic acid (mRNA) but not vasopressin mRNA in the rat hypothalamus. *Endocrinology*, **130**, 1281–88.

Day, H. E., Campeau, S., Watson Jr., S. J. and Akil, H. (1999). Expression of alpha (1b) adrenoceptor mRNA in corticotropin-releasing hormone-containing cells of the rat hypothalamus and its regulation by corticosterone. *J. Neurosci.*, **19**, 10098–106.

Dong, H. W., Petrovich, G. D. and Swanson, L. W. (2001a). Topography of projections from amygdala to bed nuclei of the stria terminalis. *Brain Res. – Brain Res. Rev.*, **38**, 192–246.

Dumont, J. E., Dremier, S., Pirson, I. and Maenhaut, C. (2002). Cross signaling, cell specificity, and physiology. *Am. J. Physiol. Cell. Physiol.*, **283**, C2–28.

Frim, D. M., Robinson, B. G., Pasieka, K. B. and Majzoub, J. A. (1990). Differential regulation of corticotropin-releasing hormone mRNA in rat brain. *Am. J. Physiol.*, **258**, E686–92.

Guardiola-Diaz, H. M., Kolinske, J. S., Gates, L. H. and Seasholtz, A. F. (1996). Negative gluco-corticoid regulation of cyclic adenosine 3′,5′-monophosphate-stimulated corticotropin releasing hormone-reporter expression in AtT-20 cells. *Mol. Endocrinol.*, **10**, 317–29.

Hallbeck, M., Larhammar, D. and Blomqvist, A. (2001). Neuropeptide expression in rat para-ventricular hypothalamic neurons that project to the spinal cord. *J. Comp. Neurol.*, **433**, 222–38.

Herman, J. P. (1995). In-situ hybridization analysis of vasopressin gene-transcription in the para-ventricular and supraoptic nuclei of the rat – regulation by stress and glucocorticoids. *J. Comp. Neurol.*, **363**, 15–27.

Herman, J. P., Tasker, J. G., Ziegler, D. R. and Cullinan, W. E. (2002). Local circuit regulation of paraventricular nucleus stress integration: glutamate-GABA connections. *Pharmacol. Biochem. Behav.*, **71**, 457–68.

Hohlweg, W. and Junkmann, K. (1932). Die hormonal-nervöse Regulierung der Funktion der Hypophysenborderlappens. *Klin. Wschr.*, **11**, 321–23.

Hoskins, R. G. (1949). The thyroid–pituitary apparatus as a servo (feedback) mechanism. *J. Clin. Endocrinol.*, **9**, 1429–31.

Itoi, K., Helmreich, D. L., Lopez-Figueroa, M. O. and Watson, S. J. (1999). Differential regulation of corticotropin-releasing hormone and vasopressin gene transcription in the hypothalamus by norepinephrine. *J. Neurosci.*, **19**, 5464–72.

Ixart, G., Alonso, G., Szafarczyk, A. *et al.* (1982). Adrenocorticotropic regulations after bilateral lesions of the paraventricular or supraoptic nuclei and in Brattleboro rats. *Neuroendocrinology*, **35**, 270–6.

Ixart, G., Conte-Devolx, B., Szafarczyk, A. *et al.* (1985). L'immunisation passive avec un immune-sérum anti-oCRF41 inhibe l'augmentation circadienne de l'ACTH plasmatique chez le rat. *CR Acad. Sci. III*, **301**, 659–64.

Jhanwar-Uniyal, M. and Leibowitz, S. F. (1986). Impact of circulating corticosterone on alpha 1- and alpha 2-noradrenergic receptors in discrete brain areas. *Brain Res.*, **368**, 404–8.

Jones, M. T. and Gillham, B. (1988). Factors involved in the regulation of adrenocorticotropic hormone/beta-lipotropic hormone. *Physiol. Rev.*, **68**, 743–818.

Kalsbeek, A., van Heerikhuize, J. J., Wortel, J. and Buijs, R. M. (1996). A diurnal rhythm of stim-ulatory input to the hypothalamo–pituitary–adrenal system as revealed by timed intrahypo-thalamic administration of the vasopressin V1 antagonist. *J. Neurosci.*, **16**, 5555–65.

Keller-Wood, M. E. and Dallman, M. F. (1984). Corticosteroid inhibition of ACTH secretion. *Endocr. Rev.*, **5**, 1–24.

Khan, A. M. and Watts, A. G. (2003). Norepinephrine rapidly elevates CRH hnRNA, c-fos mRNA, and levels of phosphorylated MAP kinases (Erk 1 and 2) in hypothalamic parvocellu-lar paraventricular neurons in vivo. *Soc. Neurosci. Absts.*

Khan, A. M. and Watts, A. G. (2004). Intravenous 2-deoxy-D-glucose injection rapidly elevates levels of the phosphorylated forms of p44/42 mitogen activated protein kinases (Erk 1/2) in rat hypothalamic parvocellular paraventricular neurons. *Endocrinology*, **145**, 351–59.

King, B. R., Smith, R. and Nicholson, R. C. (2002). Novel glucocorticoid and cAMP interactions on the CRH gene promoter. *Mol. Cell Endocrinol.*, **194**, 19–28.

Kovacs, K. J. (1998). Functional neuroanatomy of the parvocellular vasopressinergic system: transcriptional responses to stress and glucocorticoid feedback. *Prog. Brain Res.*, **119**, 31–43.

Kovacs, K. J. and Mezey, E. (1987). Dexamethasone inhibits corticotropin-releasing factor gene expression in the rat paraventricular nucleus. *Neuroendocrinology*, **46**, 365–8.

Kovács, K. J. and Sawchenko, P. E. (1996a). Sequence of stress-induced alterations in indices of synaptic and transcriptional activation in parvocellular neurosecretory neurons. *J. Neurosci.*, **16**, 262–73.

Kovacs, K. J. and Sawchenko, P. E. (1996b). Regulation of stress-induced transcriptional changes in the hypothalamic neurosecretory neurons. *J. Mol. Neurosci.*, **7**, 125–33.

Kovács, K. J., Foldes, A. and Sawchenko, P. E. (2000). Glucocorticoid negative feedback selectively targets vasopressin transcription in parvocellular neurosecretory neurons. *J. Neurosci.*, **20**, 3843–52.

Kretz, O., Reichardt, H. M., Schutz, G. and Bock, R. (1999). Corticotropin-releasing hormone expression is the major target for glucocorticoid feedback-control at the hypothalamic level. *Brain Res.*, **818**, 488–91.

Laugero, K. D., Bell, M. E., Bhatnagar, S., Soriano, L. and Dallman, M. F. (2001). Sucrose ingestion normalizes central expression of corticotropin-releasing-factor messenger ribonucleic acid and energy balance in adrenalectomized rats: a glucocorticoid-metabolic-brain axis? *Endocrinology*, **142**, 2796–804.

Leak, R. K. and Moore, R. Y. (2001). Topographic organization of suprachiasmatic nucleus projection neurons. *J. Comp. Neurol.*, **433**, 312–34.

Legradi, G., Holzer, D., Kapcala, L. P. and Lechan, R. M. (1997). Glucocorticoids inhibit stress-induced phosphorylation of CREB in corticotropin-releasing hormone neurons of the hypothalamic paraventricular nucleus. *Neuroendocrinology*, **66**, 86–97.

Lightman, S. L. and Harbuz, M. S. (1993). Expression of corticotropin-releasing factor mRNA in response to stress. *CIBA Found. Symp.*, **172**, 173–87.

Ma, X. M., Levy, A. and Lightman, S. L. (1997). Rapid changes of heteronuclear RNA for arginine vasopressin but not for corticotropin releasing hormone in response to acute corticosterone administration. *J. Neuroendocrinol.*, **9**, 723–8.

Ma, X. M. and Aguilera, G. (1999). Differential regulation of corticotropin-releasing hormone and vasopressin transcription by glucocorticoids. *Endocrinology*, **140**, 5642–50.

Ma, X. M., Camacho, C. and Aguilera, G. (2001). Regulation of corticotropin-releasing hormone (CRH) transcription and CRH mRNA stability by glucocorticoids. *Cell Mol. Neurobiol.*, **21**, 465–75.

Majzoub, J. A., Emanuel, R., Adler, G. *et al.* (1993). Second messenger regulation of mRNA for corticotropin-releasing factor. *CIBA Found. Symp.*, **172**, 30–43.

Makino, S., Gold, P. W. and Schulkin, J. (1994). Effects of corticosterone on CRH mRNA and content in the bed nucleus of the stria terminalis; comparison with the effects in the central nucleus of the amygdala and the paraventricular nucleus of the hypothalamus. *Brain Res.*, **657**, 141–9.

Malkoski, S. P., Handanos, C. M. and Dorin, R. I. (1997). Localization of a negative glucocorticoid response element of the human corticotropin-releasing hormone gene. *Mol. Cell. Endocrinol.*, **127**, 189–99.

Malkoski, S. P. and Dorin, R. I. (1999). Composite glucocorticoid regulation at a functionally defined negative glucocorticoid response element of the human corticotropin-releasing hormone gene. *Mol. Endocrinol.*, **13**, 1629–44.

Moore, C. R. and Price, D. (1932). Gonad hormone functions, and the reciprocal influence of between gonads and hypophysis with its bearing on the problem of sex hormone antagonism. *Am. J. Anat.*, **50**, 13–71.

Moore, R. Y. and Eichler, V. B. (1972). Loss of a circadian adrenal corticosterone rhythm following suprachiasmatic lesions in the rat. *Brain Res.*, **42**, 201–6.

Muglia, L. J., Jacobson, L., Weninger S. C. *et al.* (1997). Impaired diurnal adrenal rhythmicity restored by constant infusion of corticotropin-releasing hormone in corticotropin-releasing hormone-deficient mice. *J. Clin. Invest.*, **99**, 2923–9.

Plotsky, P. M. and Vale, W. (1984). Hemorrhage-induced secretion of corticotropin-releasing factorlike immunoreactivity into the rat hypophysial portal circulation and its inhibition by glucocorticoids. *Endocrinology*, **114**, 164–9.

Plotsky, P. M., Bruhn, T. O. and Vale, W. (1985). Evidence for multifactorial regulation of adrenocorticotropin secretory response to hemodynamic stimuli. *Endocrinology*, **116**, 633–9.

Reichardt, H. M., Kaestner, K. H., Tuckermann, J. *et al.* (1998). DNA-binding of the glucocorticoid receptor is not essential for survival. *Cell*, **93**, 531–41.

Ritter, S., Watts, A. G., Dinh, T. T., Sanchez-Watts, G. and Pedrow, C. (2003). Immunotoxin lesion of hypothalamically projecting norepinephrine and epinephrine neurons differentially affects circadian and stressor-stimulated corticosterone secretion. *Endocrinology*, **144**, 1357–67.

Sapolsky, R. M., Romero, L. M. and Munck, A. U. (2000). How do glucocorticoids influence stress responses? Integrating permissive, suppressive, stimulatory, and preparative actions. *Endocr. Rev.*, **21**, 55–89.

Sawchenko, P. E., Li, H. Y. and Ericsson, A. (2000). Circuits and mechanisms governing hypothalamic responses to stress: a tale of two paradigms. *Prog. Brain Res.*, **122**, 61–78.

Schneider, J. E. and Watts, A. G. (2002). Energy homeostasis and behavior. In D. W. Pfaff, Sr. ed., *Hormones, Brain, and Behavior*, Vol. 1. Academic Press, pp. 435–523.

Shelat, S. G., Fluharty, S. J. and Flanagan-Cato, L. M. (1998). Adrenal steroid regulation of central angiotensin II receptor subtypes and oxytocin receptors in rat brain. *Brain Res.*, **807**, 135–46.

Swanson, L. W. (1991). Biochemical switching in hypothalamic circuits mediating responses to stress. *Prog. Brain Res.*, **87**, 181–200.

Swanson, L. W. (2000). Cerebral hemisphere regulation of motivated behavior. *Brain Res.*, **886**, 113–64.

Swanson, L. W. and Kuypers H. G. (1980). The paraventricular nucleus of the hypothalamus: cytoarchitectonic subdivisions and organization of projections to the pituitary, dorsal vagal complex, and spinal cord as demonstrated by retrograde fluorescence double-labeling methods. *J. Comp. Neurol.*, **194**, 555–70.

Swanson, L. W. and Sawchenko, P. E. (1983). Hypothalamic integration: organization of the paraventricular and supraoptic nuclei. *Annu. Rev. Neurosci.*, **6**, 275–325.

Swanson, L. W. and Simmons, D. M. (1989). Differential steroid hormone and neural influences on peptide mRNA levels in CRH cells of the paraventricular nucleus: a hybridization histochemical study in the rat. *J. Comp. Neurol.*, **285**, 413–35.

Szafarczyk, A., Ixart, G., Malaval, F., Nouguier-Soule, J. and Assenmacher, I. (1979). Effects of lesions of the suprachiasmatic nuclei and of p-chlorophenylalanine on the circadian rhythms of adrenocorticotrophic hormone and corticosterone in the plasma, and on locomotor activity of rats. *J. Endocrinol.*, **83**, 1–16.

Tanimura, S. M. and Watts, A. G. (1998). Corticosterone can facilitate as well as inhibit CRH gene expression in the rat hypothalamic paraventricular nucleus. *Endocrinology*, **139**, 3830–37.

Tanimura, S. M. and Watts, A. G. (2000). Adrenalectomy dramatically modifies the dynamics of neuropeptide and c-*fos* gene responses to stress in the hypothalamic paraventricular nucleus. *J. Neuroendocrinol.*, **12**, 715–22.

Tanimura, S. M., Sanchez-Watts, G. and Watts, A. G. (1998). Peptide gene activation, secretion, and steroid feedback during stimulation of rat neuroendocrine CRH neurons. *Endocrinology*, **139**, 3822–9.

Thompson, R. H. and Swanson, L. W. (1998). Organization of inputs to the dorsomedial nucleus of the hypothalamus: a reexamination with Fluorogold and PHAL in the rat. *Brain Res. – Brain Res. Rev.*, **27**, 89–118.

Thompson, R. H., Canteras, N. S. and Swanson, L. W. (1996). Organization of projections from the dorsomedial nucleus of the hypothalamus: a PHA-L study in the rat. *J. Comp. Neurol.*, **376**, 143–73.

Vrang, N., Larsen, P. J., Moller, M. and Mikkelsen, J. D. (1995a). Topographical organization of the rat suprachiasmatic–paraventricular projection. *J. Comp. Neurol.*, **353**, 585–603.

Vrang, N., Larsen, P. J. and Mikkelsen, J. D. (1995b). Direct projection from the suprachiasmatic nucleus to hypophysiotrophic corticotropin-releasing factor immunoreactive cells in the paraventricular nucleus of the hypothalamus demonstrated by means of Phaseolus vulgarisleucoagglutinin tract tracing. *Brain Res.*, **684**, 61–9.

Watts, A. G. (1992). Disturbance of fluid homeostasis leads to temporally and anatomically distinct responses in neuropeptide and tyrosine hydroxylase mRNA levels in the paraventricular and supraoptic nuclei of the rat. *Neuroscience*, **46**, 859–79.

Watts, A. G. (1996). The impact of physiological stimulation on the expression of corticotropin releasing hormone and other neuropeptide genes. *Front. Neuroendocrinol.*, **17**, 281–326.

Watts, A. G. (2000). Comparative anatomy and physiology. In George Fink, Sr. ed., *The Encyclopedia of Stress*. Academic Press, San Diego, CA, USA, pp. 507–11.

Watts, A. G., Swanson, L. W. and Sanchez-Watts, G. (1987). Efferent projections of the suprachiasmatic nucleus. I. Studies using anterograde transport of *Phaseolus vulgaris* leucoagglutinin (PHA-L) in the rat. *J. Comp. Neurol.*, **258**, 204–29.

Watts, A. G. and Sanchez-Watts, G. (1995a). Region-specific regulation of neuropeptide mRNAs in rat limbic forebrain neurones by aldosterone and corticosterone. *J. Physiol. (London)*, **484**, 721–36.

Watts, A. G. and Sanchez-Watts, G. (1995b). Physiological regulation of peptide messenger RNA colocalization in rat hypothalamic paraventricular medial parvicellular neurons. *J. Comp. Neurol.*, **352**, 501–14.

Watts, A. G. and Sanchez-Watts, G. (2002). Interactions between heterotypic stressors and corticosterone reveal integrative mechanisms for controlling CRH gene expression in the rat paraventricular nucleus. *J. Neurosci.*, **22**, 6282–9.

Watts, A. G. and Swanson, L. W. (2002). Anatomy of motivational systems. In Hal Pashler and Randy Gallistell, eds., *Stevens' Handbook of Experimental Psychology, Vol. 3, Learning, Motivation, and Emotion*, 3rd edn. John Wiley & Sons, New York, NY, USA, pp. 563–632.

Watts, A. G., Tanimura, S. M. and Sanchez-Watts, G. (2004). *Crh* and *avp* gene transcription in the hypothalamic paraventricular nucleus of unstressed rats: daily rhythms and their corticosterone dependence. *Endocrinology*, **145**, 529–40.

Weiner, N. (1948). *Cybernetics*. New York: Technology Press/Wiley & Sons.

Whitnall, M. H. (1993). Regulation of the hypothalamic corticotropin-releasing hormone neurosecretory system. *Prog. Neurobiol.*, **40**, 573–629.

Wolfl, S., Martinez, C. and Majzoub, J. A. (1999). Inducible binding of cyclic adenosine 3′, 5′-monophosphate (cAMP)-responsive element binding protein (CREB) to a cAMP-responsive promoter in vivo. *Mol. Endocrinol.*, **13**, 659–69.

Yates, F. E. and Maran, J. W. (1974). Stimulation and inhibition of adrenocorticotropin release. In Knobil, E. and Sawyer, W. H., eds., *Handbook of Physiology*, Vol. IV, Part 2. *The Pituitary and its Neuroendocrine Control*, Washington. DC: American Physiological Society, pp. 367–404.

8

Glucocorticoid facilitation of corticotropin-releasing hormone in the placenta and the brain: functional impact on birth and behavior

Jay Schulkin[1], Louis Schmidt[2] and Kristine Erickson[3]

[1] Department of Physiology and Biophysics, Georgetown University, School of Medicine, Clinical Neuroendocrinology Branch, National Institute of Mental Health, American College of Obstetricians and Gynecologists, Washington DC, USA
[2] Department of Psychology, McMaster University, Canada
[3] Molecular Neuroimaging Branch, National Institute of Mental Health, Bethesda MD, USA

Introduction

Glucocorticoids (e.g. cortisol) and corticotropin-releasing hormone (CRH) are important in fetal development and eventually in parturition. However, chronically elevated glucocorticoids have both short- and long-term consequences. The cortisol/CRH system within the placenta is a positive feedback system (e.g. Robinson et al., 1988; Jones et al., 1989), similar to that of several regions in the brain that regulate the behaviors that underlie fear and anxiety (Makino et al., 1994a, b). One noted endocrine effect is the facilitation of CRH gene expression by cortisol during pregnancy. But exaggerated expression of CRH in the placenta may reflect states of adversity and an increased vulnerability to preterm delivery of the neonate (Majzoub et al., 1999).

Increased peripheral cortisol during pregnancy (and also when not pregnant) can cross the blood–brain barrier and may affect the mother's experience of stressful situations. Pregnancy is inherently a metabolically stressful condition, whether psychological expectancies are optimistic or not. Glucocorticoids, cortisol in particular, have diverse effects in the brain in the long-term regulation of gene products, one of which is CRH (Schulkin, 2003).

Additionally, findings from rat and nonhuman primate studies suggest that prenatal and early life adversity can have lifelong consequences on stress responses and, potentially, on vulnerability to physical and psychiatric disorders (Heim and Nemeroff, 2002). Elevated levels of CRH in diverse regions of the brain can signal adversity, and they are sustained by glucocorticoids.

In this chapter, we briefly review some of the evidence that surrounds the positive regulation of CRH gene expression in the placenta and the brain by glucocorticoids. Glucocorticoids play important functional roles in facilitating gene expression of CRH in both the placenta and the brain, but an exaggerated expression is an indication that something may be wrong (Schulkin, 1999), and longer-term adaptation may be compromised (McEwen, 2004). The first part of the chapter is about birth and the role of cortisol and CRH, and the second and third parts are about CRH, glucocorticoids, brain and the regulation of behavior.

Part 1 Glucocorticoids, CRH, placenta and birth

The placenta is a major vehicle in the production of diverse forms of chemical messengers, one of which is CRH (Petraglia *et al.*, 1990). The placenta functions in part as a central coordinator/regulator of maternal and fetal physiology (Figure 8.1).

In the second and third trimesters of normal human pregnancy, CRH derived from the placenta is elevated in maternal plasma. Concurrently, both fetal and maternal adrenocorticotrophic hormone (ACTH) and cortisol levels are elevated (e.g. Goland *et al.*, 1995; Erickson *et al.*, 2001). Following parturition, these plasma CRH levels rapidly decrease to typical nadir levels. Elevated secretion of placental CRH is associated with a surge of fetal glucocorticoids during the few weeks prior to normal parturition. Due to the increased CRH and glucocorticoid secretion, along with the wide variability in the level of CRH expression seen in different women, it is possible that CRH may play a role in initiating parturition (see Goland *et al.*, 1988; Wolfe *et al.*, 1988; Challis, 1995). A parallel rise in fetal cortisol production occurs during the same period, and seems, in part, to mature fetal organs in preparation out of the womb.

The human fetal pituitary system develops early in gestation and responds to low cortisol levels by secreting ACTH (Challis *et al.*, 2000). CRH messenger ribonucleic acid (mRNA) is present in placenta by 8 weeks' gestation, and there is an exponential rise in CRH levels (as much as 20 times) during the last 6 to 8 weeks of gestation. Similarly, CRH peptide levels in maternal blood are quite low until the final 8 to 10 weeks of gestation (Wolfe *et al.*, 1988; Goland *et al.*, 1988; Robinson *et al.*, 1988).

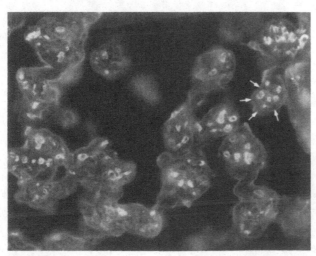

Figure 8.1   CRH immunostaining in the human placenta (courtesy of F. Petraglia and P. Sawchenko)

One possible explanation for the simultaneous rise in CRH and cortisol suggests that within the placenta the exponential rate of increase in CRH is positively related to the concentration of cortisol (Majzoub *et al.*, 1999; Challis *et al.*, 2000). Placental CRH, transported through the umbilical vein to the fetus, could stimulate the fetal pituitary–adrenal axis to produce cortisol, which would then be capable of further stimulating placental CRH production, creating a positive feedback loop. Moreover, the placental production of CRH may in part function for the fetus, reminiscent of neural function, as both a sensory and effector system in providing important sources of adaptation to environmental demands (Wadhwa *et al.*, 2001).

In several kinds of studies, positive feedback of glucocorticoids on placental CRH has been demonstrated. Glucocorticoids first were shown to increase CRH gene expression in primary cultures of placental tissue (Robinson *et al.*, 1988). The effects of CRH expression were related to the dose of glucocorticoids and may be greater in dexamethasone (DEX) compared to cortisol infusions (Jones *et al.*, 1989). The feed-forward regulation may reflect cyclic adenosine monophosphate (cAMP)-mediated CRH promoter activity (Cheng *et al.*, 2000) (Figure 8.2).

Pregnant women treated with betamethasone after 30 weeks of gestation had increased levels of CRH in plasma and placental tissue (Marinoni *et al.*, 1998). In other studies, women at 24 weeks gestation and treated with betamethasone had elevated levels of CRH (Korebrits *et al.*, 1998). Importantly, progesterone infusions decrease CRH expression in the placenta, perhaps by competing with and diminishing access of cortisol to glucocorticoid receptors to further induce CRH expression (Majzoub *et al.*, 1999). Progesterone infusions can delay parturition and withdrawal can exacerbate parturition, as a recent study has demonstrated (Meis *et al.*, 2003; Figure 8.3).

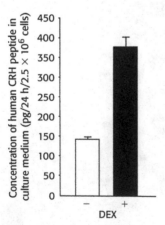

Figure 8.2   The DEX stimulates cAMP-mediated CRH promoter activity in placental tissue. Adapted from Cheng *et al.* (2000)

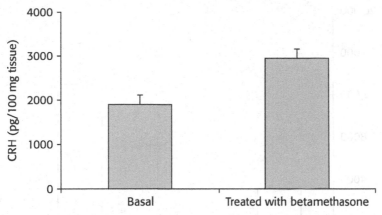

Figure 8.3   Maternal plasma levels of CRH in pregnant women at 30 weeks gestation receiving betamethasone and in control patients. Adapted from Marinoni *et al.* (1998)

This placental model is quite different from the regulation of CRH expression in the parvocellular region of the paraventricular nucleus (PVN) of the hypothalamus, which responds to cortisol with downward regulation of CRH, or negative restraint (Swanson and Simmons, 1989; Watts and Sanchez-Watts, 1995). Instead, the placental model is reminiscent of the positive feedback system of the brain's extra-hypothalamic CRH system (see below).

Diverse forms of events are associated with elevated CRH expression in the placenta: hypertension, infections, growth restriction, diabetes, multiple gestation, and psychosocial stress (Wolfe *et al.*, 1988; Goland *et al.*, 1993; 1995; Petraglia *et al.*, 1995; Hobel *et al.*, 1999). Each of these conditions creates a circumstance of increased vulnerability to early parturition and/or low-birth-weight babies. The induction of CRH gene expression by cortisol possibly accelerates the normal parturition process and fetal development. The over-expression of CRH becomes a signal of danger, perhaps, and the pregnancy begins to terminate. The positive feedback placental CRH system is one possible mechanism regulating the timing of parturition (Figure 8.4).

In cases of preterm labor, maternal cortisol concentrations are significantly higher than in mothers who carry to term (e.g. Hobel *et al.*, 1999; Erickson *et al.*, 2001). Additionally, plasma CRH levels are significantly higher and CRH-binding protein levels are significantly lower during the last 10 weeks of gestation in those who deliver preterm compared to those who carry to term. When women with various physical and psychosocial risk factors who delivered preterm were compared to those women who delivered at term with the same risk factors, the cortisol and CRH concentrations in the preterm groups were significantly higher (Erickson *et al.*, 2001). This suggests that stress during pregnancy does not necessarily result in excessive cortisol and CRH concentrations; additional vulnerability factors apparently

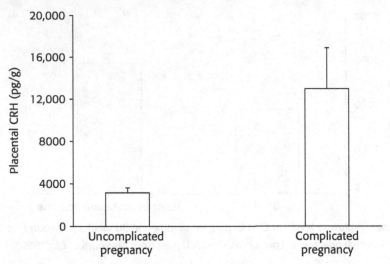

Figure 8.4   Human placental CRH in pregnancy complicated by pre-eclampsia and uncomplicated pregnancies. Adapted from Goland *et al.* (1995)

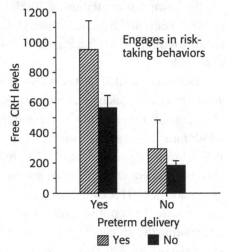

Figure 8.5   Levels of CRH in women who were risk and non-risk takers in mid pregnancy and who had or did not have a preterm delivery. Adapted from Erickson *et al.* (2001)

contribute to the expression of physical and psychosocial stressors in peripheral or placental neuroendocrine markers (Figure 8.5).

Pregnancy and neonatal development

Events in utero can have long-term physiological and behavioral consequences (e.g. Barker, 1997; Seckl, 1997; Welberg and Seckl, 2001). For example, elevated levels of salivary free cortisol concentrations in the mother during pregnancy can have a negative impact on infant motor and mental development (Buitelaar *et al.*, 2003; Huiink *et al.*, 2002), and may facilitate avoidance and shyness behaviors (Trautman *et al.*, 1995).

Psychosocial stress has been linked to low-birth-weight babies and elevated levels of CRH (e.g. Hobel *et al.*, 1999). While the data are not entirely consistent the bulk of the data suggests that diverse forms of psychological events can negatively impact reproduction in humans and other species. In one prospective study in humans, levels of stress and anxiety in the third trimester were associated with low-birth-weight babies and decreased age related births (Wadhwa *et al.*, 1993). Natural disasters, such as earthquakes have been linked to the gestational length (Glynn *et al.*, 2001). There is also evidence that levels of CRH in the maternal circulation are associated with decreased habitation to stimuli by the fetus (Sandman *et al.*, 1999).

More recent studies have noted relationships between maternal psychosocial factors. Individual differences in salivary cortisol responses in human neonates within the first 24 h of life were examined, and two findings were noted. First, salivary cortisol appears to remain moderately stable during the first 24 h of postnatal life. Second, maternal age and socioeconomic status appear to influence hypothalamic–pituitary–adrenal (HPA) axis regulation in that newborns who exhibit high-cortisol responses in the first 24 h of life had mothers who were *older*. In addition, this subset of neonates also had higher autonomic responses at birth and were rated by nurses as more distressed (Erickson *et al.* unpublished observations). Finally, neonates with both low- and high-baseline cortisol concentrations had older mothers (more than 30 years) while neonates who had moderate cortisol levels had younger mothers. The findings from this study are suggestive of maternal influences and contemporaneous relations between cortisol and negative effect in the opening hours of life.

Physiological effects of the prenatal environment include changes in programming of the central nucleus of the amygdala (CeA), and a vulnerability in the infant towards perceiving events as fearful (Welberg and Seckl, 2001). Importantly, pregnant rats treated with DEX for the entire period, or for the last third of gestation had infants that had lower body weights at birth and when these infants were tested 6–8 months later they had diminished exploratory behavior in an open field; treatment for the final third of pregnancy also resulted in deficits in forced swim test. Importantly, in these neonates amygdala CRH mRNA was elevated in both the DEX treated groups (Welberg and Seckl, 2001). The enzyme 11 beta-hydroxysteroid dehydrogenase type 2 may be particularly important for some of the effects of adult programming that perhaps result from glucocorticoid activation (Welberg *et al.*, 2000).

Glucocorticoids readily cross from the peripheral systemic circuitry into the brain. This has implications for the effects of increased circulating cortisol on the fetus and mother during pregnancy. Stress can (but not necessarily; see Erickson et al., 2001) increase glucocorticoid concentrations in the mother during pregnancy, and thus exposes the fetal developing brain to higher levels of glucocorticoids affecting early brain development. There are data in humans that repeated high levels of glucocorticoids by DEX treatment might impact size at birth (French et al., 1999). Finally, cortisol can easily cross into the brain of the mother, potentiating the extra-hypothalamic positive feedback system and increasing CRH expression in the maternal amygdala (Welberg and Seckl, 2001).

Part 2 Glucocorticoid induction of CRH in the brain, and fear-related behaviors

Glucocorticoid and other steroid receptors are part of a major class of DNA-binding factors that regulate gene transcription (Schulkin et al., 1998). Glucocorticoids are lipophillic, pass through the blood–brain barrier, and bind to intracellular high-and low-affinity corticosteroid receptors to form homodimers which then regulate gene expression by binding directly to DNA. These corticosteroid–receptor complexes regulate transcription of numerous genes in most organs of the body and brain, including several inducible transcriptional factors (Bremner et al., 1997).

Both adrenal steroids (glucocorticoids and mineralocorticoids) compete for access to the receptor sites (De Kloet, 1991); both hormones can influence CRH expression in the PVN and increase the level of CRH in the CeA (Watts and Sanchez-Watts, 1995). The effects on the developing amygdala have implications for increased fear and anxiety responses (see review by Korte, 2001) and, therefore, may impact on both infant temperament and mental health later in life.

Glucocorticoids and CRH are typically associated with the HPA axis. However, when discussing these hormones in the context of stress responses, it is important to take into consideration their activities within extra-hypothalamic regions. In regions such as the amygdala, glucocorticoids can potentiate activity, while inhibiting activity in other regions such as the hippocampus and PVN, and these glucocorticoid effects influence physiological, cognitive and behavioral domains.

Glucocorticoids are part of both positive and negative feedback systems regulating CRH expression. Within the context of positive feedback regulation, CRH and CRH mRNA expression in the CeA is increased by peripherally administered corticosterone, while at the same time CRH gene expression in the PVN are decreased (Swanson and Simmons, 1989; Makino et al., 1994a; Watts and Sanchez-Watts, 1995). Regulation of the CRH receptors in the hypothalamus and amygdala may also have different sensitivities to corticosterone (Makino et al., 1995). Glucocorticoid administration can also lead to increased CRH expression in the bed nucleus of the stria terminalis (Makino et al., 1994a, b; Watts and Sanchez-Watts, 1995), a structure that has been described as extended amygdala, and has also been associated with anxiety responses (Davis et al., 1997) (Figure 8.6).

Glucocorticoids are secreted under a number of experimental conditions in which fear, anxiety, novelty, and uncertainty are experimental manipulations (Mason, 1975; Breier, 1989). Across a number of species, including humans, glucocorticoids are secreted when there is loss of control, or the perception of loss of control (worry is associated with the loss of control) (e.g. Breier, 1989). Conversely, circulating

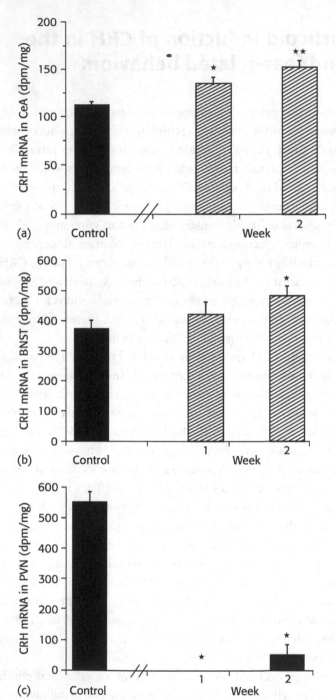

Figure 8.6   CRH mRNA levels in three regions of the brain (a) CeA, (b) bed nucleus of the stria terminalis (BNST), and (c) PVN of the hypothalamus across weeks 1 and 2 in adrenally intact rats implanted with corticosterone (see Makino *et al.*, 1994a, b for more details). dpm: disintegrations per minute

peripheral glucocorticoids are reduced when there is perceived control. Predicting the onset of an aversive signal reduces the level of circulating glucocorticoids (Mason, 1975). Within the clinical literature, one of the most consistent findings in depressed patients is elevated levels of cortisol and an enlarged adrenal cortex (e.g. Sachar et al., 1970). These findings are congruent with those of Richter (1949) who observed an enlarged adrenal gland in stressed, fearful, wild rats when compared to unstressed laboratory analogs.

The CRH is now well known to be both a peptide that regulates pituitary and adrenal function and an extra-hypothalamic peptide hormone linked to a number of behaviors, including behavioral expressions of fear (Koob et al., 1993; Kalin et al., 1994). CRH cell bodies are widely distributed in the brain (Palkovits et al., 1983; Swanson et al., 1983). The majority of CRH neurons within the PVN are clustered in the parvicellular division. Other regions with predominant CRH-containing neurons are the lateral bed nucleus of the stria terminalis and the central region of the CeA. To a smaller degree, there are CRH cells in the lateral hypothalamus, prefrontal and cingulate cortex. In brainstem regions, CRH cells are clustered near the locus coeruleus (Barringtons' nucleus) (Valentino et al., 1994; 1995), parabrachial region and regions of the solitary nucleus. Central CRH activation is consistently and reliably linked to the induction of fear in animal studies (Kalin et al., 1994; Koob et al., 1993). Intraventricular infusions of CRH, for example, are known to facilitate fear-related socially derived contextual responses, in addition to activating greater metabolic activation of the amygdala (Strome et al., 2002).

Central infusions of CRH induce or potentiate a number of fear-related behavioral responses (Takahashi et al., 1989), and infusion of CRH antagonists both within the amygdala and outside of it reduce fear-related responses (Koob et al., 1993). Startle responses are enhanced by CRH infusions (Swerdlow et al., 1989). CRH injected into the lateral ventricles increases freezing to fearful stimuli and potentiates acoustic startle in rats (Liang et al., 1992; Koob et al., 1993). Conversely, administration of a CRH antagonist reduces freezing and anxious behavior on several tests or symptoms of fear (Koob et al., 1993), and attenuates fear-potentiated startle (Swerdlow et al., 1989). An increase (or sensitization) in CRH in the brain occurs after abuse, maternal deprivation, and exposure to other stressful situations in macaques (Habib et al., 1999). A severe social stressor in macaques is the addition of an unknown intruder in an adjacent cage. This results in behaviors associated with anxiety and fear such as body tremors, grimacing and teeth gnashing, and CRH expression is increased in this situation (Habib et al., 2000). Administration of a CRH antagonist reduces the fear and anxiety displays, increases exploratory behaviors, and reduces the production of CRH during the stressful situation (Habib et al., 2000). Importantly, lesions of the CeA, and not the PVN, disrupt CRH-potentiated conditioned fear responses (Liang et al., 1992). That is, only lesions of the

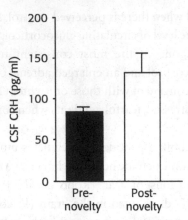

CSF CRH (pg/ml)

Pre-
novelty

Post-
novelty

Figure 8.7   Levels of CRH in the CSF of macaques in response to a familiar (pre-novelty) and unfamiliar (post-novelty) object. Adapted from Habib *et al.* (2000)

amygdala and not of the hypothalamus disrupt the behavioral response, suggesting that CRH induced or facilitated fearful behaviors are generated through extra-hypothalamic brain regions independently of the role of CRH in the HPA axis (Figure 8.7).

High levels of systemic glucocorticoids are associated with fear (or the perception of adverse events) in a number of species (e.g. Mason, 1975; Breier, 1989; Jones *et al.*, 1992), and may be essential for the formation for some forms of fear conditioning (Pugh *et al.*, 1997). In one set of experiments rats (adrenal intact) were pretreated with corticosterone to investigate whether it facilitated conditioned fear-induced freezing (Coordimas *et al.*, 1994). All rats received conditioning trials in which the unconditioned stimulus (footshock) was presented concurrently with the conditioned stimulus (auditory tone). Several days after the trials the rats were treated with corticosterone. The same treatment of corticosterone that increased CRH gene expression in the CeA and bed nucleus of the stria terminalis also facilitated conditioned fear-induced freezing in rats (Coordimas *et al.*, 1994).

In a subsequent study (Thompson *et al.*, 2004), contextual fear conditioning was investigated in groups of rats that were chronically treated with corticosterone or given a vehicle treatment. CRH expression was differentially regulated in the CeA and the parvocellular region of the PVN. One week after the completion of the conditioning and the last corticosterone injection, the rats were tested for the retention of conditioned fear. The corticosterone treated rats displayed more fear conditioning than the vehicle treated rats. The data suggest that repeated high levels of corticosterone could facilitate the retention of contextual fear conditioning, perhaps by the induction of CRH gene expression in critical regions of the brain such as the amygdala.

As noted above, CRH facilitates startle responses. This response does not depend on the adrenal glands because centrally delivered CRH facilitates startle responses in the absence of the adrenal glands (Lee *et al.*, 1994). In that study, Lee *et al.* demonstrated that high chronic plasma levels of corticosterone in adrenal intact rats facilitated CRH-induced startle responses (Lee *et al.*, 1994). Perhaps what occurs normally is that the glucocorticoids, by increasing CRH gene expression, increase the likelihood that something will be perceived as a threat, which results in a startle response. Thus, a dose of CRH, given intraventricularly, did not produce a startle response, but when the adrenal intact rats were maintained at high levels of corticosterone for several days prior to the CRH injection, the same dose did produce a startle response.

Implants of corticosterone directly into the amygdala of rats increased CRH expression in the CeA and reduced their open field exploratory behavior (Shepard *et al.*, 2000). Typically, rats initially are hesitant to explore new environments, and the induction of CRH in the CeA following corticosterone delivery to the amygdala exacerbated this characteristic. In addition, corticosterone implants directly into the CeA increased levels of CRH expression in the parvocellular region of the PVN of the hypothalamus (Shepard *et al.*, 2003).

An important study further demonstrated that the CRH response in the amygdala of sheep to a natural (dog) and unnatural (footshock) stressor is regulated by glucocorticoids (Cook, 2002). Following acute exposure to a dog for 6 min, both venous and amygdala levels of cortisol increased after 10–30 min. Amygdala CRH had a large increase during exposure to the dog and a second peak 10–30 min later corresponding to the increase in cortisol. Similar dual peaks of CRH release also were found with footshock. Administration of a glucocorticoid receptor antagonist blocked the second CRH peak in the amygdala without affecting the first peak. These data indicate that the initial response of CRH in the amygdala to an acute fearful stimulus is independent of cortisol, but the second delayed peak is cortisol dependent. In addition, and most interesting, the initial CRH response to a stressor following repeated inescapable exposure to the dog came under the control of cortisol. Sheep were given 7 days of repeated exposure to the dog, either with the ability to escape or not to escape from the dog. On the eighth day, the sheep were given a footshock. While venous and amygdala cortisol levels in response to the footshock were identical in escape and non-escape groups, both peaks of CRH release in the amygdala were higher in the repeated non-escape group compared to the escape group and became regulated by cortisol (Figure 8.8).

We interpret these findings to indicate that during normal acute danger, CRH in the amygdala increases rapidly to participate in mounting fear responses. This response is similar to effects of exogenously applied CRH and is not under the control of glucocorticoids. However, with repeated stress, glucocorticoids sensitize the

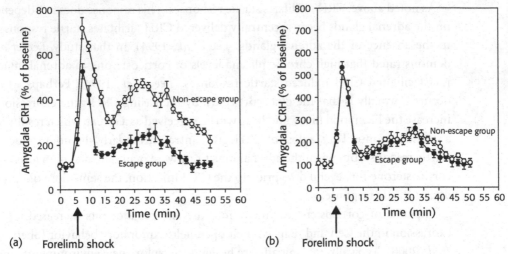

Figure 8.8   Facilitated CRH response in the amygdala of sheep to a stressor (footshock) following inescapable exposure to a dog is blocked by a glucocorticoid receptor antagonist. (a) The CRH (collected by microdialysis) in the amygdala of sheep exposed to a footshock is greater following inescapable experience with dog, and (b) Mifepristone, a glucocorticoid receptor antagonist, blocks the effects of inescapable exposure to a dog. Adapted from Cook (2002)

amygdala CRH cells so they release exaggerated amounts of CRH to the adverse event. The psychological stressor of inescapable, repeated danger produces an up-regulation of the CRH amygdala system. Taken together with other experimental data, these results demonstrate that high levels of glucocorticoids increase CRH mRNA expression in the CeA (Swanson and Simmons, 1989; Makino *et al.*, 1994a, b; Watts and Sanchez-Watts, 1995; Thompson *et al.*, 2004).

The CRH receptors within the amygdala are largely found in the lateral but not in the central region of the amygdala; the central nucleus produces the peptide, the lateral region contains the receptors (e.g. Makino *et al.*, 1995; Behan *et al.*, 1996). It should be noted that the basal lateral region of the amygdala is essential for most forms of fear (Le Doux, 2000).

CRH in the central nucleus is produced under diverse conditions; CRH receptor antagonists decrease the behavioral effects of CRH production in the CeA (Roozendaal *et al.*, 2002). The basal lateral region is importantly involved in memory consolidation of aversive events. Infusion of glucocorticoids into this region of the amygdala facilitates the memory of aversive events. CRH type I (see below) receptor blocker infusions into the basal lateral region reduce the expression of the aversive memory and CRH gene expression in the CeA (Roozendaal *et al.*, 2002). Thus, the effect of cortisol on memory consolidation may perhaps affect CRH gene expression in the CeA, or elsewhere in the brain (e.g. lateral bed nucleus of the stria terminalis).

Part 3 Glucocorticoids and postnatal development

There appear to be both pre- and postnatal critical periods in development, and these critical periods differ among the species. In some species (e.g. rats), the sensitivity to glucocorticoids and the regulation of the HPA axis varies with age (Levine, 1975; 2000; Levine et al., 2000). Alteration of corticosterone levels during critical stages of postnatal development has effects on behavior. For example, rats deprived of corticosterone between 10 and 14 days post partum do not express the normal fear of unfamiliar objects; infusion of corticosterone either systemically or centrally restores or facilitates the behavioral responses (Takahashi and Kim, 1994). Perhaps this occurs via the induction of CRH gene expression in the brain. However, excessive CRH injections in neonatal rats resulted in compromised brain function and vulnerability to diverse forms of behavioral dysfunction (Brunson et al., 2001).

Indeed, early life events have long-term consequences for both brain and behavior and alter CRH expression in the brain (Meaney et al., 1993; Levine, 2000). For example, adult rats, deprived of maternal closeness for 3 h a day for a 2-week period as pups, were found to have higher levels of CRH mRNA expression in the PVN, CeA and the lateral bed nucleus of the stria terminalis as adults than those separated for only 15 min a day (Plotsky, 1996; Levine, 2000). These maternal-deprived rats were also more likely to develop helpless behavior in uncontrollable aversive contexts suggesting that these rats were excessively stressed or fearful. Interestingly, their systemic levels of corticosterone as adults were not different from normal rats, but the central state of exaggerated fear induced by the early experience was long-lasting.

Infant monkeys reared by mothers experiencing unpredictable foraging conditions had higher CRH in cerebrospinal fluid (CSF) in adulthood than infant monkeys reared by mothers that had either a predictable overabundance or a predictable scarcity of food. The studies show that unpredictability in early life, and not just chronic hardship, is associated with persistently higher CRH levels in the CSF in adulthood, up to 5 years later (Coplan et al., 2001). Perhaps the induction of CRH gene expression by cortisol partially explains why this occurs.

The lateral bed nucleus of the stria terminalis, a region of the brain rich in CRH cell bodies (Swanson and Simmons, 1989; Makino et al., 1994a, b; Watts and Sanchez-Watts, 1995), has been linked to general anxiety (Davis et al., 1997). Infusing CRH in this region potentiates anxious arousal (Davis et al., 1997). Importantly, glucocorticoids are known to facilitate increases in CRH gene expression in the lateral region of the bed nucleus of the stria terminalis (Makino et al.,

1994a, b; Watts and Sanchez-Watts, 1995). The bed nucleus might be considered the primary central ganglia of the PVN; it massively projects and is known to regulate CRH PVN release (Herman and Cullinan, 1997). Moreover, the central nucleus and other regions of the amygdala have access to the PVN largely through the amygdala innervation of the bed nucleus of the stria terminalis (Herman *et al.*, 2003). Therefore, perhaps the induction of CRH during these environmental events contributes to the sense of unease, the exaggerated sense of arousal, alertness, and uncertainty in the animal.

Temperamental shyness, cortisol, and CRH

Kagan and his colleagues have been instrumental in describing the origins and developmental course of temperamental shyness in children over the last two decades. More specifically, Kagan's group has been interested in variations in normal children's reactions to novelty. Kagan's group has noted that a subset of normally developing infants and children (5–10%) exhibit extreme fear and wariness to the presentation of novel social and nonsocial stimuli, and this subset can be described as behaviorally inhibited. Kagan *et al.* (1987; 1988) speculated that individual differences in infant reactivity to novelty may be linked to sensitivity in forebrain circuits involved in the processing and regulation of emotion, and they argued that children who become easily distressed and subdued during the presentation of novel stimuli may have a lower threshold for arousal in forebrain areas, particularly the CeA. This hypothesis is based largely on findings from studies of animals in which the amygdala plays an important role in the regulation and maintenance of conditioned fear, as noted above.

Conceptually, shyness in humans might reflect a preoccupation with the self in response to real or imagined social encounters (Kagan *et al.*, 1988; Schmidt and Schulkin, 1999). Although a large percentage (90%) of the population has reported experiencing shyness at some point in their lives, a smaller percentage (5–10%) of individuals are characterized by temperamental or dispositional shyness. Temperamental shyness is an early emerging form of shyness that is linked to early infant reactions to novelty, associated with a number of distinct psychophysiological responses at rest and in response to social stress, remains modestly preserved through the young adult years, and is predictive of social and emotional difficulties.

Preschool-aged children with temperamental shyness generally have increased levels of cortisol (Kagan *et al.*, 1988; Gunnar *et al.*, 1989; Schmidt *et al.*, 1997; Figure 8.9(a)). They are more fearful in response to novel social events. It was suggested some time ago that this exaggerated fear might reflect a 'hyperactive amygdala' (Kagan *et al.*, 1988; see also Rosen and Schulkin, 1998). Children at 21 months of age were assessed as having an inhibited or uninhibited temperament, and

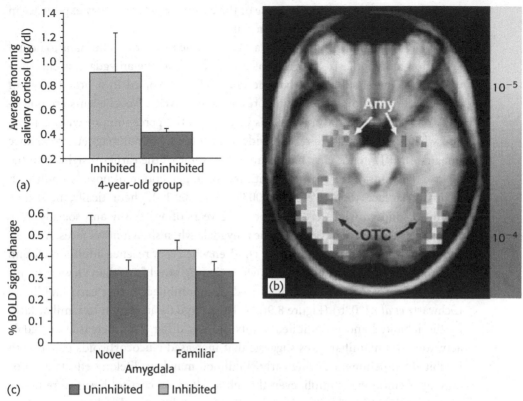

Figure 8.9   (a) Levels of cortisol in children that were determined to be shy and wary. Adapted from Schmidt *et al.* (1997), (b) Colorized group statistical map superimposed on coronal group averaged T1 structural image in Talairach space. Significant fMRI signal changes (arrows) are shown in the right (peak *P* value = 2.5 × 10^{-5}; Talairach coordinates *x, y, z* = 21, −6.5, −14) and left (*P* = 4.2 × 10^{-4}; *x, y, z* = −21.5, −6.7, −18) amygdalae (Amy) and occipito-temporal cortex (OTC), and (c) Percent (%) blood oxygenation level-dependent (BOLD) signal change (versus fixation) in Amy to novel versus familiar faces in adult subjects who were inhibited and uninhibited in the second year of life. One standard error of the mean is indicated. Adapted from Schwartz *et al.* (2003a)

behavioral and physiological assessments of these children at 5½ years of age suggested that cortisol levels were discriminative between the two temperamental extremes. Additionally, at 7½ years of age, those described as shy and timid in the initial assessment were quiet and socially avoidant in novel social situations suggesting that this temperamental category is stable over time (Kagan *et al.*, 1988). This has important health implications, as shy children with high levels of cortisol are vulnerable to allergic symptoms (Bell *et al.*, 1990; Kagan *et al.*, 1991), vascular disease (Bell *et al.*, 1993) and anxiety disorders (Van Ameringen *et al.*, 1998; Kagan and Snidman, 1999), perhaps because of the chronic worry that they experience in social contexts or in unfamiliar environments.

Linking behavioral, physiological, and endocrine measures in humans to neural activation in hypothesized regions of interest, such as the amygdala, is currently underway. One should note that the amygdala is involved in a broad array of behavioral regulation, including the response to novelty. Novel events are potentially dangerous, and the amygdala is involved in the perception of what is novel and what is familiar. More recent evidence, using functional magnetic resonance imaging (fMRI) in humans, has expanded on some of the earlier insights into the diverse functions of the amygdala with regard to perception of novel stimuli such as unfamiliar faces (Schwartz *et al.*, 2003a; Figure 8.9(b)). Theoretically, these same inhibited children who were described at 2 years of age as shy and socially wary should reveal greater activation of the amygdala when shown novel faces. A longitudinal study of these shy and fearful children when they reached adulthood found that amygdala activation was greater when viewing novel faces than viewing familiar faces, compared to those categorized as uninhibited during early childhood (Schwartz *et al.*, 2003b) (Figure 8.9(c)). The amygdala activation to familiar faces by the inhibited and uninhibited adults did not differ. The increased amygdala activation to unfamiliar faces suggests that increased glucocorticoids paired with inhibited temperament during early childhood may have lifelong effects on processing of emotional stimuli, even though at 7½ years cortisol levels were not as discriminating of the inhibited and uninhibited children as they had been during earlier assessments (Kagan *et al.*, 1988).

Prefrontal cortex and temperament, cortisol, and CRH

The prefrontal cortex is tied to temperamentally fearful and distressed infants and behaviorally inhibited toddlers; these children exhibit a pattern of greater relative right frontal electroencephalography (EEG) activation at rest and heightened startle responses to a stranger approach at 9 months of age (Schmidt *et al.*, 1997; 1999a). These temperamentally fearful and distressed infants who develop shyness later in childhood are also characterized by elevated basal and reactive salivary cortisol (Gunnar *et al.*, 1989; 1996).

The pattern of frontal brain activity and salivary cortisol responses in temperamentally shy children is preserved up through the school age years. For example, we have noted that children who were classified as extremely shy and socially wary at age 4 exhibited elevated morning salivary cortisol (Schmidt *et al.*, 1997) and greater relative right frontal EEG activation at rest (Schmidt *et al.*, 1997; Davidson and Rickman, 1999) compared with their socially outgoing counterparts. Temperamentally shy children also exhibit a greater increase in right, but not left, frontal EEG activity and heart rate in response to social challenge compared with their non-shy counterparts at age 7

(Schmidt *et al.*, 1999a) and they display a relatively lower decrease from baseline levels on salivary cortisol reactivity measures (Schmidt *et al.*, 1999a). Six-month-old human infants who show withdrawal behaviors displayed the same right-greater-than-left frontal activation and higher basal and reactive cortisol concentrations found in non-human primates (see below Buss *et al.*, 2003).

Turning to nonhuman primates, a subset of young rhesus monkeys can be characterized as anxious and fearful by observing their behavioral reactions to stressful situations. These monkeys freeze for longer periods of time than other rhesus monkeys not characterized by fearful behavioral responses and have high levels of cortisol (Champoux *et al.*, 1989). These characteristics can be induced in macaques by manipulating rearing conditions. When macaques are raised in an artificial environment with their peers, instead of in a more naturalistic environment with their parents and extended family, alterations in behaviors and in hormones like cortisol and CRH are observed. In adult rhesus monkeys, high levels of cortisol and high levels of CRH from the CSF are associated with behavioral inhibition (Habib *et al.*, 2000; Kalin *et al.*, 2000).

A subset of these macaques not only have higher levels of CRH and cortisol than other monkeys, but they also demonstrate greater fearful temperament and greater activation of the right hemisphere. Increased relative right hemisphere activation has been linked to withdrawal and negative perception of events (Davidson and Rickman, 1999; Kalin *et al.*, 2000). Differences in temperamental expression to a number of unconditioned fear-related stimuli may reflect frontal neocortical activation (Kalin *et al.*, 2001). Ibotenic acid lesions (cell body destroyed and fibers left intact) of the macaque amygdala left a number of unconditioned behavioral trait-like responses intact (Kalin *et al.*, 2001), in addition to the normal asymmetry associated with trait-like dispositions (Figure 8.10).

Much of the research on the role of prefrontal cortical regions in emotional behavior, affective experience and temperament, characterizes emotion into an approach and withdrawal dichotomy. EEG studies indicated that during reward and punishment paradigms, reward trials were associated with greater left hemisphere activation while punishment trials were associated with greater right hemisphere activation (Davidson, 2000). Extending these EEG findings, individual differences in baseline frontal lobe asymmetry suggested that greater right frontal activation might be associated with a more negative affective style, and vice versa with greater baseline left-than-right frontal activation. Frontal cortex responses to reward and punishment interact with underlying baseline asymmetries in activation (Davidson *et al.*, 1990). When these EEG recordings were performed with children, the generalization was upheld, showing that those children who displayed social competence had greater relative left frontal activation, while those who were characterized as withdrawn had greater right frontal activation (e.g. Schmidt *et al.*, 1997; 1999a). Greater

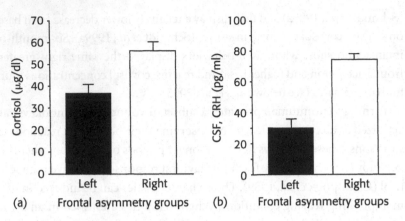

Figure 8.10 (a) Levels of systemic cortisol, and (b) CSF, CRH in left and right frontal brain activation in macaques who were more fearful, and demonstrated greater right prefrontal activation. Adapted from Kalin *et al.* (1998a; 2000)

right frontal electrical activity is stable over time in nonhuman primates, and is correlated with more defensive responses and elevated cortisol concentrations (Kalin *et al.*, 1998b). The CSF CRH concentrations are also elevated and stable over time in monkeys with extreme right frontal activation (Kalin *et al.*, 2000).

Interestingly, the medial prefrontal cortex (anterior cingulate) also plays a part in the glucocorticoid response to stress. When the cingulate is lesioned in rats, restraint stress leads to increased plasma ACTH and corticosterone levels, and corticosterone implants to the cingulate significantly decrease plasma corticosterone in response to stress (Diorio *et al.*, 1993; see also Sullivan and Gratton, 2002). However, these manipulations do not affect glucocorticoid levels in the absence of stress.

The prefrontal cortex is divisible into several functional areas, and the medial and orbital prefrontal (OMPFC) regions appear to be particularly important for emotional regulation (Davidson, 2000). The OMPFC is reciprocally connected to the amygdala (Amaral and Price, 1984), and in primates glucocorticoid receptors are distributed in the prefrontal cortex to a much greater extent than they are in rodents (Sanchez *et al.*, 2000). CRH receptors are expressed in this region of the brain, and postmortem studies in suicide patients who were diagnosed with severe depression indicated decreases in CRH receptor distribution (Nemeroff *et al.*, 1988). The following section discusses the implications of altered cortisol and CRH to increased vulnerability to psychiatric disorders.

Elevated cortisol, CRH, and vulnerability to affective disorders

Increased exposure to stress or uncertainty during early life may produce a vulnerability to developing affective disorders. Research on affective disorders such as depression and anxiety indicate neural activation and neuroendocrine patterns similar to those observed in those exposed to suboptimal conditions pre- or postnatal. However, when reviewing this literature, keep in mind that there is also a significant genetic contribution to the vulnerability to mood disorders. Therefore, those with genetic vulnerability may require little to no early exposure to environmental factors to develop psychiatric disorders, while others who are exceptionally resilient may experience extreme traumas early in life and emerge relatively unscathed.

Many investigators have found increased functional activity in the amygdala of patients with depression (Drevets et al., 2002). This increased amygdala activation correlated with negative affect in a sample of medication-free depressives (Abercrombie et al., 1998) and was also seen in patients suffering from a number of anxiety disorders (see Davis and Whalen, 2001). Prefrontal cortex activity is also correlated with anxiety and depression (Davidson, 2000). These effects are largely lateralized in both amygdala and prefrontal cortex (Davidson, 2000; Drevets et al., 2002). Often in depression, particularly in those with co-morbid anxiety (Gold et al., 1988), hypercortisolemia, hyperactivity in the HPA axis, and high levels of CRH in CSF are found (Nemeroff et al., 1984; Arborelius et al., 1999; Holsboer, 2000). Melancholic depressives (those with hyperarousal, fear, and anhedonia symptoms) reportedly show a positive correlation between abnormally high levels of cortisol and high but normal levels of CSF, CRH (Wong et al., 2000) indicating a lack of negative feedback control of CRH by cortisol. In addition to this apparent dysfunction of negative feedback in the HPA axis, elevated levels of cortisol may involve sustained hyperactivity in the amygdala via feed-forward processes. One study has found a significant positive correlation ($r = 0.69$) between glucose metabolism in the amygdala measured by [F-18]2-deoxy-2-fluoro-D-glucose (FDG) positron emission tomography (PET) and plasma cortisol levels in both unipolar and bipolar depressives (Drevets et al., 2002). There is now some evidence that cortisol infusions increase glucose metabolism in the amygdala (Erickson et al., unpublished). It is intriguing to speculate that the cause of first depressive episode in patients who also have enlarged amygdala (Frodl et al., 2002) may be increased chronic levels of glucocorticoids and blood flow in the amygdala (Figure 8.11).

Although the research has developed along two separate paths, activity in the amygdala in a number of different anxiety disorders has been shown to be highly reactive to triggers that evoke anxious reactions (Davis and Whalen, 2001), and the HPA axis is hyper-responsive in anxiety disorders, particularly post-traumatic stress disorder (PTSD) (Mason et al., 1988; Yehuda et al., 1991; Yehuda, 2002). PTSD patients tend to have lower basal hypocortisolemia than normals (Mason et al., 1988; Yehuda, 2002), though not always, but increased reactivity of the HPA axis to cortisol, suggesting that CRH- and ACTH-secreting cells are sensitized to

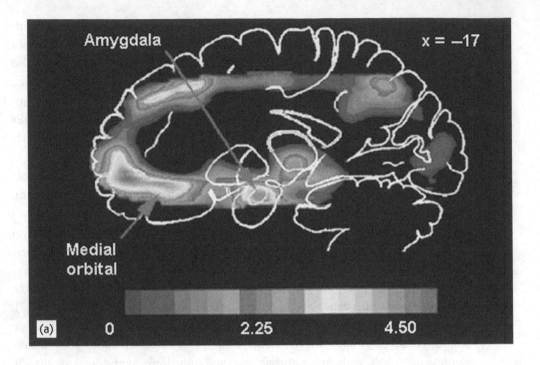

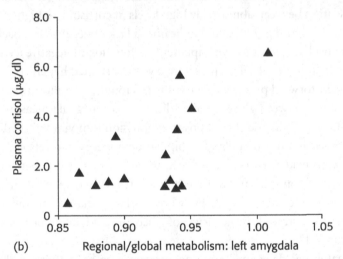

Figure 8.11 Amygdala and prefrontal cortex activation in depression. (a) Areas of abnormally increased CBF in familial major depressive disorder (MDD). Analyses show areas of increased CBF in depressed patients relative to controls in the amygdala and medial orbital cortex. Anterior is to the left, and (b) Relationship between plasma cortisol concentrations measured immediately prior to the PET radiotracer injection and normalized glucose metabolism in the left amygdala for an MDD sample ($n = 15$). Adapted from Drevets *et al.* (2002)

cortisol in PTSD patients (Yehuda, 2002). Indeed, CRH has been found to be elevated in CSF of PTSD patients (Bremner *et al.*, 1997; Baker *et al.*, 2001). Individuals with generalized social phobia, another type of anxiety disorder, hyper-secreted cortisol during a public performance involving a mental arithmetic test (Condren *et al.*, 2002). The amygdala research demonstrates a similar phenomenon. PTSD and social phobic patients have normal resting (non-provoked) levels of amygdala activity, but the amygdala is highly responsive to anxiety provocation (Rauch *et al.*, 1996; Shin *et al.*, 1997; Schneider *et al.*, 1999; Rauch *et al.*, 2000).

Finally, behavioral inhibition in childhood, characterized by increased cortisol levels and right frontal EEG recordings, is associated with increased risk for anxiety disorders in adulthood (e.g. Schmidt *et al.*, 1997; 1999a, b; Rosenbaum *et al.*, 2000; Biederman *et al.*, 2001; Buss *et al.*, 2003). Behavioral inhibition is more likely to manifest in children whose parents are diagnosed with social phobia and depression (Rosenbaum *et al.*, 2000). In addition, there is evidence that infants of mothers with mood and anxiety disorders show neural characteristics different from those of psychiatrically healthy mothers in the absence of overt behavioral differences. For example, infants of mothers with panic disorder show elevated salivary cortisol and disturbed sleep although they did not show higher behavioral reactivity, behavioral inhibition, or ambivalent or resistant attachment to the mothers. The neurophysiological differences observed in these infants might be important early indicators of risk (Warren *et al.*, 2003).

Conclusions

Glucocorticoids have both permissive, suppressive and stimulatory effects on diverse end organ systems (Sapolsky, 2000). Most well known are the suppressive effects, particularly at the level of the PVN projections to the pituitary gland. Less well known are the stimulatory effects on diverse tissue with regard to CRH in the placenta and in several regions of the brain, particularly those regions involved in emotional behavior and emotional regulation. Chronic exposure to stress or stressful situations results in increased glucocorticoid concentrations and the facilitation of CRH gene expression in these regions (Schulkin *et al.*, 1998; Dallman *et al.*, 2003). Animals that have higher levels of glucocorticoids as a result of selective breeding or through glucocorticoid infusions tend to act more fearful (Jones *et al.*, 1992). Glucocorticoids are secreted in diverse events that require the expenditure of energy (Dallman *et al.*, 2003). While glucocorticoids are certainly not the molecules of fear and anxiety, they are associated with fear, anxiety, and trauma – all of which are metabolically demanding events.

In the human placenta, while not definitely demonstrated, one function of glucocorticoids in normal pregnancy is to make CRH available to promote the timing of parturition; this process can be accelerated, perhaps as the result of adverse environmental conditions. Chronic alterations of CRH by diverse events, including nutritional needs, hypertension and psychosocial stress (e.g. Hobel *et al.*, 1999), can render women vulnerable to low-birth-weight infants and preterm delivery of their offspring. Glucocorticoids are also increased, and exposure to elevated glucocorticoids prenatally can alter amygdala development by increasing CRH expression in the CeA (Welberg *et al.*, 2000). This suggests potential lifelong consequences and vulnerabilities resulting from prenatal glucocorticoid exposure. In extra-hypothalamic sites in the brain that underlie the behavioral regulation of fear, CRH plays an important role in the fear response, and glucocorticoids play an important role in sustaining fear-related behavioral responses. High cortisol levels, due to genetic and/or early environmental factors, may induce long-lasting hyper-excitability in central CRH gene expression. Elevated levels of CRH are tied to increased salience of environmental stimuli (Merali *et al.*, 2003) which can result in hypervigilance and a vulnerability for exaggerated fear responses. Interestingly, CRH type I receptor antagonists delay early parturition in sheep (Chan *et al.*, 1998) and can reduce fear-related behavioral responses in macaques and rats (Deak *et al.*, 1999; Habib *et al.*, 2000), indicating another link between placental and amygdala CRH.

The neural circuit that includes the amygdala, bed nucleus of the stria terminalis and regions of the prefrontal cortex contributes to the behavioral regulation of emotional responses, particularly fear. The CRH induction by glucocorticoids may underlie the fear responses. The CRH has been localized in regions of the prefrontal cortex, and glucocorticoids may regulate CRH in this region (Swanson, personal communication; unpublished observations) in addition to the amygdala and bed nucleus of the stria terminalis.

Corticotropin-releasing gene expression can also be altered by postnatal events (e.g. Brunson *et al.*, 2001). Diverse experiments have suggested that glucocorticoids are important in adapting to fearful events, and the susceptibility of HPA and extra-hypothalamic regions to alterations during early life may be evolutionarily adaptive. In nonhuman primates, exposure to variable foraging conditions has long-term effects on neuroendocrine systems (Coplan *et al.*, 2001), and macaques raised by peers instead of by their mothers also show long-term changes in behavioral and neuroendocrine responses to stress. These alterations are maladaptive in humans, and may create increased vulnerability to psychiatric disorders.

Fear of unfamiliar objects is a basic adaptation, perhaps exaggerated in vulnerable individuals who have been shown to have higher levels of glucocorticoids (which has been demonstrated in a number of species, (Kagan *et al.*, 1988; Cavigelli and McClintock, 2003)). Heightened levels of arousal and fear responses to strangers and novel situations found in shy human infants also persist at least into later child-hood. These children can have exaggerated cortisol and autonomic physiological responses (Kagan *et al.*, 1988; Gunnar *et al.*, 1996; Schmidt *et al.*, 1997). Indeed, excessively shy children display both exaggerated startle responses and high salivary cortisol levels (Schmidt *et al.*, 1997). Temperamental shyness is also associated with increased amygdala and right frontal activation (e.g. Schmidt *et al.*, 1997; Davidson *et al.*, 2003). In addition, extremely shy, socially withdrawn children may be vulner-able to anxiety disorders and perhaps to depression throughout their lives (Hirshfeld *et al.*, 1992; Schwartz *et al.*, 1999). The induction of CRH gene expression by glucocorticoids may contribute to the central state that underlies fear- and anxiety-related behavioral responses. These events, namely the induction of elevated levels of CRH gene expression, are adaptive in the short term; in the long run (both from prenatal and postnatal events), they may result in long-term aberrations in CRH gene expression and vulnerability to excessive anxious behaviors.

REFERENCES

Abercrombie, H. C., Schaefer, S. M. *et al.* (1998). Metabolic rate in the right amygdala predicts negative affect in depressed patients. *Neuroreport*, 9(14), 3301–7.

Amaral, D. G. and Price, J. L. (1984). Amygdalo-cortical projections in the monkey (*Macaca fascicularis*). *J. Comp. Neurol.*, 230, 465–96.

Arborelius, L., Owens, M. J. *et al.* (1999). The role of corticotropin-releasing factor in depression and anxiety disorders. *J. Endocrinol.*, 160(1), 1–12.

Baker, D. G., West, S. A., Nicholson, W. E. *et al.* (1999). Serial CSF corticotropin-releasing hormone levels and adrenocortical activity in combat veterans with posttraumatic stress disorder. *Am. J. Psychiatr.*, 156, 585–8.

Barker, D. J. (1997). The fetal origins of coronary heart disease. *Acta Paediatr. Suppl.*, 422, 78–82.

Behan, D. P., Grigoridalis, D. E., Lovenberg, T. *et al.* (1996). Neurobiology of corticotropin releasing factor (CRF) receptors and CRF-binding protein: implications for the treatment of CNS disorders. *Mol. Psychiatr.*, 1, 265–77.

Bell, I. R., Jasnoski, M. L., Kagan, J. and King, D. S. (1990). Is allergic rhinitis more frequent in young adults with extreme shyness? A preliminary study. *Psychosom. Med.*, 52, 517–25.

Bell, I. R., Martino, G. M., Meredith, K. E. *et al.* (1993). Vascular disease risk factors, urinary free cortisol, and health histories in older adults: shyness and gender interactions. *Biol. Psychol.*, 35, 37–49.

Biederman, J., Hirshfeld-Becker, D. R. *et al.* (2001). Further evidence of association between behavioral inhibition and social anxiety in children. *Am. J. Psychiatr.*, 158(10), 1673–9.

Breier, A. (1989). Experimental approaches to human stress research: assessment of neurobiological mechanisms of stress in volunteers and psychiatric patients. *Biol. Psychiatr.*, 26, 438–62.

Bremner, J. D., Innis, R. B. *et al.* (1997). Positron emission tomography measurement of cerebral metabolic correlates of yohimbine administration in combat-related posttraumatic stress disorder. *Arch. Gen. Psychiatr.*, **54**(3), 246–54.

Bremner, J. D., Licinio, J. *et al.* (1997). Elevated CSF corticotropin-releasing factor concentrations in posttraumatic stress disorder. *Am. J. Psychiatr.*, **154**(5), 624–9.

Brunson, K. L., Avishai-Eliner, S. *et al.* (2001). Neurobiology of the stress response early in life: evolution of a concept and the role of corticotropin releasing hormone. *Mol. Psychiatr.*, **6**(6), 647–56.

Buitelaar, J. K., Huizink, A. C., Mulder, E. J., deMedina, P. G. and Visser, G. H. (2003). Prenatal stress and cognitive development and temperament in infants. *Neurobiol. Aging*, **24**, 67–8.

Buss, K. A., Schumbacher Malmstadt, J. R. and Dolski, I. (2003). Right frontal brain activity, cortisol and withdrawal behavior in 6-month old infants. *Behav. Neurosci.*, **117**, 17–30.

Cavigelli, S. A. and McClintock, M. L. (2003). Fear of novelty in infant rats predicts adult corticosterone dynamics and an early death. *Proc. Natl. Acad. Sci. USA* (in press).

Challis, J. R. (1995). CRH, a placental clock and preterm labour. *Nat. Med.*, **1**(5), 416.

Challis, J., Sloboda, D. *et al.* (2000). Fetal hypothalamic–pituitary adrenal (HPA) development and activation as a determinant of the timing of birth, and of postnatal disease. *Endocr. Res.*, **26**(4), 489–504.

Champoux, M. B. *et al.* (1989). Hormonal effects of early rearing conditions in infant rhesus monkeys. *Am. J. Primatol.*, **19**, 111–18.

Chan, E. C., Falconer, J., Madsen, G. *et al.* (1998). A corticotropin-releasing hormone type I receptor antagonist delays parturition in sheep. *Endocrinology*, **139**, 3357–60.

Cheng, Y. H., Nicholson, R. G., King, B. *et al.* (2000). Glucocorticoid stimulation of corticotropin releasing hormone gene expression requires cyclic adenosine 3′, 5′-monophosphate regulatory element in human primary placental cytrophoblast cells. *J. Clin. Endocrinol. Metab.*, **85**, 1937–46.

Cook, C. J. (2002). Glucocorticoid feedback increases sensitivity of the limbic system in stress. *Physiol. Behav.*, **75**, 456–64.

Coordimas, K. J., LeDoux, J. E., Gold, P. W. and Schulkin, J. (1994). Corticosterone potentiation of learned fear. In R. DeKloet, E. C. Azmita and P. W. Landfield, eds., *Brain Corticosteroid Receptor*, New York: Academic Press.

Coplan, J., Smith, E. *et al.* (2001). Variable foraging demand rearing: sustained elevations in cisternal cerebrospinal fluid corticotropin-releasing factor concentrations in adult primates. *Biol. Psychiatr.*, **50**(3), 200–4.

Dallman, M. F., Pecoraro, N., Akana, S. F. *et al.* (2003). Chronic stress and obesity: a new view of 'comfort food'. *Proc. Natl. Acad. Sci. USA*, **100**, 11696–701.

Davidson, R. (2000). Affective style, psychopathology and resilance: brain mechanisms and plasticity. *Am. Psychol.*, **55**, 1193–214.

Davidson, R. J. and Rickman, M. (1999). Behavioral inhibition and the emotional circuitry of the brain: stability and plasticity during the early childhood years. In L. A. Schmidt and J. Schulkin, eds., *Extreme Fear, Shyness, and Social Phobia*, New York: Oxford University Press.

Davidson, R. J., Ekman, P., Saron, C. D., Senulis, J. A. and Friesnen, W. V. (1990). Approach-withdrawal and cerebral asymmetry: emotional expression and brain physiology. *Int. J. Pers. Soc. Psychol.*, **58**, 330–41.

Davis, M. and Whalen P. J. (2001). The amygdala: vigilance and emotion. *Mol. Psychiatr.*, **6**(1), 13–34.

Davis, M., Walker, D. L. *et al.* (1997). Roles of the amygdala and bed nucleus of the stria terminalis in fear and anxiety measured with the acoustic startle reflex. Possible relevance to PTSD. *Ann. NY Acad. Sci.*, **821**, 305–31.

Deak, T., Nguyen, K. T., Ehrlich, A. L. *et al.* (1999). The impact of a non-peptide corticotropin-releasing hormone antagonist antalarmin on behavioral and endocrine response to stress. *Endocrinology*, **140**, 79–86.

De Kloet, E. R. (1991). Brain corticosteroid receptor balance and homeostatic control. *Front. Neuroendocrinol.*, **12**, 95–164.

Diorio, D., Viau, V. *et al.* (1993). The role of the medial prefrontal cortex (cingulate gyrus) in the regulation of hypothalamic–pituitary–adrenal responses to stress. *J. Neurosci.*, **13**(9), 3839–47.

Drevets, W. C., Price, J. L. *et al.* (2002). Glucose metabolism in the amygdala in depression: relationship to diagnostic subtype and plasma cortisol levels. *Pharmacol. Biochem. Behav.*, **71**(3), 431–47.

Erickson, K., Thorsen, P. *et al.* (2001). Preterm birth: associated neuroendocrine, medical, and behavioral risk factors. *J. Clin. Endocrinol. Metab.*, **86**(6), 2544–52.

French, N., Hagan, R., Evans, S. F. *et al.* (1999). Repeated antenatal corticosteroids: size at birth and subsequent development. *Am. J. Obstet. Gynecol.*, **180**, 114–21.

Frodl, T., Meisenzahl, E., Zetzsche, T. *et al.* (2002). Enlargement of the amygdala in patients with a first episode of major depression. *Biol. Psychiatry*, **51**(9), 708–14.

Glynn, L. M., Wadhwa, P. D., Dunkel-Schetter, C., Chicz-Demet, A. and Sandman, C. A. (2001). When stress happens matters: effects of earthquake timing on stress responsivity in pregnancy. *Am. J. Obstet. Gynecol.*, **184**, 637–42.

Goland, R. S., Wardlaw, S. L. *et al.* (1988). Biologically active corticotropin-releasing hormone in maternal and fetal plasma during pregnancy. *Am. J. Obstet. Gynecol.*, **159**(4), 884–90.

Goland, R. S., Jozak, S., Warren, W. B. *et al.* (1993). Elevated levels of umbilical cord plasma corticotropin-releasing hormone in growth-retarded fetuses. *J. Clin. Endocrinol. Metab.*, **77**, 1174–9.

Goland, R. S., Tropper, P. J., Warren, W. B. *et al.* (1995). Concentrations of corticotropin-releasing hormone in the umbilical cord blood of pregnancies complicated by pre-eclampsia. *Reprod. Fertil. Develop.*, **7**, 1227–30.

Gold, P. W., Goodwin, F. K. and Chrousos, G. P. (1988). Clinical and biochemical manifestation of depression: relation to the neurobiology of stress (part 2 of 2 parts). *New England Journal of Medicine*, **319**, 348–53.

Gunnar, M. R., Mangelsdorf, S., Larson, M. and Hertsgaard, L. (1989). Attachment, temperament, and adrenocortical activity in infancy: a study of psychoendocrine regulation. *Develop. Psychol.*, **25**, 355–63.

Gunnar, M. R., Brodersen, L. *et al.* (1996). Stress reactivity and attachment security. *Develop. Psychobiol.*, **29**(3), 191–204.

Habib, K. E., Weld, K. P., Schulkin, J. *et al.* (1999). Cerebrospinal fluid levels of corticotropin-releasing hormone positively correlate with acute and chronic social stress in non-human primates. *Presented at Society for Neuroscience Annual Meeting*, Miami Beach: Florida.

Habib, K. E., Weld, K. P., Rice, K. C. *et al.* (2000). Oral administration of a corticotropin-releasing hormone receptor antagonist significantly attenuates behavioral, neuroendocrine, and autonomic responses to stress in primates. *Proc. Natl. Acad. Sci. USA*, **97**, 6079–84.

Heim, C. and Nemeroff, C. B. (2002). Neurobiology of early life stress: clinical studies. *Semin. Clin. Neuropsychiat.*, **7**(2), 147–59.

Herman, J. P. and Cullinan W. E. (1997). Neurocircuitry of stress: central control of the hypothalamo–pituitary–adrenocortical axis. *Trend. Neurosci.*, **20**(2), 78–84.

Herman, J. P., Figueiredo, H., Mueller, N. K. *et al.* (2003). Central mechanisms of stress ingegration: hierarchical circuitry controlling hypothalamic–pituitary adrenocortical responsiveness. *Front. Neuroendocrinol.*, **24**, 151–80.

Hirshfeld, D. R., Rosenbaum, J. F. *et al.* (1992). Stable behavioral inhibition and its association with anxiety disorder. *J. Am. Acad. Child Adolesc. Psychiatr.*, **31**(1), 103–11.

Hobel, C. J., Dunkel-Schetter, C., Roesch, S. C., Castro, L. C. and Arora, C. P. (1999). Maternal plasma corticotropin-releasing hormone associated with stress at 20 weeks' gestation in pregnancies ending in preterm delivery. *Am. J. Obstet. Gynecol.*, **180**, S257–63.

Holsboer, F. (2000). The corticosteroid receptor hypothesis of depression. *Neuropsychopharmacology*, **23**(5), 477–501.

Huiink, A. C., de Medina, P. G., Mulder, E. J., Visser, G. H. and Buitelaar, J. K. (2002). Psychological measures of prenatal stress as predictors of infant temperament. *J. Am. Acad. Child Adolesc. Psychiatr.*, **41**, 1078–85.

Jones, S. A., Brooks, A. N. and Challis, J. R. G. (1989). Steroids modulate corticotropin-releasing hormone production in human fetal membranes and placenta. *Clin. Endocrinol. Metab.*, **68**, 825–30.

Jones, R. B., Satterlee, D. G. and Ryder, F. H. (1992). Fear and distress in Japanese quail chicks of two lines genetically selected for low or high adrenocortical response to immobilization stress. *Horm. Behav.*, **26**, 385–93.

Kagan, J. and Snidman, N. (1999). Early childhood predictors of adult anxiety disorders. *Biol. Psychiatr.*, **46**, 1536–41.

Kagan, J., Reznick, J. S. *et al.* (1987). The physiology and psychology of behavioral inhibition in children. *Child Develop.*, **58**(6), 1459–73.

Kagan, J., Resnick, J. S. and Snidman, N. (1988). Biological bases of childhood shyness. *Science*, **240**, 167–71.

Kagan, J., Snidman, N., Julia-Sellers, M. and Johnson, M. O. (1991). Temperament and allergic symptoms. *Psychom. Med.*, **53**, 332–40.

Kalin, N. H., Takahashi, L. K. and Chen, F. L. (1994). Restraint stress increases corticotropin releasing hormone mRNA content in the amygdala and the paraventricular nucleus. *Brain Res.*, **656**, 182–6.

Kalin, N. H., Larson, C., Shelton, S. E. and Davidson, R. J. (1998a). Asymmetric frontal brain activity, cortisol, and behavior associated with fearful temperament in rhesus monkeys. *Behav. Neurosci.*, **112**, 286–92.

Kalin, N. H., Shelton, S. E., Rickman, M. and Davidson, R. J. (1998b). Individual differences in freezing and cortisol in infant and mother rhesus monkeys. *Behav. Neurosci.*, **112**, 251–4.

Kalin, N. H., Shelton, S. E. and Davidson, R. J. (2000). Cerebrospinal fluid corticotropin-releasing hormone levels are elevated in monkeys with patterns of brain activity associated with fearful temperament. *Biol. Psychiatr.*, **47**, 579–85.

Kalin, N. H., Shelton, S. E., Davidson, R. J. and Kelley, A. E. (2001). The primate amygdala mediates acute fear but not the behavioral and physiological components of anxious temperament. *J. Neurosci.*, **21**, 2067–74.

Koob, G. F. *et al.* (1993). The role of corticotropin releasing hormone in behavioral responses to stress. In K. Chadwick, J. Marshj and K. Ackrill, eds., *Corticotropin Releasing Factor*, New York: Wiley.

Korebrits, C., Ramirez, M. M. *et al.* (1998). Maternal corticotropin-releasing hormone is increased with impending preterm birth. *J. Clin. Endocrinol. Metab.*, **83**(5), 1585–91.

Korte, S. M. (2001). Corticosteroids in relation to fear, anxiety and psychopathology. *Neurosci. Biobehav. Rev.*, **25**, 117–42.

Le Doux, J. E. (2000). Emotion circuits in the brain. *Annu. Rev. Neurosci.*, **23**, 155–84.

Lee, Y., Schulkin, J. and Davis, M. (1994). Effect of corticosterone on the enhancement of the acoustic startle reflex by corticotropin releasing hormone. *Brain Res.*, **666**, 93–8.

Levine, S. (1975). Psychosocial factors in growth and development. In L. Levi, ed., *Society, Stress, and Disease*, London: Oxford University Press.

Levine, S. (2000). Modulation of CRF gene expression by early experience. *Neuropsychopharmacology*, **23**, S77.

Levine, S., Dent, G. and De Kloet, E. R. (2000). Stress-hyporesponsive period. *Encylop. Stress*, **3**, 518–26.

Liang, K. C., Melia, K. R., Campeau, S. *et al.* (1992). Lesions of the central nucleus of the amygdala but not the paraventricular nucleus of the hypothalamus block the excitatory effects of corticotropin-releasing factor on the acoustic startle response. *J. Neurosci.*, **19**, 2313–20.

Majzoub, J. A., McGregor J. A. *et al.* (1999). A central theory of preterm and term labor: putative role for corticotropin-releasing hormone. *Am. J. Obstet. Gynecol.*, **180**(1 Pt 3), S232–41.

Makino, S., Gold, P. W. and Schulkin, J. (1994a). Corticosterone effects on corticotropin-releasing hormone mRNA in the central nucleus of the amygdala and the parvocellular region of the paraventricular nucleus of the hypothalamus. *Brain Res.*, **640**(1–2), 105–12.

Makino, S., Gold, P. W. and Schulkin, J. (1994b). Effects of corticosterone on CRH mRNA and content in the bed nucleus of the stria terminalis; comparison with the effects in the central nucleus of the amygdala and the paraventricular nucleus of the hypothalamus. *Brain Res.*, **657**(1–2), 141–9.

Makino, S., Schulkin, J., Smith, M. A. *et al.* (1995). Regulation of corticotropin-releasing hormone receptor messenger ribonucleic acid in the rat brain and pituitary by glucocorticoids and stress. *Endocrinology*, **136**, 4517–25.

Marinoni, E., Korebrits, C., Di Iorio, R., Cosmi, E. V. and Challis, J. R. (1998). Effect of betamethasone in vivo on placental corticotropin-releasing hormone in human pregnancy. *Am. J. Obstet. Gynecol.*, **178**, 770–8.

Mason, J. W. (1975). Emotions as reflected as patterns of endocrine integration. In L. Levi, ed., *Emotions: Their Parameters and Measurements*, New York: Raven Press.

Mason, J. W., Giller, E. L. *et al.* (1988). Elevation of urinary norepinephrine/cortisol ratio in posttraumatic stress disorder. *J. Nerv. Ment. Dis.*, **176**(8), 498–502.

McEwen, B. S. (2004). Protection and damaging effects on the mediators of stress adaptation: allostasis and allostatic load. In J. Schulkin, ed., *Allostasis, Homeostasis and the Costs of Physiological Adaptation*, Cambridge: Cambridge University Press.

Meaney, M. J., Bhatucgar, S., Larocque, S. *et al.* (1993). Individual differences in the hypothalamic pituitary adrenal stress response and the hypothalamic CRF system. *Ann. NY Acad. Sci.*, **697**, 70–85.

Meis, P. J., Kiebanoff, M., Thom, E. *et al.* (2003). Prevention of recurrent preterm delivery by 17 alpha-hydroxyprogesterone caproate. *New Engl. J. Med.*, **348**, 2379–455.

Merali, Z., Michaud, D., McIntosh, J., Kent, P. and Anisman, H. (2003). Differential involvement of amygdaloid CRH systems in the salence and valence of the stimuli. *Progr. Neuropsychopharmacol. Biol. Psychiatr.*, **27**, 1201–12.

Nemeroff, C. B., Widerlöv, E., Bissette, G. *et al.* (1984). Elevated concentrations of CSF corticotropin releasing factor-like immunoreactivity in depressed outpatients. *Science*, **26**, 1342–4.

Nemeroff, C. B., Owens, M. J., Bissette, G., Andorn, A. C. and Stanley, M. (1988). Reduced corticotropin-releasing factor binding sites in the frontal cortex of suicide victims. *Arch. Gen. Psychiatr.*, **45**, 577–9.

Nemeroff, C. B., Krishnan, K. R., Reed, D. *et al.* (1992). Adrenal gland enlargement in major depression: a computed tomographic study. *Arch. Gen. Psychiatr.*, **49**, 384–7.

Palkovits, M., Brownstein, M. J. and Vale, W. (1983). Corticotropin releasing hormone immunoreactivity in hypothalamus and extrahypothalamic nuclei of sheep brain. *Neuroendocrinology*, **37**, 302–5.

Petraglia, F., Volpe, A., Genazzani, A. R. *et al.* (1990). Neuroendocrinology of the human placenta. *Front. Neuroendocrinol.*, **11**, 6–37.

Petraglia, F., Aguzzoli, L., Florio, P. *et al.* (1995). Maternal plasma and placental immunoreactive corticotropin-releasing factor concentrations in infection-associated term and pre-term delivery. *Placenta*, **16l**, 157–64.

Plotsky, P. M. (1996). Early environmental regulation of forebrain glucocorticoid receptor gene expression: implications for adrenocortical responses to stress. *Develop. Neurosci.*, **18**, 49–72.

Pugh, C. R., Tremblay, D., Fleshner, M. and Rudy, J. W. (1997). A selective role for corticosterone in fear conditioning. *Behav. Neurosci.*, **111**, S303–11.

Rauch, S. L., van der Kolk, B. A. *et al.* (1996). A symptom provocation study of posttraumatic stress disorder using positron emission tomography and script-driven imagery. *Arch. Gen. Psychiatr.*, **53**(5), 380–7.

Rauch, S. L., Whalen, P. J. *et al.* (2000). Exaggerated amygdala response to masked facial stimuli in posttraumatic stress disorder: a functional MRI study. *Biol. Psychiatr.*, **47**(9), 769–76.

Richter, C. P. (1949). Domestication of the norway rat and its implications for the problem of stress. *Proc. Assoc. Res. Nerv. Ment. Dis.*, **29**, 19–30.

Robinson, B. G., Emanuel, R. L. *et al.* (1988). Glucocorticoid stimulates expression of corticotropin-releasing hormone gene in human placenta. *Proc. Natl. Acad. Sci. USA*, **85**(14), 5244–8.

Roozendaal, B., Brunson, K. L., Holloway, B. L., McGaugh, J. L. and Baram, T. Z. (2002). Involvement of stress-released corticotropin-releasing hormone in the basolateral amygdala in regulating memory consolidation. *Proc. Natl. Acad. Sci.*, **99**, 13908–13.

Rosen, J. B. and Schulkin, J. (1998). From normal fear to pathological anxiety. *Psychol. Rev.*, **105**, 325–50.

Rosenbaum, J. F., Biederman, J. *et al.* (2000). A controlled study of behavioral inhibition in children of parents with panic disorder and depression. *Am. J. Psychiatr.*, **157**(12), 2002–10.

Sachar, E. J., Hellman, L., Fukushima, d. K. and Gallagher, T. F. (1970). Cortisol production in depressive illness: a clinical and biochemical clarification. *Arch. Gen. Psychiatr.*, **23**, 289–98.

Sanchez, M. M., Young, L. J., Plotsky, P. M. and Insel, T. R. (2000). Distribution of corticosteroid receptors in the rhesus brain: relative absence of glucocorticoid receptors in the hippocampal formation. *J. Neurosci.*, **20**, 4657–68.

Sandman, C. A., Wadhwa, P. D., Chicz-DeMet, A., Porto, M. and Garite, T. J. (1999). Maternal corticotropin-releasing hormone and habituation in the human fetus. *Develop. Psychobiol.*, **34**, 163–73.

Sapolsky, R. M. (2000). Glucocorticoids and hippocampal atrophy in neuropsychiatric disorders. *Archiv. of Gen. Psychiatr.*, **57**, 925–35.

Schmidt, L. A. and Schulkin, J. (1999). *Extreme Fear, Shyness and Social Phobia*, Oxford: Oxford University Press.

Schmidt, L. A., Fox, N. A., Rubin, K. J. *et al.* (1997). Behavioral and neuroendocrine responses in shy children. *Develop. Psychobiol.*, **30**, 127–40.

Schmidt, L. A., Fox, N. A., Schulkin, J. and Gold, P. W. (1999a). Behavioral and psychophysiological correlates of self-presentation in temperamentally shy children. *Develop. Psychobiol.*, **35**, 119–35.

Schmidt, L. A., Fox, N. A., Sternberg, E. M. *et al.* (1999b). Adrenocortical reactivity and social competence in seven year-olds. *Pers. Indiv. Differ.*, **26**, 977–85.

Schneider, F., Weiss, U. *et al.* (1999). Subcortical correlates of differential classical conditioning of aversive emotional reactions in social phobia. *Biol. Psychiatr.*, **45**(7), 863–71.

Schulkin, J. (1999). CRH signals adversity in both the placenta and the brain: regulation by glucocorticoids and allostatic overload. *J. Endocrinol.*, **161**, 340–56.

Schulkin, J. (2003). *Rethinking Homeostasis*, Cambridge: MIT Press.

Schulkin, J., Gold, P. W. and McEwen, B. S. (1998). Induction of corticotropin-releasing hormone gene expression by glucocorticoids: implication for understanding the states of fear and anxiety and allostatic load. *Psychoneuroendocrinology*, **23**(3), 219–43.

Schwartz, C. E., Snidman, N. *et al.* (1999). Adolescent social anxiety as an outcome of inhibited temperament in childhood. *J. Am. Acad. Child Adolesc. Psychiatr.*, **38**(8), 1008–15.

Schwartz, C. E., Wright, C. I. *et al.* (2003a). Inhibited and uninhibited infants 'grown up': adult amygdala response to novelty. *Science*, **300**, 1952–3.

Schwartz, C. E., Wright, C. I. *et al.* (2003b). Differential amygdalar response to novel versus newly familiar neutral faces: a functional MRI probe developed for studying inhibited temperament. *Biol. Psychiatr.*, **53**(10), 854–62.

Seckl, J. R. (1997). Glucocorticoids, feto-placental 11 beta-hydroxysteroid dehydrogenase type 2, and the early life origins of adult disease. *Steroids*, **62**, 89–94.

Shepard, J. D., Barron, K. W. and Myers, D. A. (2000). Corticosterone delivery to the amygdala increases corticotropin-releasing hormone mRNA in the central nucleus of the amygdala and anxiety-like behavior. *Brain Res.*, **851**, 288–95.

Shepard, J. D., Barron, K. W. and Myers, D. A. (2003). Sterotaxic localization of corticosterone to the amygdala enhances hypothalamic–pituitary adrenal responses to behavioral stress. *Brain Res.*, **963**, 203–13.

Shin, L. M., Kosslyn, S. M. *et al.* (1997). Visual imagery and perception in posttraumatic stress disorder. A positron emission tomographic investigation. *Arch. Gen. Psychiatr.*, **54**(3), 233–41.

Strome, E. M., Trevor-Wheler, G. H., Higley, J. D. *et al.* (2002). Intracerebroventricular CRH increases limbic glucose metabolism and has social context dependent behavioral effects in nonhuman primates. *Proc. Natl. Acad. Sci.*, **99**, 15749–54.

Sullivan, R. M. and Gratton, A. (2002). Prefrontal cortical regulation of HPA function in the rat and implications for psychopathology. *Psychoneuroendocrinology*, **27**, 99–114.

Swanson, L. W. and Simmons, D. M. (1989). Differential steroid hormone and neural influences on peptide mRNA levels in CRH cells of the paraventricular nucleus: a hybridization histochemical study in the rat. *J. Comp. Neurol.*, **285**, 413–35.

Swanson, L. W., Sawchenko, P. E., Rivier, J. and Vale, W. W. (1983). Organization of ovine corticotropin releasing hormone immunoreactive cells and fibers in the rat brain: an immunohistochemical study. *Neuroendocrinology*, **36**, 165–86.

Swerdlow, N. R., Briton, K. T. and Koob, G. F. (1989). Potentiation of acoustic startle by corticotropin-releasing factor (CRF) and by fear are both reversed by alpha-helical CRF (9–41). *Neuropsychopharmacology*, **2**, 285–92.

Takahashi, L. K., Kalin, N. H., Vanden-Burgt, J. A. and Sherman, J. E. (1989). Corticotropin-releasing hormone modulates defensive-withdrawal and exploratory behavior in rats. *Behav. Neurosci.*, **3**, 648–54.

Takahashi, L. K. and Kim, H. (1994). Intracranial action of corticosterone facilitates the development of behavioral inhibition in the adrenalectomized preweanling rat. *Neurosci. Lett.*, **176**, 272–6.

Tanimura, S. M. and Watts, A. G. (1998). Corticosterone can facilitate as well as inhibit corticotropin-releasing hormone gene expression in the rat hypothalamic paraventricular nucleus. *Endocrinology*, **139**, 3830–6.

Thompson, B. L., Erickson, K., Schulkin, J. and Rosen, J. B. (2004). Repeated corticosterone administration facilitates retention of contextual fear conditioning and increases CRH mRNA expression in the amygdala. *Behav. Brain Res.*, **149**, 209–15.

Trautman, P. D., Meyer-Bahlburg, H. F., Postelnek, J. and New, M. I. (1995). Effects of early prenatal dexamethasone on the cognitive and behavioral development of young children: results of a pilot study. *Psychoneuroendocrinology*, **20**, 439–49.

Valentino, R. J. *et al.* (1994). Evidence for widespread afferents to Barrington's nucleus, a brainstem region rich in CRF neurons. *Neuroscience*, **62**, 123–45.

Valentino, R. J., Pavcovich, L. A. and Hirata, H. (1995). Evidence for corticotropin-releasing hormone projections from Barrington's nucleus to the periaqueductal gray and dorsal motor nucleus of the vagus in the rat. *J. Comp. Neurol.*, **363**, 402–22.

Van Ameringen, M., Mancini, C. *et al.* (1998). The relationship of behavioral inhibition and shyness to anxiety disorder. *J. Nerv. Ment. Dis.*, **186**(7), 425–31.

Wadhwa, P. D., Sandman, C. A., Porto, M., Dunkel-Schetter, C. and Garite, T. J. (1993). The association between prenatal stress and infant birth weight and gestational age at birth: a prospective investigation. *Am. J. Obstet. Gynecol.*, **169**, 858–65.

Wadhwa, P. D., Sandman, C. A. *et al.* (2001). The neurobiology of stress in human pregnancy: implications for prematurity and development of the fetal central nervous system. *Progr. Brain Res.*, **133**, 131–42.

Warren, S. L., Gunnar, M. R. *et al.* (2003). Maternal panic disorder: infant temperament, neurophysiology, and parenting behaviors. *J. Am. Acad. Child Adolesc. Psychiatr.*, **42**(7), 814–25.

Watts, A. G. and Sanchez-Watts, G. (1995). Region-specific regulation of neuropeptide mRNAs in rat limbic forebrain neurones by aldosterone and corticosterone. *J. Physiol.*, **484**(Pt 3), 721–36.

Welberg, L. A., Seckl, J. R. and Holmes, M. C. (2000). Inhibition of 11 beta-hydroxysteroid dehydrogenase, the foeto-placental barrier to maternal glucocorticoids, permanently programs amygdala GR mRNA expression and anxiety-like behavior in the offspring. *Eur. J. Neurosci.*, **12**, 1047–54.

Welberg, L. A. and Seckl, J. R. (2001). Prenatal stress, glucocorticoids and the programming of the brain. *J. Neuroendocrinol.*, **13**, 113–28.

Wolfe, C. D., Patel, S. P. *et al.* (1988). Plasma corticotrophin-releasing factor (CRF) in normal pregnancy. *Br. J. Obstet. Gynaecol.*, **95**, 997–1002.

Wong, M. L., Kling, M. A. *et al.* (2000). Pronounced and sustained central hypernoradrenergic function in major depression with melancholic features: relation to hypercortisolism and corticotropin-releasing hormone. *Proc. Natl. Acad. Sci. USA*, **97**(1), 325–30.

Yehuda, R. (2002). Current status of cortisol findings in post-traumatic stress disorder. *Psychiatr. Clin. North Am.*, **25**(2), 341–68, vii.

Yehuda, R., Giller, E. L. *et al.* (1991). Hypothalamic–pituitary–adrenal dysfunction in posttraumatic stress disorder. *Biol. Psychiatr.*, **30**(10), 1031–48.

Index